It is estimated that up to thirteen percent of hospital admissions result from the adverse effects of diagnosis or treatment, and that almost seventy percent of iatrogenic complications are preventable. The obligation to 'do no harm' has been central to medical conduct since ancient times, yet iatrogenic illness – literally, illness or injury that is induced by the physician – has now come to be recognized as a significant risk factor in health care delivery.

The authors examine the emerging concept of iatrogenic illness in the context of historical developments in medical science, practice and legislation, particularly in the United States. They integrate history, philosophy, medical ethics, and empirical data to examine the concept and phenomenon of medical harm, covering such issues as appropriateness of care, acceptable risk, and practitioner accountability. There are chapters on nosocomial infection, adverse drug effects, and unnecessary surgery, and the book concludes with recommendations for limiting iatrogenic harm. Essential reading for medical ethicists, physicians, and those involved in health care policy and administration, this stimulating and highly readable book will be of interest to all providers of health care, and many of their patients.

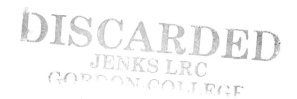

MEDICAL HARM

MEDICAL HARM:

Historical, Conceptual, and Ethical Dimensions of Iatrogenic Illness

VIRGINIA A. SHARPE
The Hastings Center, New York

ALAN I. FADEN
Georgetown University, Washington DC, USA

CAMBRIDGE
UNIVERSITY PRESS

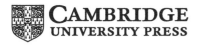

PUBLISHED BY THE PRESS SYNDICATE OF THE UNIVERSITY OF CAMBRIDGE
The Pitt Building, Trumpington Street, Cambridge CB2 1RP, United Kingdom

CAMBRIDGE UNIVERSITY PRESS
The Edinburgh Building, Cambridge CB2 2RU, United Kingdom
40 West 20th Street, New York, NY 10011-4211, USA
10 Stamford Road, Oakleigh, Melbourne 3166, Australia

First published 1998

Printed in the United Kingdom at the University Press, Cambridge

Typeset in Times 10/13 pt [VN]

A catalogue record for this book is available from the British Library

Library of Congress Cataloguing in Publication data
Sharpe, Virginia A. (Virginia Ashby), 1959–
    Medical harm: historical, conceptual, and ethical dimensions of
iatrogenic illness / Virginia A. Sharpe, Alan I. Faden.
        p.   cm.
    Includes biliographical references and index.
    ISBN 0 521 57133 2 (hardback)
    1. Iatrogenic diseases.   2. Surgery, Unnecessary.   3. Drugs–Side
effects.   I. Faden, A. I.   II. Title.
    [DNLM]: 1. Iatrogenic Disease–prevention & control.   2. Ethics,
Medical.   3. Delivery of Health Care.   QZ 42 S532m   1998]
RC90.S46   1998
615.5–dc21
DNLM / DLC
for Library of Congress   97–11814   CIP

ISBN 0 521 57133 2 hardback
ISBN 0 521 63490 3 paperback

This book is dedicated with love to
Patricia M. Sharpe and Alton R. Sharpe, Jr., M.D.
and
to the memory of Leon Lable Faden, a loving and supportive
father whose untimely death was likely of iatrogenic origin.

Contents

Acknowledgments

Many people generously contributed their time and their intelligence to this project. We would especially like to thank Susan Stocker, Dan Davis, Martin Pernick, Edmund Pellegrino, Margaret Little, David Degrazia, Elaine Larson, Kenneth DeVille, Victoria Pedrick, Kenneth Dretchen, and our colleagues at the Kennedy Institute of Ethics.

We would also like to thank Coleen MacNamara, Andrei Selishev, and Elizabeth Wellner whose technical support both in research and in manuscript preparation was invaluable.

Finally, we would like to thank the Charles E. Culpeper Foundation whose generous support of Dr. Sharpe through the Culpeper Scholarship in the Medical Humanities made this project possible.

Introduction

'Tis impossible to separate the chance of good from the risk of ill.
David Hume

The phrase 'medical harm' seems paradoxical. It defies our expectations about medicine; our expectations that medicine will benefit, rather than harm us and that individual and institutional providers will improve rather than diminish our health. But iatrogenic illness – literally, illness that is 'induced by the physician' – has come to be recognized as a significant source of patient risk. In the United States, it has been estimated that during hospitalization, as many as a third of patients suffer from complications related to their medical or nursing care.[1] Between 5% and 13% of hospital admissions result from the adverse effects of diagnosis or treatment.[2] The 1991 Harvard Medical Practice Study concluded that almost 70% of iatrogenic complications are preventable and affect more than 1.3 million hospitalized patients annually.[3] During the fee for service era, patients were believed to be at considerable risk for *unnecessary* treatments.[4] Today, there is growing concern regarding the risks associated with economically-motivated denials of *necessary* care.[5]

In the last half of the twentieth century, attention to the problem of medically induced illness in the United States has come from a number of sources including the medical and legal professions, federal agencies and consumer advocacy groups.

It was in the 1950s and 1960s, after the enormous post-war expansion in pharmacological therapies, that the occurrence of iatrogenic complications – particularly adverse drug reactions – began to receive attention in the medical literature. From the professional point of view at this time, iatrogenic adverse effects were regarded as the inevitable price of medical progress; 'the price we must pay for the modern management of disease,'[6] and were defined as the sequelae of *sound and sanctioned* medical practice. The earliest studies based on this narrow definition found that roughly one out of every 20 patients suffered from a major toxic reaction while receiving hospital care.[7]

Iatrogenic illness has been viewed quite differently from the perspective of medical malpractice law. In the 1950s the average number of claims per physician per year in the United States was 1 in 100. In the 1970s that number had grown ten-fold to 10 in 100. Since then, the total number of claims has roughly doubled.[8] The story told in malpractice verdicts against providers is one not of the inevitable downsides of conscientious care but, rather, of the most egregious harms following from a violation of professional standards. From the point of view of tort law, it is the blameworthiness of negligent injury or illness that stands out as the most significant dimension of medical harm.

Since the late 1960s, iatrogenic illness has also been the focus of governmental agencies. The late 1960s and early 1970s saw the establishment of the Hospital Infections Branch of the Center for Disease Control (CDC)[9] and the Task Force on Prescription Drugs under the US Department of Health Education and Welfare (HEW).[10] The establishment of these two bodies was prompted by two disquieting episodes in the recent history of medical harms. The CDC investigation and surveillance of nosocomial infection (infection contracted in the hospital) was prompted by a pandemic of staphylococcal infections sweeping hospitals in the United States. Statistics at the time revealed that over half of the infected patients became infected after admission to the hospital.[11] Subsequent data demonstrated that in 1970 only about 10% of hospitals in the United States had any sort of infection control program.[12] By the 1980s, nosocomial infection was identified as the fifth leading cause of hospital death and infection control had become an integral part of hospital quality management.

The HEW Task Force on Prescription Drugs was, in part, a response to the thalidomide disaster in which infants exposed to the drug *in utero* were born with deformed or missing limbs. The thalidomide experience triggered the establishment of national and international post-marketing drug surveillance systems. In recent years, the Food and Drug Administration (FDA) in the United States has introduced the MEDWatch program to facilitate the reporting of serious adverse drug and device events by health providers and manufacturers.[13] While these regulatory strategies have addressed the public health implications of drug-induced illness, governmental attention to another type of iatrogenic harm – unnecessary surgery – has had a slightly different focus.

In 1967, a British study on surgical rate variation determined that surgeons in the United States performed twice as many operations per capita as their British counterparts.[14] These data were followed in 1974 by a presurgical screening study of American union members. This study found that in almost one-quarter of cases, a second opinion failed to support a recommendation for surgery.[15] On the basis of these data the US House of Representatives convened a subcommittee on unnecessary surgery. Extrapolating from the presurgical screening study data, the subcommittee, in 1974, concluded that 2.4 million or 17.6% of surgical interventions in the United States were unnecessary, resulting in costs of 3.9 billion dollars.[16] With the prospect of fewer unnecessary surgeries and enormous anticipated savings, the Department of Health, Education, and Welfare and many private insurers and employers promptly instituted second opinion programs. Thus, in the case of unnecessary surgery, the focus has tended since the 1970s to be on the direct aggregate economic costs of the phenomenon rather than on its human costs in morbidity, mortality, pain, suffering, or loss of livelihood to individuals. In other words, unnecessary surgery has typically been understood in terms of unnecessary expenditures rather than in terms of iatrogenic harm.

It is the consumer advocacy literature that has emphasized the patient's perspective on iatrogenic harm. Reports of the dangers associated with drugs and devices, including thalidomide, the Dalkon Shield, Diethylstil bestrol (DES), coupled with a growing distrust of institutions and traditional forms of authority in the 1960s and 1970s gave rise to a host of books intended not only to galvanize health consumers but also to educate them about particular heath care risks.[17]

One of the most influential books of this period was Ivan Illich's *Medical Nemesis*.[18] In this and other works, Illich harshly criticized social institutions for augmenting the problems that they were originally intended to solve. In classical Greek mythology, Nemesis was divine retribution against mortal hubris that presumed the ability to acquire the attributes of the gods.[19] For example, because of their attempt to transform their mortal natures, Prometheus and Sisyphus were condemned by Nemesis to a self-defeating existence of progress turned in on itself. Likewise, argues Illich, the medical industry and those of us who naïvely subject ourselves to its machinations have created a self-reinforcing iatrogenic loop where the supposed remedies have themselves become pathogenic. In its most general sense, Illich's term *iatrogenesis* meant the paradoxical counterproductivity in human societies that paralyzes autonomous action. *Clinical iatrogenesis*, the by-product of modern bureaucratized medicine, comprises 'all clinical conditions for which remedies, physicians or hospitals are the pathogens,' or 'sickening agents.'[20] In the book, Illich enumerated the general and specific dangers of clinical care and the medicalization of life and death. Above all, he encouraged patients and people generally to become more independent and self-reliant in the task of health.

During this period of increased, and sometimes highly charged, attention to patient harms, the definition of iatrogenic illness in the medical literature became more inclusive of harms associated with contraindicated and substandard care as well as physician and nursing error. The subtitle of Moser's *Diseases of Medical Progress*[21] reveals the transformation that was occurring in the professional literature during this period. In its first edition in 1959, the book's subtitle was *A Survey of Diseases and Syndromes Unintentionally Induced as a Result of Properly Indicated, Widely Accepted Therapeutic Procedures*. By its third edition, 10 years later, the subtitle reflects a broader and more circumspect view of the problem: *A Contemporary Analysis of Illness Produced by Drugs and other Therapeutic Procedures*.

Studies during the 1960s and 1970s also began to distinguish iatrogenic complications according to severity, including not only serious but also moderate and minor adverse effects in their definitions. One study, for example, defined an iatrogenic adverse effect as any 'complication resulting from reactions to medication or procedures, physical injury or accident, psychological decompensation, nosocomial infections, and medical or nursing errors – including errors of omission.'[22] In this study, a 38% complication rate was reported in hospitalized patients, twice that reported in studies limited to adverse effects of *sound* medical care and eight times as high as studies that reported only 'major toxic events.'

In recent years, the preventability of iatrogenic adverse events has emerged as one of the most pressing questions in the study and improvement of health care quality. In the Harvard Medical Practice Study (HMPS) of acute care, nonpsychiatric hospitals in New York State, over 30,000 patients' charts were reviewed for the occurrence of iatrogenic adverse events.[23] Based on the study findings, it has been estimated that almost 4% of hospitalized patients each year suffer from a hospital-related injury and that more than two-thirds of these events are preventable.

Because adverse drug events (ADEs) constituted the largest percentage of iatrogenic complications in their study (19%), authors of the HMPS have recently done two further investigations of preventable ADEs in 4031 hospitalized medical and surgical adult patients.[24] Of the life-threatening and serious ADEs, 42% were judged to be the result of preventable error. What is striking about these most recent studies is their identification of system failures as major factors contributing to preventable error. The most common systems failures were in drug knowledge dissemination, drug dose and identity checking, and patient information availability. The lesson of these studies of ADEs is that their occurrence is more directly related to defects or breakdowns in the complex processes that comprise tertiary care than to individual incompetence. This is also the lesson from recent studies on the prevention and control of nosocomial infection. Data from the multi-site Study on the Efficacy of Nosocomial Infection Control (SENIC)[25] has revealed that over 30% of the three million annual hospital infections in the United States are preventable through programs that emphasize active surveillance of processes in medical, surgical, and nursing care. The most successful prevention measures are not those that target individual providers but those that discern the complex relationships between the agent, source, and route of transmission, the environment, and the host of infection. With the implementation of organized surveillance and control activities, SENIC found that a hospital's infection rates could be reduced by one-third.

Recently reported events highlight the significance of system failures in the occurrence of iatrogenic harm. In the case of Betsy Lehman, a Boston woman, who died from an overdose of chemotherapeutic agents, the four-fold error in drug dosage went unnoticed by at least a dozen nurses, doctors, and pharmacists at Dana Farber Cancer Institute. This happened despite the fact that a similar error had resulted in a life-threatening complication for a different patient two days earlier.[26] Subsequent investigation of Dana Farber's quality assurance procedures revealed that in 5% of cases, one patient's records were found in another patient's file; nurses who administered high doses of chemotherapy to 27 patients did not have access to detailed instructions; and reports of medication errors were collected but not reviewed.

In the case of Willie King, a Florida man who had the wrong leg amputated, the misidentification of the patient's leg began with an entry error in the hospital's computer system, and was repeated on the operating room schedule and blackboard. When the surgeon entered the operating suite, the incorrect leg was already draped and sterilized.[27] It was not until the surgery was well underway that a surgical nurse realized the error.

In both cases, the patient's outcome was directly attributable to breakdowns in communication and in the processes of care.

Attention from all of these different quarters has raised awareness about the occurrence of iatrogenic illness. It also has raised fundamental questions about how we do, and how we should, reflect on the problem of medical harm. These questions cannot be strictly practical, for the fact of harm to individuals, and especially within a context such as medicine where the presumptive obligation is one of benefit, carries with it enormous ethical significance. How, for example, are we to understand iatrogenic harm in light of the practitioner's ancient obligation to 'do no harm'? How, in light of the evidence that most preventable harms are the result of system failures, are we to understand accountability? The ethical dimensions of medical harm are linked, moreover, to important conceptual questions. What and whose values should inform the definition of medical harm? If, as is increasingly the case, assessments of harm (and benefit) are understood in terms of the 'appropriateness' of care, what and whose values should inform the definition of appropriateness? Further, as third-party payers increasingly influence clinical decision making, what and whose values will determine what constitutes an acceptable risk? These fundamentally normative issues are inescapably embedded in the practical and policy questions surrounding medical harm, its prevention, and compensation. We believe that explicit attention to these normative questions should be central to practical and policy deliberations. In this book, a framework is provided for reflecting on these normative questions. We do so, by situating these normative concerns within an historical context that illuminates the forces that have shaped the twentieth century perception of medical harm. In the remainder of this introduction we look particularly at nineteenth century America to provide the historical context from which the themes of this book are drawn.

Although the term 'iatrogenic illness' was not coined until the early twentieth century, medical harm is in no sense a modern notion. The seventeenth century BC Code of Hammurapi describes penalties for harmful physician error depending upon the social status of the patient.[28] The Hippocratic corpus also contains references to the subject, the most notable of which are the injunction 'to help or at least to do no harm,'[29] and the physician's pledge to use his treatments 'to help the sick, but never with a view to injury and wrongdoing.'[30] In the first century AD, Pliny the Elder cautions his compatriots against physicians because, he says, they not only learn their skills at the expense of their patients' lives, they also cast blame on the patient for the harms that befell him during his treatment.[31] The theme of the physician-poisoner was commonplace in classical Roman literature and the paradox of the murderous healer was the subject matter of a great many rhetorical exercises.[32] In this same vein, Al-Ruhawi, an Islamic physician of the Middle Ages makes use of the ambiguous Greek term *pharmakon*, which had the double meaning: remedy/poison. As he explains, the virtuous and skillful physician is like a nourishing remedy while the ignorant or unskilled practitioner is 'like poison' to the patient.[33] In the seventeenth century, the philosopher Leibniz referred to hospitals as *Seminaria mortis* – places where the seeds of death are sown.[34] Throughout the eighteenth century, the German city of Halle was apparently a center for the study of iatrogenic illness.[35] One work originating from this region was the 1728 treatise on 'Doctors as the Cause of Illness,' which presents case histories that demonstrate the harmful effects of bloodletting.[36] Other texts throughout the seventeenth and eighteenth centuries detailed the harms associated with the uses and misuses of medications such as mercury, phosphorus, arsenic, opium, and digitalis.[37] One layperson's response to the use of calomel (mercurous chloride) as a 'cure-all' in febrile illness showed some awareness of the serious harm of mercury poisoning:

Since calomel's become their boast,
How many patients have they lost,
How many thousands they make ill,
Of poison with their calomel.[38]

These historical references not only bear witness to the phenomenon of medical harm but also reflect its normative character within a particular cultural context. In the Code of Hammurapi, for example, the blameworthiness of such a harm or the degree of censure was relative to the status of the victim. If a free citizen died while in the physician's care, the physician's hand or fingers were to be cut off. If the patient were a slave, the physician was required to pay recompense to the owner.[39] The Hippocratic injunction 'to help the sick, but never with a view to injury and wrongdoing,' is reflective of Pythagorean teleology that interpreted the technical and moral demands of the craftsman according to the proper end of the craft – in this case, patient benefit. The signal importance of this orientation to the proper end of medicine transcended even the social dichotomy between freemen and slaves. The Oath goes on to specify that the physician should abstain from mischief, injustice, and sexual relations with free and slave alike. It has also been argued that the Hippocratic injunction to 'do no harm' reflected the physician's status as a craftsman whose livelihood was dependent on the good will of his customers.[40] The precarious economic position of the doctor, in other words, added to his incentive to avoid harm to patients.

In nineteenth century America, the notion of medical harm was textured by cultural attitudes towards Providence, by debates on the relative power of the medical 'Art' vs. 'Nature' as a healing force, and by corresponding beliefs regarding the proper goal of therapy and the moral responsibility of the physician. The notion of medical harm was also shaped by political forces: substantial rhetoric regarding 'brutal' and 'murderous' practices and medical 'quackery' was deployed by competing therapeutic schools vying for professional prominence.

In the early nineteenth century, therapeutics in the United States was characterized by a debate between those who championed Benjamin Rush's 'heroic' application of the art of medicine and those such as Jacob Bigelow who defended the healing powers of nature. Heroic medicine was based more or less explicitly on the theory of counter-irritation: because the body was believed to house only one affliction at a time, the proper therapy for routing out a serious disease was a remedy of even greater potency. Thus, the more virulent the remedy, the better its chances of counteracting disease. This reasoning provided the justification for toxic doses of calomel (mercurous chloride), serial bloodletting, and violent blistering – all of which had been, for example, administered to George Washington upon his death bed in 1899.[41] Natural healing, by contrast, was based on the belief that most diseases would, if left alone, resolve themselves. By letting nature take its course, Bigelow asserted, 'the amount of death and disaster in the world would be less.'[42] This conflict in medical epistemology translated into a moral conflict as well. In keeping with the epistemological distinction between 'Art' and 'Nature', a moral distinction was made between harms of omission and harms of commission. According to the heroic healers, the harms associated with therapeutic intervention were necessary and thus justified. Harms of omission were, however, reprehensible. This sentiment is captured in one Ohio physician's declaration in 1849 that the doctor's duty is not 'to stand by and do nothing . . . [but] to study every disease and interfere.'[43] The failure to administer calomel in desperate cases was regarded as abandonment of the patient.[44]

Natural healers, or 'nature-trusters', by contrast, saw medical intervention as an inherently harmful affront to the natural order. Restraint was laudable, intervention was culpable. J. Marion Sims, one of the nineteenth-century's most famous gynecological surgeons said that at the time of his graduation from medical school in 1835 medical practice was heroic and murderous.

I knew nothing about medicine, but I had sense enough to see that doctors were killing their patients, that medicine was not an exact science, that it was wholly empirical and that it would be better to entrust entirely to Nature than to the hazardous skill of the doctors.[45]

We find this same sentiment expressed by Thomas Jefferson in a letter to one of Rush's contemporaries:

[T]o an unknown disease, there cannot be a known remedy. Here then, the judicious, the moral, the humane physician should stop. Having been so often a witness to the salutary efforts which nature makes to re-establish the disordered functions, he should rather trust to their action, than hazard the interruption of that, and a greater derangement of the system by conjectural experiments on a machine so complicated and so unknown as the human body, and a subject so sacred as a human life[46]

In a less diplomatic frame of mind, Jefferson observed about heroic healers that this 'inexperienced and presumptuous band of medical tyros let loose upon the world, destroys more of human life in one year, than all the Robinhoods, Cartouches & Macheaths do in a century.'[47]

Notwithstanding these different theories of disease and therapeutics, practitioners on both sides of the debate sought to defend their actions with reference to the principles of Christian and gentlemanly rectitude. The Christian gentleman was guided in his actions by virtuous intentions. Thus, in the Christian practitioner, bad outcomes could not logically be the result of bad faith. The force of this appeal often became the tool of one's detractors. By casting aspersions on someone's moral character, one could effectively undermine faith in his therapeutic competence.

In the mid to late nineteenth century, therapeutic breakthroughs such as the acceptance of anesthesia, the germ theory of disease, and surgical antisepsis and asepsis, revolutionized medical practice. Humoral theories of disease and constitutional approaches to therapy were largely supplanted in the late nineteenth and early twentieth centuries by discrete explanatory systems based in pharmacological specificity, immunology, physiology, and laboratory science. The successes of medical science and technology, especially in the field of surgery, offered legitimacy to the emerging medical profession. Rigorous educational standards were adopted for medical training, licensure laws were reestablished and a unified profession institutionalized and safeguarded its authority through various forms of self-regulation. During this period, a fragmented mix of 'regular' and sectarian practitioners eager to incriminate one another, gave way to a consolidated profession of regulars under the aegis of the American Medical Association (AMA) and state medical societies. The AMA's 1847 Code of Ethics was essential in establishing and maintaining this new professional solidarity. It did so not only by prohibiting consultation with 'irregulars' but also by condemning in its members any public criticism of the work of a colleague.

With the rise of scientific medicine, empirical evidence began to displace theoretical dogma as the arbiter of therapeutic efficacy. In this same period, belief in direct Providence as the cause of 'misfortune' gave way to belief in human culpability and responsibility as earthly sources of harm and remediation. The growth of the insurance industry in the mid nineteenth century was one manifestation of this shift. Another was the rise in medical malpractice cases when patients looked to the courts for redress.[48] Rather than give themselves over to fate, or to an uncritical naturalism, Americans began to insure themselves against the risks of daily life and to seek accountability in the actions of others. As these cultural influences came together, both the benignity of natural processes and the ministrations of physicians were opened to question. The moral distinction between acts and omissions in medicine gave way to a conservative therapeutic middle course wherein the physician's duty was to minimize total harm regardless of its source.[49]

The period of professional consolidation and therapeutic triumph raised the expectations of both practitioners and the public regarding the benefits of medical care. Among the public, higher expectations led to intensified demands and dissatisfaction when treatments failed or patients experienced unfavorable results. Between 1830 and 1900, medical malpractice cases in the United States increased more than 2000%.[50] Among practitioners, inflated expectations about medicine's potential inhibited the development of realistic standards of care. Finally, physicians – chilled by the upsurge in malpractice cases – looked to statistics for an accurate assessment of therapeutic efficacy. Frank Hamilton's work on fracture treatment provided evidence – for use both in court and in practice – on what benefits might be reasonably expected from these interventions.[51] This represented one of the first systematic efforts in what is today known as outcomes research.

The adoption of experimental and statistical techniques as a basis for therapeutic decision making and evaluation was not, however, immediate or wholehearted. Evidence of the instability surrounding the notion of scientific standards in medical practice is found in the tension between the growing acceptance of a philosophy of conservative medicine and surgery in the last half of the nineteenth century and the fact that during the same period, practitioners from vastly different therapeutic camps (sectarians and regulars) were allowed to provide expert testimony interchangeably at each other's malpractice trials.[52] Likewise, the theory of regional therapeutics – echoed in the locality rule in medical malpractice[53] – that medicine should be practiced and assessed according to *local* standards and to particularities of constitution and meteorology – suggested that, despite the growing application of scientific medicine and the calculation of relative harms and benefits, society and practitioners were still far from accepting the premise of universal and objective scientific standards.

Most fundamentally, scientific medicine and the statistical assessment of effectiveness presented a threat to the professional identity and morality of the American practitioner. Science refuted not only many of the traditional therapies that doctors had to offer, but also it challenged the very idea of professional judgment. James Jackson, Jr., articulated the conflict that many scientifically-trained practitioners must have felt – 'As a Doctor,' he said, 'I believe in the use of many remedies which, as a scientific man, I am not entirely persuaded to see useful.'[54] Although science was vital to the consolidation of authority by the regular profession, it also demanded that practitioners forsake or at least reconfigure the moral world view that had heretofore defined their practice.

In the prescientific era, the absence of a confirmed germ theory, generally-held convictions about Providence and theories of healing, such as counter-irritation, had together, exempted the physician from moral blame associated with the considerable harms induced by blistering, bleeding, purging, and fatal infection. When the empirical investigations by Louis on bloodletting and amputation and by Semmelweis on puerperal fever established the ineffectiveness or outright harm of emblematic practices, physicians vociferously defended the heretofore established connection between the physician's character and the effectiveness of treatment.[55] Responding to O. W. Holmes' charge that obstetricians were themselves responsible for maternal death from childbed fever, C. D. Meigs countered with what he equally believed to be unassailably true, namely, that 'a gentleman's hands are clean.'[56] Likewise, when the Surgeon General of the US Army restricted the use of calomel, citing a high incidence of mercury poisoning among treated soldiers, the AMA denounced the policy as 'a most grievous offense against the dignity, usefulness and humanity of our profession.'[57] Finally, when experimental science began to replace Christian and gentlemanly rectitude as the basis for therapeutic evaluation,[58] practitioners were forced to confront the dawning possibility that they were morally culpable for the harms associated with medical care. In his discussion of the rise of 'conservative medicine,' Pernick points out that statistical assessment brought with it a new moral norm. The physician's duty was now to 'minimize total harm' as determined through a proportional calculus of the pain and suffering associated with both disease and treatment.

Throughout the last third of the nineteenth century, the moral authority of the physician in America was increasingly seen as a function of scientific expertise. In fact, in 1882, the more scientifically inclined members of the AMA challenged the continued relevance of the 1847 Code of Ethics saying that those 'who trusted in the natural laws revealed by experimental science no longer needed the artificial laws embodied in codes of professional ethics.'[59] This revolt was a reaction to the AMA's regulatory and punitive use of the Code to exclude 'irregulars' from practice. Those who embraced the promise of scientifically-based therapeutics believed that science rather than professional ethics should be the ultimate judge of proper practice. Although the moral *authority* of the physician was increasingly associated with scientific expertise, the physician's moral *responsibility*, was, from the point of view of medical harm, interestingly divided.

First, from the mid-nineteenth century, the practitioner's responsibility was divided between loyalty to patient and to profession – The AMA Code of Ethics articulated simultaneously the physician's duty not only to advance patient welfare but also to safeguard the newly established brotherhood of regulars by upholding professional etiquette. As Shryock has observed, 'etiquette forbade criticism of the work of an inferior or careless colleague, while the welfare of possible patients seemed to demand it.'[60] Secondly, from the mid-nineteenth century, the practitioner's responsibility was divided between a duty to the individual patient (the object of the healer's ministrations) and the 'average' patient (the object of science). As science, with its emphasis on universal norms became an authoritative source of medical knowledge, the individual patient was displaced as the focus of professional attention and identity. With disease now understood as deviation from a normal state (measurable by new technologies such as the thermometer and the stethoscope), rather than as a disturbance of natural balance, the individual patient became increasingly unimportant as a reporter of clinical signs.[61] Harms and benefits began to be regarded as *objective* facts determinable only by the expertise of the physician. Assessments of therapeutic efficacy were also animated by the ideal of scientific universalism. As a result, physicians now judged the effectiveness of treatment by focusing on the average or statistical patient, rather than on the sick individual.

Debates about the moral probity of this focus called into question the nature of medicine and the identity of the practitioner. Was the clinician's responsibility the normalization of physiological processes or the care of the sick patient? Could the physician justify imposing on a patient the risks associated with interventions such as anesthesia administration? Charles Meigs spoke for those who maintained that their professional duty depended on the *specific* rather than the *relative* value of a therapy. 'What sufficient motive have I,' Meigs asked, 'to risk the life or death of even one in a thousand [of my patients]?'[67]

In Part I we show how these two sources of tension in professional responsibility (between allegiance to profession and to patient and between dedication to scientific objectivity and the subjectivity of the individual patient) have been defining features of the perception of medical harm in the United States in the nineteenth and twentieth centuries.

In Chapter 1 we show how the tradition of personal accountability was maintained under the socially-sanctioned policy of professional self-regulation. How, in other words, a physician's allegiance to the profession guaranteed him considerable discretion in his practice and freedom from formal oversight. We also discuss how Ernest Codman's efforts to reform hospital quality explicitly in terms of patient benefit fundamentally challenged this norm of personal accountability. As Codman saw it, under his 'end-result system,' documented competence would replace individual conscience as the basis of clinical evaluation.

In Chapter 2 we discuss how different medical epistemologies, that is, different conceptions of health and disease from humoralism to experimental medicine, have influenced the meaning of harm and benefit and, by extension, the health care providers' perception of their obligations of beneficence and nonmaleficence.

In Chapter 3 we examine how public concern about patient harms, both in therapy and research, gave rise to new forms of accountability in medicine. In particular, we show how the post World War II utilitarian justification for iatrogenic harm was replaced in the 1960s and 1970s by a more critical conception of moral accountability, one responsive to the emerging call for patient rights.

In Part II we provide a conceptual and ethical analysis of medical harm. In Chapter 4, we examine the philosophical basis for the duty to 'do no harm' and argue that this obligation is best sustained by a fiduciary rather than by a market-based, contractual model of the healing relationship.

In Chapter 5 we examine how this duty is specified in the notion of due care. We look particularly at due care in the establishment of standards, in the selection of treatment, in provider-patient communication and in the delivery of care.

In Chapter 6 we provide a conceptual analysis of medical harm, looking specifically at its meaning in terms of source, object, and scope. Recognizing the limitations of the term 'iatrogenic' illness, we offer the term 'comiogenic' to capture the diversity in sources of medical harm. In addition, we examine the values that inform the concept of harm in patient care. Building on our analysis of the moral basis of medicine, we argue that a more patient-centered ethos will regard the individual patient's values as central not only to determinations of benefit and risk but also to occurrent harm.

On the basis of these observations, we provide a framework for the moral evaluation of medical harm and the imposition of risk. We consider conditions under which comiogenic harm or the imposition of risk may be justified and conditions under which they may be excused. Our discussion of potential excusing conditions for comiogenic harm makes reference to recent empirical work on the complex etiology of medical mistakes and quality failures. We argue that a model of collective agency and accountability may provide a more fruitful basis for comiogenic harm prevention than do traditional models restricted merely to individual agency and accountability.

Whereas in Part II we look specifically at moral norms as the fundamental mechanisms of accountability in health care, in Part III we look at formal and regulatory mechanisms as applied to nosocomial infection control, the prevention of adverse drug effects and the regulation of unnecessary surgery. In Chapters 7, 8, and 9 we examine recent data on the scope and incidence of these specific types of medical harm. We examine the potential of epidemiologic methods and systems analysis in the prevention of drug harms and hospital infections.

In Chapter 10 we examine the concept of appropriateness in patient care. As the literature on unnecessary surgery makes clear, assumptions regarding which treatments are necessary and which are not depend on an understanding of clinical appropriateness. The shift to appropriateness research in health care comes at a time when other, that is, 'non-clinical' values, in particular, those of the patient and those of third-party payers, play a central role in the process of health care decision making. In addition to questions of evidentiary justification, determinations of appropriateness now inevitably touch on questions of the desirability and cost-worthiness of treatment. In this chapter, we identify four sources of value that give meaning to appropriateness in patient care: the clinical point of view, the point of view of the individual patient, the point of view of the third-party payer, and the social point of view.

Finally, in Chapter 11 we offer a number of general and specific recommendations on how iatrogenic harms might be limited in the future. Specifically, we point to the value of adopting active surveillance strategies; initiating systems analysis; modifying the education of physicians and other health care providers; and enhancing the focus on the evidentiary basis of medical practice.

Endnotes

1 See Table A.1.
2 See Table A.2.
3 Brennan TA, Leape LL, Laird NM, et al. Incidence of adverse events and negligence in hospitalized patients. Results of the Harvard Medical Practice Study I. *N Engl J Med* 1991; 324(6):370–6.
4 Consumer Reports. Wasted health care dollars. *Consumer Reports* 1992; 57(7):435–48.
5 Rich S. Managed care, once an elixir, goes under the legislative knife: Cost-cutting focus feared harmful to patients. *Washington Post* September 25, 1996, p. A1.
6 Barr DP. Hazards of modern diagnosis and therapy – the price we pay. *JAMA* 1956; 159:1452–6.
7 Schimmel EM. The hazards of hospitalization. *Ann Intern Med* 1964; 60:100–10. Barr DP (see No. 6).
8 Danzon PM. *New Evidence on the Frequency and Severity of Medical Malpractice Claims.* Santa Monica: RAND, 1986, p. 16. Weiler PC, Hiatt HH, Newhouse JP, et al. *A Measure of Malpractice: Medical Injury, Malpractice Litigation and Patient Compensation.* Cambridge, MA: Harvard University Press, 1993, p. 4.
9 Williams REO. Summary of the conference. In Brachman PS, Eickhoff TC, eds. *Proceedings of the International Conference on Nosocomial Infections.* Chicago: AHA, 1971, pp. 318–21.
10 US Department of Health, Education and Welfare. *Task Force on Prescription Drugs: Report and Recommendations.* Committee Print of the US Congress, Senate Subcommittee on Monopoly of the Senate Select Committee on Small Business, 90th Congress, 2nd session, 1968.
11 White FMM. Nosocomial infection control: Scope and implications for health care. *Am J Infect Control* 1981; 9:66.
12 Eickhoff TC. The third dicennial international conference on nosocomial infections: Historical perspective. The landmark conference in 1970. *Am J Med* 1991; 91:3B–5S.
13 Kessler DA (for the Working Group). Introducing MEDWatch: A new approach to reporting medication and device adverse effects and product problems. *JAMA* 1993; 269:2765–8.
14 Bunker JP. Surgical manpower: A comparison of operations and surgeons in the United States and in England and Wales. *N Engl J Med* 1970; 282:135–44.
15 McCarthy EG, Widmer GW. Effects of screening by consultants on recommended elective surgical procedures. *N Engl J Med* 1974; 291:1331–5.
16 US Congress, House Subcommittee on Oversight and Investigation. *Cost and Quality of Health Care: Unnecessary Surgery.* Washington DC: USGPO, 1976.
17 Knowles J. (ed.). *Doing Better and Feeling Worse: Health Care in the United States.* New York: W.W. Norton, 1977. Krause EA. *Power and Illness: The Political Sociology of Health and Medical Care.* New York: Elsevier, 1977. Millman M. *The Unkindest Cut: Life in the Backrooms of Medicine.* New York: William Morrow & Co Inc, 1977. Stroman DF. *The Quick Knife: Unnecessary Surgery.* New York: Kennikat, 1979. Lipp M. *The Bitter Pill: Doctors, Patients and Failed Expectations.* New York: Harper and Row; 1980.

Inlander CB, Levin LS, Weiner E. *Medicine on Trial*. New York: Prentice Hall, 1988.

18 Illich I. *Medical Nemesis: The Expropriation of Health*. New York: Pantheon Books; 1976.

19 Illich, p. 34 (see No. 18).

20 Illich, p. 27 (see No. 18).

21 Moser RH. *Diseases of Medical Progress*. Springfield, Ill.: Chas. Thomas, 1959, 3rd edn, 1969.

22 Reichel W. Complications in the care of five hundred elderly hospitalized patients. *J Am Geriatr Soc* 1965; 13:973–81.

23 Brennan TA, et al. (see No. 3).
Leape LL, Brennan TA, Laird N, et al. The nature of adverse events in hospitalized patients. Results of the Harvard Medical Practice Study II. *N Engl J Med* 1991; 324(6): 377–84.

24 Bates DM, Cullen DJ, Laird N, et al. for the ADE Prevention Study Group. Incidence of adverse drug events and potential adverse drug events: Implications for prevention. *JAMA* 1995; 274:29–34.
Leape LL, Bates DW, Cullen DJ, et al. for the ADE Prevention Study Group. Systems analysis of adverse drug events. *JAMA* 1995; 274:35–43.

25 Haley RW, Culver DH, White JW, et al. The efficacy of infection surveillance and control programs in preventing nosocomial infections in US hospitals. *Am J Epidemiol* 1984; 121:182–205.

26 Associated Press. Report details errors at Cancer Institute. *Washington Post*, May 31, 1995, p. A20.

27 Doctor who cut off wrong leg is defended by colleagues. *New York Times*, September 17, 1995, p. A28.

28 'Medicine' *Encyclopedia Brittanica*. Chicago: Encyclopedia Brittanica, 1988, vol. 23, p. 886.

29 Epidemics I. In *Hippocrates*. (Trans., WHS Jones. Loeb Classical Library.) Cambridge, MA: Harvard University Press, 1923–1988, vol. X, p.165.

30 The Oath. In *Hippocrates*. (Trans., WHS Jones. Loeb Classical Library.) Cambridge, MA: Harvard University Press, 1923–1988, vol. 1, p. 299.

31 Pliny Secundus, *Natural History*, cited in Illich I. *Medical Nemesis*, p. 29n.

32 Ratzan RM, Ferngren GB. A Greek progymnasma on the physician-poisoner. *J Hist Med Allied Sci* 1993; 48:157–70.

33 Levey M. *Medical Ethics of Medieval Islam, with Special Reference to al-Ruhawi's Practical Ethics of the Physcian*. Philadelphia: American Philosophical Society, 1967, ch. XVI.

34 Ackerknecht EH. Zur Geschichte der iatrogenen Krankheiten. *Gesnerus* 1970; 27(1):57–63.

35 Ackerknecht EH (see No. 34).

36 Ackerknecht EH (see No. 34).

37 Ackerknecht EH. Zur Geschichte der iatrogenen Erkrankungen des Nervensystems. *Therapeutische Umschau* 1970; 27(6):345–6.

38 Davies DM. *Textbook of Adverse Drug Reactions*. 4th edn. Oxford: Oxford University Press, 1991, p.2.

39 'Medicine' *Encyclopedia Brittanica* (see No. 28). Similar disparities in redress for medical harm existed in the pre Civil War south.
For a discussion of harm to slaves versus harm to whites see Savitt TL. *Medicine and Slavery: The Disease and Health Care of Blacks in Antebellum Virginia*. Urbana, IL: University of Illinois Press, 1978.

40 Risse G. Medical care. In BynumWF, Porter R, eds. *Companion Encyclopedia of the History of Medicine*. New York: Routledge, 1993, ch.4 (pp. 45–77).
41 Rothstein WG. *American Physicians in the Nineteenth Century: From Sects to Science*. Baltimore: Johns Hopkins Press, 1992, p. 55.
42 Starr P. *The Social Transformation of American Medicine*. New York: Basic Books, 1982, p. 55.
43 Warner JH. *The Therapeutic Perspective: Medical Practice, Knowledge and Identity in America 1820–1885*. Cambridge, MA: Harvard University Press, 1986, p. 19.
44 Rothstein WG, p.50 (see No. 41).
45 Rothstein WG, p. 62 (see No. 41).
46 quoted in Sullivan RB. Sanguine practices: A historical and historiographic reconsideration of heroic therapy in the age of Rush. *Bull Hist Med* 1994; 68:225.
47 Quoted in Rothstein WG, p. 44–5 (see No. 41).
48 DeVille KA. *Medical Malpractice in Nineteenth-Century America: Origins and Legacy*. New York: NYU Press, 1990.
49 Pernick MS. The calculus of suffering in nineteenth-century surgery. *Hastings Ctr Rep*. 1983; 13:26–36.
50 DeVille KA, p. 3 (see No. 48).
51 Cassedy JH. *American Medicine and Statistical Thinking*. Cambridge, MA: Harvard University Press, 1984.
52 DeVille KA. *Medical Malpractice in Nineteenth–Century America*.
53 *Small v. Howard* 128 Mass 131 (1880).
54 Warner JH, p. 26 (see No. 43).
55 Baker R, Porter D, Porter R (eds). *The Codification of Medical Morality: Historical and Philosophical Studies of the Formalization of Western Medical Morality in the Eighteenth and Nineteenth Centuries*. Volume 1: *Medical Ethics and Etiquette in the Eighteenth Century*. Boston: Kluwer Academic Publishers, 1993.
56 Meigs CD. *On the Nature, Signs and Treatment of Childbed Fever*. Philadelphia: 1859.
57 Konold D. *A History of American Medical Ethics 1947–1912*. Madison: State Historical Soc. of Wisconsin, 1962, p.35.
58 Burns CR. *Medical Ethics in the U.S. Before the Civil War*. Ann Arbor: University Microfilms, 1973.
59 Warner JH. Ideals of science and their discontents in late 19th century American medicine. *Isis* 1991; 82:468.
60 Shryock RH. *The Development of Modern Medicine*. New York: Knopf, 1947, p. 267.
61 Warner JH (see No. 59).
62 Pernick M. *A Calculus of Suffering: Pain, Professionalism and Anesthesia in Nineteenth Century America*. New York: Columbia University Press, 1985.

PART I

1

Divided loyalties:
harm to the profession vs. harm to the patient

Recent scholarship in the history and sociology of American medicine provides a compelling account of how the professional authority of physicians was consolidated in the mid-nineteenth and early twentieth centuries. This consolidation occurred both by chance and by design. The introduction of surgical antisepsis (and later asepsis) and of diagnostic technologies such as the stethoscope, and X-ray as well as diagnostic tests, enhanced the credibility of the 'regular' physician and distinguished his abilities from the less demonstrative ones of homeopaths and botanics. This was also the most dramatic period of hospital growth in the United States. In 1873, there were 178 hospitals and by 1910 there were more than 4000.[1] The role of physicians – and especially surgeons – was essential to this growth, for it was surgeons who provided the patients to fill the ever increasing number of hospital beds. By the late 1920s, surgical admissions outnumbered medical admissions by almost two to one.[2] Further, as the public began to respond to the promise of surgical cures, the availability of surgical resources provided the all important argument for the advantage of hospital over home care. During this period, the hospital as a social institution was changing dramatically. In the early 1800s, hospitals were essentially charitable institutions, indeed, almshouses for the 'deserving poor'. A patient's admission to the hospital was based on an assessment by hospital trustees of the moral character of the potential 'inmate'. At the close of the nineteenth century, hospital admissions were based increasingly on medical diagnosis with physician referral accounting for three-quarters of admissions.[3] Professional consolidation was significantly aided by the establishment of the American Medical Association (AMA) and its foundational Code of Ethics.

In this chapter we examine how the mechanisms of professional solidarity: the Code of Ethics; the growth of local medical societies and the important symbiosis between hospitals and doctors challenged the physician's loyalty to patient welfare. We show how allegiance to the profession guaranteed the physician considerable discretion in his practice and freedom from formal oversight. We also discuss how efforts to reform hospital quality around the principle of patient benefit fundamentally challenged this norm of personal accountability which had played a key role in the achievement of professional consolidation.

The ethics of consolidation

In the early years of the nineteenth century, medical practice was largely unregulated. The hospital was not yet an essential locus of medical training, nor was it the context in which the majority of care was provided. Moreover, scientific medicine with its important therapeutic breakthroughs had not yet distinguished the 'regular' practitioner. Physicians were highly competitive and their success was based largely on their personal reputations. In this context, the ferocity of diatribes by sectarian and regular practitioners against one another served only to increase the vulnerability of the individual physician. Establishment of the AMA in 1847 was a self-conscious strategy on the part of orthodox practitioners to protect and champion their collective interests. As the first president of the Association understood it, with the establishment of a national organization, the profession 'comes forward in the majesty of its might to vindicate its rights and redress its wrongs.'[4]

The AMA's Code of Ethics, which was adopted at the time of the Association's founding, provided a rallying point in this strategy to consolidate the regular profession and to foster cooperation over competition. Regarding disputes over ethics and etiquette, the profession was instructed to maintain a 'special reserve toward the public.' Publicity regarding professional disputes, the Code observed, would reflect badly not only on the individual physicians involved, but, more importantly would 'bring discredit on the faculty.[5] The Code's mandate regarding intraprofessional duties also served to strengthen the ties between orthodox practitioners. Physicians had an obligation to treat each other and their families free of charge. Competition and professional rivalry were suppressed by the prohibition against advertisement, which the Code asserts is 'derogatory to the dignity of the profession.' Finally, the 1847 Code's consultation clause was a powerful means of placing sectarian practitioners – and by implication, anyone who consulted with them – outside the bounds of ethical practice. This was achieved by the use of misleading rhetoric implying that 'regular' practitioners could be counted on to have had an education in the sciences. 'No one,' says the Code,[6]

can be considered as a regular practitioner or a fit associate in consultation, whose practice is based on exclusive dogma, to the rejection of the accumulated experience of the profession, and of the aids actually furnished by anatomy, physiology, pathology and organic chemistry.

To prevent misinterpretations of this ominous warning, the AMA ruled unanimously in 1885 that under no circumstances – including emergency situations – could regular physicians consult with sectarians.[7]

The effectiveness of the AMA's 1847 Code can no doubt be accounted for in large part because its more self-serving aims are articulated in and alongside an expansive rhetoric expressing the ideal of patient welfare. 'A physician should not only be ever ready to obey the calls of the sick, but his mind ought also to be imbued with the greatness of his mission, and the responsibility he habitually incurs in its discharge.'[8] Moreover, he should treat his patients with 'attention, steadiness, and humanity' and should not abandon those whose afflictions are incurable but should stand by to relieve their 'pain and mental anguish'.[9]

Nowhere was the beneficent mission of the profession expressed so righteously as in the Code's condemnation of 'quackery.' 'The ease, the health and the lives of those committed to the charge [of physicians],' says the Code, 'depend on their skill, attention and fidelity.'[10] It is, therefore, 'the duty of physicians, who are frequent witnesses of the enormities committed by quackery, and injury to health and even destruction of life caused by the use of quack medicines, to expose the injuries sustained by the unwary from the devices and pretensions of artful empirics and impostors.'[11]

This ennobling rhetoric fits seamlessly with the profession's political aim of confederation against sectarians. When the ideals of patient welfare and the prevention of patient harms posed a threat to the profession's own interests, however, they were not so passionately embraced.

The tension between the physician's obligation to the patient and to the interests of the profession was manifested in a number of different areas. Reporting on professional deficiencies was one. In many passages of the 1847 Code, oblique reference is made to circumstances of professional disagreement or to the incompetence or deficiency of colleagues. In each passage (all of which appear in the section 'The Duties of Physicians to Each Other, and to the Profession at Large') discretion and silence are the rule. In consultation, for example, 'all discussions should be held as secret and confidential. Neither by words nor manner should any of the parties to a consultation assert or insinuate that any part of the treatment pursued did not receive his assent.'[12] Furthermore, the consulting physician should not make any hint or insinuation that 'could impair the patient's confidence in the attending physician or negatively affect his reputation.'[13]

Association members were also cautioned against any negative appraisal of their peers based on a patient's unsuccessful outcome – the Code argued that 'want of success' in a particular case is 'no evidence of a lack of professional knowledge or skill.'[14] Although a poor outcome is *insufficient* grounds for a determination of a provider's ineptitude, such evidence clearly does not *rule out* the possibility of professional incompetence. Despite this fact, the Code makes no provisions for good-faith reporting of deficiencies in a regular colleague. There are a number of explanations for this omission. First and most obvious is the Association's reluctance to engender among its members the same attitude and atmosphere of distrust that it garnered against sectarians and the use of quack remedies. A second explanation is that the AMA did not, by reason either of circumstance or intention, have any formal mechanisms for investigating such charges. Indeed, given the absence of standards for either medical education or practice at the time, such an investigation would have been difficult to undertake. Where the job of regulation fell to the state medical societies, ethical restrictions proved largely unenforceable. A third, related explanation is linked to the gentlemanly ideal of self-scrutiny that held sway from the eighteenth to the early twentieth century. A gentleman was defined not by his class but by his moral virtues of integrity, honesty, generosity, courage, graciousness, politeness, and consideration for others.[15] Within this tradition, the honorable man was understood to be his own worst critic. He was one who could be counted on to acknowledge his errors and to prevent their occurrence in the future. Or as the Code states in its first paragraph: the obligations of the physician 'are the more deep and enduring because there is no tribunal, other than his own conscience, to adjudge penalties for carelessness and neglect.'[16] This tradition of gentlemanly honor was carried over from Thomas Percival's influential 1803 treatise, *Medical Ethics or A Code of Institutes and Precepts adapted to the Professional Conduct of Physicians and Surgeons*.[17] Regarding medical mistakes, Percival counsels physicians against self-deception, saying that their errors of omission and commission should be 'brought to mental view.'[18] He does not go on to suggest, however, that medical mishaps should be included in the record or disclosed to colleagues. Within the tradition of gentlemanly honor inherited from Percival, the AMA was entirely consistent in respecting and safeguarding the physician's moral autonomy. Character, rather than empirical standards, provided the basis for evaluation and, in deference to the ideal of personal integrity, the job of evaluation was left to each individual. Once established as a peer and thus presumably as a gentleman, the regular physician was spared the demeaning and meddlesome intrusions of his professional colleagues.[19] In fact, the demand for personal autonomy influenced the AMA to revise the Code in 1903 from an 'enforcement' to an 'advisory' document. In support of this less authoritarian role, one medical editor declared that 'character must be the foundation upon which ethical action is to be built. Proper conduct among men and affairs must be left to the man, his tact, his judgment, his education and his experience.'[20]

Even if we assume that the majority of practitioners were conscientious about learning from their mistakes, we can see that this model of accountability was seriously flawed. It did little for the patient at whose expense the insight might be gained. It contributed nothing to the general knowledge of therapeutic safety and effectiveness. And it shielded the practitioner from direct professional censure. In theory and in practice, this model of accountability has played an important role in maintaining the silence that has historically shrouded the phenomenon of iatrogenic illness. Interestingly, recent sociological studies of physicians' perceptions of their own accountability reveal that by and large, physicians and physicians-in-training continue to believe that they are answerable only to themselves.[21] As we will see, Ernest Codman's effort to institute a system of hospital oversight was a direct challenge to this tradition of personal accountability. As such, the effort was, during its time, largely unsuccessful.

Medical malpractice and the growth of local medical societies

Medical malpractice in the late nineteenth century proved to be another area in which the physician's obligations to patient welfare on the one hand, and to professional solidarity on the other, came into conflict. In the early part of the nineteenth century, malpractice was rare in part because there existed few objective standards by which practice could be evaluated. Indeed, as De Ville points out, the then dominant theory of medical specificity – that drugs worked differently in different people – made malpractice charges largely unsupportable.[22] As the nineteenth century progressed, however, so did scientific medicine. By mid-century, knowledge in such areas as the treatment of fractures and dislocations had advanced to the point where objective assessment was possible. Objective evidence elevated the stature of regular physicians who could now lay claim to a scientifically informed practice. It also, however, made them more vulnerable to external evaluation, particularly in the non-clinical setting of the courtroom. Between 1830 and 1900, medical malpractice cases in America increased more than 20-fold.[23] Responding to this on-slaught, the profession banded together under the aegis of local medical societies which had grown in strength and number since 1878.

During the latter part of the nineteenth and the early years of the twentieth century, local medical societies provided malpractice insurance and defense services to its members. The 1880 ruling in *Small* v. *Howard* established the 'locality rule' as the standard of evaluation in malpractice cases[24] and thereby guaranteed the growing authority of local societies. One practical effect of the locality rule was that it became almost impossible for a patient to get testimony against a member of the local society – now the arbiter of professional standards.[25] Indeed, in 1887, the Michigan state society ruled it unethical to volunteer testimony against one's professional colleagues.[26]

Local medical society membership brought with it the benefits not only of malpractice insurance and defense, but also of patient referrals and hospital privileges. In addition, it was a prerequisite for membership in the national association. Further, the success of the medical societies in de-fending cases against their members resulted in lower malpractice insurance rates for those within the society. Without membership, however, these advantages were hard if not impossible to obtain. As Starr observes, as 'the local medical fraternity became the arbiter of a doctor's position and fortune . . . he could no longer choose to ignore it.'[27]

As the practitioner's survival became increasingly dependent on the organized profession and the good will of colleagues, the patient's interests became increasingly obscured in the area of malpractice. The general sentiment was expressed in 1897 in the *Boston Medical and Surgical Journal*. 'Doctors have to protect each other, not to the extent of doing wrong, but to cover up any misfortune of their brethren so far as they can, in order that the general respect of the profession be preserved.'[28] As Konold points out, this protection extended to concealing mistakes in diagnosis and treatment. The author of a 1909 study of abdominal surge-ries reported 60 cases in which surgeons had left a foreign object in the abdominal cavity without 'damage to their reputations . . . Although the resulting infections often killed the patient, physicians did not ordinarily report accidents of this sort.'[29]

The upsurge in malpractice claims also became a significant factor influencing physician's treatment decisions. What became known in the 1970s as 'defensive medicine' seems to have had its origins in this period. In the case of fracture treatment, new methods of bone setting often resulted in visible imperfection – for example, the repaired leg healing shorter than the patient's other leg. Such imperfections could be pointed to as evidence of malpractice. Recognizing their vulnerability, some physicians were motivated to use amputation – an outdated and more dangerous procedure – that left behind no potentially damning evidence. As one historian observes, in the case of fractures, 'the best treatment for the patient was not necessarily the safest treatment for the physician.'[30]

Medical education reform

During the latter part of the nineteenth century, medical education became another area of emergent tension between the physician's obligation to patient welfare and to professional interest. Before the 1870s, medical education in the United States was almost entirely lacking in standards. Medical schools were fairly inexpensive to operate and were very profitable to their faculty who might personally collect $15 a year from each student.[31] Very few schools offered clinical training and might demand no more than a year of study from their students. Due to the ease of obtaining a medical degree and the haphazard requirements, between 1790 and 1850, the number of physicians in the United States rose from five to forty thousand – a rate much faster than the growth of the population.[32] The competence of medical school graduates during this period was, at best, questionable and was made even more suspect by the financial incentives of the schools to crank out greater and greater numbers of graduates. At one Ohio college, the school's receipt of the graduation fee was contingent on the student's passing the final examination – a potentially perverse incentive for the examining board.[33] It is perhaps, then, no accident that, during the Civil War, the Army rejected as incompetent 80% of all Ohio applicants for surgical positions.

In its 1847 Code, the AMA declared that a 'regular medical education' was a necessary and authorizing precondition for practice. In fact, it was the 'first duty' of the patient to select as a medical advisor only one who had received a 'regular professional education.'[34] Having made such a claim, and indeed having implied that regular practitioners were distinguished by their 'scientific' education, the profession was compelled to establish some formal educational standards. As Konold notes, the AMA struggled with the problem unsuccessfully for its first 25 years. During that time, delegates twice rejected a constitutional amendment that would have restricted Association membership to medical college graduates. The passage of such an amendment would, of course, have meant the exclusion of a large proportion of the existing membership. Many medical schools were equally reluctant to support educational reforms because they rightly believed that more rigorous requirements would threaten their very existence.

In the last quarter of the nineteenth century, progress in laboratory medicine, the growing importance of the hospital as a clinical classroom, and isolated but momentous curricular reforms at Harvard and Johns Hopkins began to yield the educational reforms that the AMA had been unable to accomplish during the previous 25 years. The course of medical study was extended to three years, basic science was added to didactic lectures, and students were required to pass not simply the majority but, rather, *all* of their courses. Johns Hopkins became the first medical school in the United States to require a college degree for admission. In 1870, Charles Eliot, the President of Harvard, had declared that 'the ignorance and general incompetency of the average graduate of American Medical Schools, at the time when he receives the degree which turns him loose upon the community, is something horrible to contemplate.'[35] This observation was underscored in 1906 by the newly established AMA Council on Medical Education. The Council had inspected the 160 extant medical schools and had found one-quarter to be sub-standard and one-fifth to be irredeemable. As Starr points out, although these results were disclosed at an AMA meeting, they were never made public. Publication would not only have generated ill will toward the Association but, as we have seen, would also have violated the admonitions concerning discretion in its own Code.[36]

As an alternative, the AMA invited the disinterested Carnegie Foundation for the Advancement of Teaching to undertake a similar investigation. They agreed, and in 1910 produced what has come to be known as the Flexner Report. The report was the culminating event in a series of changes that established national standards for medical education – standards that sought to link science and clinical practice.

Flexner's survey revealed, among other findings, a profession overcrowded with poorly educated and poorly trained surgeons. Lack of skill and fierce competition in the glutted surgical market resulted in fee splitting, inadequate laboratory analysis of tissues, and unnecessary surgery.[37] At this same time, hospitals and physicians – especially surgeons – were developing a symbiotic relationship. The surgeon benefited from the prestige and clinical opportunities associated with a hospital appointment. The hospital's benefit was principally financial – and it was a double benefit. The hospital offered no monetary compensation to accompany a surgeon's hospital privileges and yet, benefited financially when the affiliated physician referred patients to the hospital for treatment.

In 1912, catalyzed by Flexner's indictment of American medical education and his call for medical education reform, the Clinical Congress of Surgeons of North America initiated a plan for comparable reforms in surgical practice and the quality of hospital care. This plan was undertaken by Ernest A. Codman, chairman of the Committee on Hospital Standardization, and Edward Martin, whose Clinical Congress led directly to the formation of the American College of Surgeons (ACS) in 1913.

Ernest Codman and the 'end-result system'

During the early part of the twentieth century, surgeons and hospitals increasingly relied on the prestige of science to advance their reputations and interests. Codman challenged members of the medical establishment to demonstrate that their practices and outcomes were indeed compatible with the rigorous medical science they espoused. 'Will we put the methods of science to work in the evaluation of our own practices,' he asked, or,

must we admit that no matter how much we read, study, practice and take pains, when it comes to a show-down of the results of our treatment, no one could tell the difference between what we have accomplished and results of some genial charlatan ...?[38]

As a remedy, Codman offered the 'end-result system,' which was based, he said, 'on the common-sense notion that every hospital should follow *every* patient it treats, long enough to determine whether or not the treatment has been successful, and then to inquire 'if not, why not?' with a view to preventing similar failures in the future.'[39]

Codman's work is significant for a study of medical harm for a number of reasons. It was one of the earliest systematic attempts to determine and address the causes of adverse patient outcomes. As such, it was one of the first efforts in the United States to systematize health care quality improvement through data based on the processes and outcomes of care. Its emphasis on the public reporting of deficiencies in medical work made it one of the first and most forceful challenges to the tradition of personal accountability in medicine. Codman's work is significant as well because the end-result system explicitly identified patient benefit as the ultimate criterion of hospital efficiency. In this way, Codman's reform efforts, represented an attempt to harness the methods of science to serve the ancient obligations to benefit and to do no harm. Finally and more specifically, Codman's work was the point of departure for investigations into one particular type of medical harm – unnecessary surgery. In what follows we describe Codman's efforts to identify and prevent patient harms through his end-result system. In later chapters we explore some of the implications of Codman's work for our understanding of health care quality, unnecessary surgery, and the aims of medicine.

In his end-result system, Codman aimed to achieve hospital and surgical quality by a number of interrelated means. The centerpiece of the end-result system was a complete patient record that included the following information:[40]

(1) The symptoms or conditions for which [the patient] seeks relief.
(2) The diagnosis of the pathologic conditions which the doctor who gives the treatment believes to be the cause of the symptoms, and on which he bases his treatment.
(3) The general plan or important points of the treatment given.
(4) The complications which followed before the patient left the hospital.
(5) The diagnosis which proved correct or final at discharge.
(6) The results each year afterward.

The complete patient record was also to include an assessment of why a treatment was unsuccessful. The assessment was to be based on the following classifications:[41]

(1) Errors due to lack of technical knowledge or skill.
(2) Errors due to lack of surgical judgment.
(3) Errors due to lack of care or equipment.
(4) Errors due to lack of diagnostic skill.
(5) The patient's unconquerable disease.
(6) The patient's refusal of treatment.
(7) The calamities of surgery or those accidents and complications over which we have no known control.

The data collected in these categories could also serve an auditing function to evaluate, compare, and establish benchmarks for the performance of physicians and of hospitals.

The end-result system also offered a framework for prevention. Physician error could be controlled to a certain degree by such organizational strategies as credentialing and surgical assignments based on demonstrated competence. For adverse outcomes whose causes were unknown, prevention required not only scrupulous study but also the acknowledgment of uncertainty by both the profession and the public. 'Improvement is sure to follow,' Codman observed optimistically, 'for it is the error of which we are ignorant that we persist in carrying with us.'[42]

The end-result system was no theoretical dogma. Codman had followed its prescriptions for five years at his own private Boston hospital and published his results. In fact, one historian suggests that Codman's original motivation for clinical improvement may have come from his own personal experience of the possibly unnecessary death of a patient under his care.[43] Whereas Codman's own experience may have been sufficient to galvanize him in his quest for quality improvement, the translation of this plan from Codman's private hospital to the entrenched and highly politicized context of larger community and academic hospitals proved sufficiently heterodox to be unrealizable.

Codman's end-result system was unorthodox in a number of ways. The prevailing custom of hospital accounting assessed efficiency in purely financial terms, that is, in terms of monies subscribed and monies spent in different departments, numbers of patients treated and the per capita expense. Codman proposed to assess hospital efficiency in *therapeutic* rather than *fiscal* terms.[44] The real product of a hospital, he argued, is not its revenues but its success or failure in benefiting its patients. All of the business of a hospital from education to administration to medical publications, he said, must be judged by the standard of patient benefit. To the extent that a patient is harmed by a delay in recovery due to surgical wound infection, by an unnecessary or inappropriate operation, or by preventable death, the hospital product is a 'waste product.'[45]

Codman's system was unorthodox as well because it required formal and systematic evaluation of performance and thus fundamentally challenged the moral and professional autonomy of the physician. Under the end-result system, documented competence would replace individual conscience as the basis of clinical evaluation. With a clear understanding of the effrontery that his proposal presented to professional honor, Codman declared that to physicians, the 'comparison of achievements . . . would be as odious as a comparison of incomes.'[46] His reference to income was not accidental. Codman's plan also placed hospital administrators in the very awkward position of assessing the performance of the physicians to whom they offered no compensation but on whom they depended for patient income. When he was unable to get institutional administrators to support his plan Codman observed 'that the reason was MONEY; in other words, the staffs are not paid, and therefore cannot be held accountable.'[47] In his challenge to hospital trustees, Codman asserted that the conferral of hospital privileges must no longer be based upon the social or political prestige that the physician might bring to the hospital, but rather on his documented ability to benefit patients.[48]

Codman's unorthodox proposals were accompanied by equally unorthodox rhetoric. His most spectacular denunciation of resistance to the assessment of patient outcomes – particularly in the case of his own Massachusetts General Hospital – came in the form of a notorious eight foot (*ca.* 2.4 m) cartoon unveiled at a 1915 meeting on hospital efficiency in Boston. In the cartoon, Codman depicts the Back Bay community of Boston as an ostrich with its head buried in a mound of humbuggery, laying 'golden surgical eggs' such as appendicitis for the eager physicians at Massachusetts General. The trustees of the hospital are shown wondering whether candid outcomes reporting would stifle their lucrative enterprise: would the golden goose-ostrich, 'still be willing to lay, if we let her know the truth about our patients?' The word 'humbug' was carefully chosen by Codman to turn the tables on those members of the profession who prided themselves on their crusades against supposed quackery.[49] Anticipating the uproar that followed, Codman had already resigned his post at Massachusetts General.

It was only in 1916, when the ACS decided to incorporate Codman's Committee on Hospital Standardization, that his proposals began to receive serious consideration. The momentum of this effort was frustrated, however, by World War I. When the movement for surgical and hospital reform was renewed after the war, the program of hospital standardization advocated by the ACS had become significantly diluted. The new 'Minimum Standard for Hospitals' omitted the two most controversial features of the proposal and those that were most dear to Codman himself: the analysis of patient outcomes and the reporting of preventable error.[50] One explanation for the ACS's rejection of these direct measures of surgical and hospital performance may lie in the findings of the College's first broad study of surgical care. On the basis of objective criteria, J.G. Bowman, the director of the College, undertook a survey of cases of chronic appendicitis in 'good' hospitals and in 'poor' ones. His stated goal was to determine 'if any unnecessary surgical operations were performed, if incompetent surgeons were practicing, and/or if lax, lazy or incomplete diagnoses were made.'[51] According to one commentator, 'the facts elicited by the first survey were so shocking that the survey committee ordered the individual survey reports destroyed forthwith.'[52] Although none of these study data survive, it was reported that only 89 (13%) of the 692 hospitals investigated in these first years by the College met reasonable criteria of quality.

The Minimum Standard, that was ultimately adopted by the College, provides some evidence that when the ACS began its oversight, hospitals lacked even the most rudimentary standards of institutional structure and functioning. The Minimum Standard, which provided the basis of hospital evaluation from 1918 to 1952, required hospitals to: (1) institute medical staff organization, (2) restrict staff membership to competent and professional physicians, (3) oversee the establishment of policies regarding staff meetings and the analysis of clinical practice, (4) establish systematic and accessible medical recordkeeping, and (5) provide diagnostic and therapeutic facilities.[53] The intensive focus on needed structural guidelines seems to have supplanted the original and more contentious question of a hospital's rates of unnecessary operations and surgical failures.

Although it was significantly diluted in the Minimum Standard, this early work by Codman's ACS Committee on Standardization led directly to the formation in 1952 of the Joint Commission on Accreditation of Hospitals, now the Joint Commission on Accreditation of Healthcare Organizations or JCAHO. This professional association has become the largest accrediting body and overseer of hospital quality in the United States.

Endnotes

1 Rosenberg CE. *The Care of Strangers: The Rise of America's Hospital System.* New York: Basic Books, 1987, p. 341.
   Starr P. *The Social Transformation of American Medicine.* New York: Basic Books, 1982, p. 73 (note 50).
2 Rosenberg CE, p. 150 (see No. 1).
3 Rosenberg CE, p. 247 (see No. 1).
4 Cited in Konold DE. *A History of American Medical Ethics: 1847–1912.* Madison: State Historical Society of Wisconsin, 1962, p. 9.
5 American Medical Association, *Code of Medical Ethics*, 2nd edn. New York: William Wood & Company, 1868. (Cited hereafter as AMA Code, 1847.)
6 As we will see, this implication was manifestly false and the AMA spent considerable energy in its first 25 years attempting precisely to establish the educational standards whose existence was implied in the Code.
7 Konold DE, p. 25 (see No. 4).
8 AMA Code, 1847, p. 1 (see No. 5).
9 AMA Code, 1847, p. 7 (see No. 5).
10 AMA Code, 1847, p. 4 (see No. 5).
11 AMA Code, 1847, p. 38 (see No. 5).
12 AMA Code, 1847, p. 25 (see No. 5).
13 AMA Code, 1847, p. 27 (see No. 5).

14 AMA Code, 1847, p. 30 (see No. 5).
15 Himmelfarb G. *The De-Moralization of Society*. New York: Knopf, 1995, p. 46.
16 AMA Code, 1847, p. 3 (see No. 5).
17 Percival T. *Medical Ethics or A Code of Institutes and Precepts adapted to the Professional Conduct of Physicians and Surgeons*. Manchester: S. Russell, 1803. Regarding the review of one's cases, Percival counsels physicians to 'let no self-deception be permitted in the retrospect; and if errors either of omission or comission, are discovered, it behooves that they should be brought fairly and fully to mental view. Regrets may follow, but criminality will thus be obviated. For good intentions and the imperfections of human skill which cannot anticipate the knowledge that events alone disclose, will sufficiently justify what is past provided the failure be made conscientiously subservient to future wisdom and rectitude in professional conduct' (p.107).
18 Percival T, p. 107 (see No. 17).
19 Baker takes a different view, arguing that the codification of medical morality by Percival and later by the AMA in fact exchanged the traditional moral autonomy of the gentleman for collective standards of medical and moral propriety. That is, in the formation of codes, individual autonomy was replaced by collective autonomy. While it is true that the codes by their very nature were intended to impose general standards, the AMA standards were tolerable precisely because they still, fundamentally sanctified personal accountability.
    See Baker R. Deciphering Percival's code. In Baker R, Porter D, Porter R, eds. *The Codification of Medical Morality: Historical and Philosophical Studies of the Formalization of Western Medical Morality in the Eighteenth and Nineteenth Centuries. Volume 1: Medical ethics and etiquette in the eighteenth century*. Boston: Kluwer Academic Publishers, 1993, p. 179–211.
20 Konold DE, p. 69 (see No. 4).
    Engelhardt has pointed out that a similar standard of accountability was predominant in the Hippocratic era as well. As the Hippocratic text *On Laws* observes: 'medicine is the only art which our states have made subject to no penalty save that of dishonor.' *See* Engelhardt HT. *The Foundations of Bioethics*, 2nd edn. New York: Oxford, 1996) p. 166.
21 Mizrahi T. Managing medical mistakes: ideology, insularity and accountability among internists in-training. *Soc Sci Med* 1984; 19:135–146.
22 DeVille KA. *Medical Malpractice in Nineteenth-Century America: Origins and Legacy*. New York: NYU Press, 1990, p. 69.
23 DeVille KA, p. 3 (see No. 22).
24 *Small* v. *Howard* 128 Mass 131 (1880).
25 Starr P, p. 111 (see No. 1).
26 Konold DE, p. 49 (see No. 4).
27 Starr P, p. 111 (see No. 1).
28 Konold DE, p. 49 (see No. 4).
29 Crossen HS. Abdominal surgery without detached pads or sponges. *Am J Obstet* 1909; 59:58–75 & 250–284, cited in Konold, p. 49 (see No. 4).
30 DeVille KA, p. 154 (see No. 22).
31 Rothstein WG. *American Physicians in the Nineteenth Century: From Sects to Science*. Baltimore: Johns Hopkins Press, 1992, p. 94.
32 Starr P, p.64 (see No. 1).
33 Rothstein WG, p. 94 (see No. 31).

34 AMA Code, 1847, pp. 8–9 (see No. 5).

35 Quoted in Starr P, p. 113 (see No. 1).

36 Starr P, p. 118 (see No. 1).

37 Lembcke PA. Evolution of the medical audit. *JAMA* 1967; 199:534–50.

38 Meeting announcement for January 6, 1915 in Codman EA. *The Shoulder.* Malabar, FL: RE Kreiger, 1984 (first published 1934), p. xxiii.

39 Codman EA, p. xii (see No. 38).

40 Codman EA. *A Study in Hospital Efficiency as Demonstrated by the Case Report of the First Five Years of a Private Hospital.* Boston: n.p., n.d (probably 1916). Reprinted, Oakbrook Terrace: Joint Commission on Accreditation of Health care Organizations, 1996, p. 55.

41 Codman EA, p. 59 (see No. 40).

42 Codman EA, p. 58 (see No. 40).

43 Reverby S. Stealing the golden eggs: Ernest Amory Codman and the science and management of medicine. *Bull Hist Med* 1981; 55:156–71 (see pp. 157–8).

44 Reverby S. Stealing the golden eggs, p. 160 (see No. 43). Codman EA, p. xxiii (see No. 38).

45 Codman EA. The product of the hospital. *Surg Gynecol Obstet* 1914; 18(4):491–6 (see p. 495).

46 Codman EA, p. xxxv (see No. 40).

47 Meeting announcement for January 6, 1915 in Codman EA, p. xxiv (see No. 40).

48 Codman EA. A study in hospital efficiency as represented by product. *Trans Am Gynecol Soc* 1914; 39:92.

49 Reverby S, p. 161 (see No. 43).

50 Moore FD. Social biology and applied sociology: Cannon and Codman Fifty years later. *Harvard Med Alum Bull* 1975; 49(3):12–21.

51 Bowman JG. Hospital standardization series: General hospitals of 100 or more beds. Report for 1919. *Bull Am Coll Surg* 1920; 4:3–36.

52 Lembcke PA. Evolution of the medical audit. *JAMA* 1967; 199:545.

53 Bowman JG, p. 4 (see No. 51).

2

Medical epistemology, medical authority and shifting interpretations of beneficence and nonmaleficence

When Ernest Codman identified patient benefit as the ultimate standard and measure of the quality of care, he provided no explicit argumentation to justify his claim. Most likely, he saw it as self evident since his position reflected one of the most fundamental ethical commitments of medicine since the time of Hippocrates. The Hippocratic referents for the obligation to benefit the patient (beneficence) and to avoid patient harm (nonmaleficence) are found in the *Oath* and the *Epidemics*. In the *Oath*, the Hippocratic physician vows 'to use my treatment to help the sick according to my ability and judgment, but never with a view to injury and wrong-doing.' and to come 'to whatever houses I may visit . . . for the benefit of the sick . . .'[1] In *Epidemics I*, the physician is instructed to 'make a habit of two things – to help, or at least to do no harm.'[2]

In order to make historical sense of medical harm and the shifting interpretations of beneficence and nonmaleficence we examine the tradition of humoralism and its gradual displacement by scientific medicine in the nineteenth and twentieth centuries. We find, in each of these therapeutic traditions a paternalistic cast to the interpretation of these duties. Whereas the medical paternalism of the early nineteenth century may have been relatively unproblematic from the patient's point of view (since patient and physician had a common understanding of disorders and their treatments) the paternalism accompanying scientific medicine is grounded in the presumed epistemic authority of the physician. In practical terms, this presumption has profoundly shaped the patient–physician relationship insofar as it has given physicians the prerogative to define both benefit and harm. This presumption has proved to be the principal target of contemporary medical ethics and the stimulus for the advancement of patient autonomy. We look at the charitable paternalism of the nineteenth century and the scientific paternalism of the twentieth century to understand and demonstrate how definitions of benefit and harm (and thus perceptions of the obligations of beneficence and nonmaleficence) are closely tied to particular medical epistemologies. We also examine how a utilitarian conception of benefit invoked for promotion of public or common goods comes into tension with the conception of individual benefit central to the traditional ethos of healing.

Medical epistemology and medical practice

In the Hippocratic era, the art of medicine was practiced on the basis of humoral theory. Illness was conceived as the result of an imbalance or disturbance in the body's humors or fluids. Methods of treatment and prophylaxis were thus oriented to restoring or preserving humoral equilibrium. In the Hippocratic texts *On Disease IV*, and *On the Nature of Man*, the humors are identified as blood, bile, phlegm, and water or black bile each of which corresponds to a particular season. Not only did the Hippocratic writers emphasize a correlation between humoral and seasonal change, they also linked the excesses and deficiencies characteristic of illness to climate and geographical location. These linkages enhanced the diagnostic – or explanatory – power of humoral epistemology and provided a basis for a holistic therapeutics. Hippocratic diagnosis required a comprehensive understanding of the individual patient and his or her familial and environmental context. In earlier, primitive diagnosis and therapy, disease was largely understood as a manifestation of possession by some supernatural force. The healer was a priest or magician who sought to combat demonic possession with other and more supernaturally powerful potions.[3] The Hippocratic physician was, by contrast, a craftsman, whose effectiveness depended not on any supernatural connection but rather on working *with* nature and tailoring his art to the individual patient in his or her circumstances. The effectiveness of Hippocratic therapeutics was also attributable to its simplicity and accessibility to laypersons who might equally treat themselves or join with the physician in determining the treatment plan.[4]

Like other craftsmen of the period, the average Hippocratic physician held a very low social position.[5] From the patient's perspective, physicians were not regarded as authorities and their knowledge was not accorded automatic deference. Nor was the physician revered as a spiritual authority. From the patient's point of view, the physician earned both respect and income only by proving his ability through demonstrated technical skill, proper decorum, and successful treatments. According to Gunter Risse, it

was precisely the physician's dependence on personal character and reputation to earn a living that made him especially eager to benefit the patient
and to avoid iatrogenic harm.[6]

The epistomic and cultural origins of Hippocratic medical ethics find a
number of parallels in the medical ethics of eighteenth and nineteenth
century America. As historian Charles Rosenberg has pointed out, between the fifth century BC and the turn of the nineteenth century, 'medical
therapeutics [had] changed remarkably little.'[7] Humoralism remained the
dominant theoretical basis for diagnosis and treatment well into the nineteenth century and physicians still depended largely on the implicit association between character, reputation and efficacy to promote their services.
In addition, in the nineteenth century the dominant code of ethics in the
United States was, as in ancient times, as much an effort to raise the status
of the medical profession as it was an articulation of the moral ideals
governing patient care.

The influence of humoral epistemology in the early nineteenth century
reflected a shared belief system between practitioners and patients. Both
healer and patient regarded the body as 'a system of dynamic interaction
with its environment.'[8] Health was understood as a moment of equilibrium
in this dynamic interchange. Disease was an imbalance in the organism
that manifested itself in the excess or deficiency of bodily secretions. Since
the time of Galen in the 2nd century AD, humoralism had provided an
increasingly comprehensive explanatory framework for human disorders.
The humors were thought to correspond not only to the seasons of the
year, but also to the developmental phases of life, to temperaments, and
even, in the early Christian era, to the disciples Peter, Paul, Mark and
John.[9]

In the America of the eighteenth and early nineteenth centuries, this
shared holistic perception of health and disease resulted in a collaborative
method of diagnosis and therapy. In addition, with the senses as the only
diagnostic tools of the period, (the stethoscope was not introduced until
the mid-1800s, and the thermometer not until the late 1860s) doctors,
patients, and patients' families could all offer important information on
perspiration, urination, menstruation, and other phenomena associated
with the patient's condition. Each observer could ascertain whether the
particular remedy – diuretic, narcotic, cathartic, or emetic – achieved the
expected and desired modification. According to Rosenberg, in this era,
the effectiveness of therapy was evaluated in terms, above all else of its
production of a particular physiological effect. If the patient's condition
was one of overstimulation, then depletive therapy, such as bleeding or

purgation, would be required to produce calm. To the extent that the therapy delivered this effect, it was said to 'work' and produce, therefore, some degree of satisfaction for healer and patient. Within this framework, the physician's primary responsibility, both technical as well as moral, was to play an *active* role in adjusting and stabilizing the natural flow of bodily secretions.

Holistic rationalism and heroic medicine

In the late eighteenth and early nineteenth centuries, therapeutic activism found its most extreme expression in the so-called 'heroic medicine' championed by John Brown, Benjamin Rush, and others. When we look back on the history of iatrogenic harm in American medicine, it is this period that stands out most vividly for the violence of its remedies. Believing the Philadelphia yellow fever epidemic of 1793 to be the result of 'morbid excitement,' Rush countered with depletive therapies such as calomel, which might produce four or five large evacuations a day, and copious blood-letting whereby often up to five pints (*ca.* 2.84 liters) or half the total volume of blood would be lost in one day.[10] The virulence of Rush's therapeutics engendered so much fear and outrage that one newspaper editor decried it as 'one of those great discoveries which has contributed to the depopulation of the earth.'[11] Indeed, medical historian Robert Sullivan has argued that the term 'heroic medicine' was itself applied as a pejorative by detractors of Rush's methods who hoped thereby to distance themselves from practices that were becoming increasingly unacceptable in the early 1800s.[12] One Louisiana physician maintained that heroic therapeutics was just as horrible as the heroism of war, for both are achieved only by 'the slaughter of our fellow creatures.'[13]

It is important to point out that even as they administered their noxious remedies, practitioners such as Rush maintained an unfailing commitment to the duty of patient benefit. Rush's decision to remain in Philadelphia and continue treating patients during the yellow fever epidemic is only one manifestation of this commitment. In a 1793 letter to his wife, Rush expressed not only his belief in the propriety of his drastic remedies but also his acceptance of the ultimate power of divine Providence as an explanation for his therapeutic failures:

I feel the distress of my fellow citizens the more from my being unable to assist them, and from my hearing constantly of some of them being murdered by large and ill-timed doses of bark and wine. But I must not arraign the conduct of divine providence. 'When obedient nature knows His will A doctor or disease alike can kill.'[14]

To understand how heroic therapy was consistent with the obligations to benefit the patient and to do no harm, it is helpful to look at the imperatives behind the theory that emerged as heroic medicine's most powerful rival – therapeutic skepticism.

Skeptical empiricism and therapeutic nihilism

Opposition to activist, interventionist therapies increased throughout the early years of the nineteenth century. Patients, fearful of the traumas associated with copious bleeding and toxic doses of calomel and tartar emetic, began to seek out milder remedies from new homeopathic and hydropathic practitioners. The shift to milder remedies was also a function of the skeptical empiricism that American medical students imported from Paris in the 1800s.

Arguing against the Galenic rationalist tradition which was the basis of humoralism, the empiricists maintained that the truth was to be found not in theories (like humoralism) but in (observable) things. Accordingly, they advocated scrupulous clinical observation as the authoritative method-ological basis of medical practice.[15] The commitment to empiricism was epitomized by Pierre Louis' 'numerical' method. By the statistical assess-ment of diseases and their treatments, Louis set out to determine the efficacy of traditional therapeutics. This early effort at outcomes research confirmed the suspicion that such orthodox practices as bloodletting and the widespread use of tartar emetic and calomel were at best useless and at worst positively harmful.[16] The practical correlate of these discoveries was a *therapeutic* skepticism: empiricists increasingly espoused a less interven-tionist, and, therefore, they believed, a less harmful approach to patient care. The healing powers of nature were recommended over those of the art of medicine and the program for therapeutics was supportive rather than interventionist. This shift was captured by Gabriel Andral, a skeptic confrère of Louis, who reversed the classic therapeutic maxim 'better something doubtful than nothing,' to read: 'better nothing than something doubtful.'[17]

When this chary approach to therapeutics was imported to the United States, it collided with the established tradition of active, interventionist practice championed by Benjamin Rush. As medical historian Martin Pernick has pointed out, these two approaches to patient care represented, not simply two rival methods of cure but two competing visions of the doctor's professional role and ethical duties . . . The natural healers' version of professional duty portrayed the doctor's role as simply to help the patient avoid anything that might interfere with nature's healing power . . . The scientific claim that nature heals [the *vis medicatrix naturae*] shaded easily into the ethical fallacy that nature is good . . . In this view, medical interference with nature was not simply harmful, it was immoral. Natural healing held a physician ethically responsible only for the damage done by medicine.[18]

Rush, by contrast, specifically condemns the Hippocratic belief in the healing powers of nature and the physician as nature's servant as impediments to the progress of medicine. 'It is impossible,' says Rush, 'to calculate the mischief which Hippocrates has done by first marking nature with his name, and afterwards, letting her loose upon sick people. Millions have perished by her hands in all ages and countries.'[19] In Rush's estimation,

the first duty of a doctor was action – 'heroic' action – to fight disease. Rush regarded a physician who killed a patient through overdosing as perhaps overzealous, but one who allowed the patient to die through insufficiently vigorous therapy was both a murderer and a quack.[20]

Each of these medical philosophies manifests a commitment to patient benefit. They differ, however, in their interpretations of benefit and therefore, necessarily of harm. In each case, complex cultural and religious forces influenced how benefit was understood. As the heroic practitioner understood it, benefit meant giving priority to the value of saving life over that of preventing suffering. As such, the heroic physician eschewed attempts to alleviate suffering if they posed risk to life. Amputation, which produced gruesome pain, hemorrhage, and often fatal shock, vividly illustrates the practical consequences of this understanding. Their belief in the virility of the American pioneer spirit, in the peculiar harshness of Americans – as contrasted with European – illness, and in pain itself as a positive therapeutic mechanism whose severity might counteract illness, allowed heroic physicians to justify the humanity of their practices. 'Severe pain,' it was argued, 'should never be an obstacle to the performance of life preserving operations.'[21]

Natural healers, by contrast, reflected nineteenth century Romanticism in their conception of nature as a beneficent force. In addition, some natural healers imbued the suffering associated with illness (or 'disordered nature') as spiritually cleansing. Finally, rather than combating illness with contrary forces (heat with cold, lassitude with stimulation, excitation with depletion) natural healers trained in homeopathy sought to treat 'like with like'. Benefit was to be found not in opposition to nature but in conformity with it.

By the 1830s, natural healing had begun to displace heroic medicine as the dominant therapeutic paradigm in the United States. It was accompanied by a new ethical paradigm that identified the principle of non-maleficence (literally not *doing* harm) as the physician's primary duty. It is in this skeptical climate that we find the origin of the expression *primum non nocere* or '*first* do no harm.' Although the injunction is often mistakenly attributed to Hippocrates (whose *Epidemics I*, charged physicians to '*at least* do no harm'), Worthington Hooker in his 1849 treatise *Physician and Patient,* credits its first use to A.-F. Chomel, preceptor to Pierre Louis.[22] The phrase *primum non nocere* thus seems to have been a natural outgrowth of combined beliefs about the inefficacy and danger of traditional therapeutics and the benignity and beneficence of natural processes. To avoid causing harm to one's patient, one must forgo active intervention in favor of a facilitation of nature's own curative capacities. This epistemological shift, which was branded as 'therapeutic nihilism' by its detractors, fundamentally challenged the professional identity and morality of the American practitioner. If, as the axiom *primum non nocere* implies, the physician must unconditionally avoid direct harm to the patient, then most medical interventions would, as interventions, be prohibited on moral grounds.

Statistical empiricism and therapeutic moderation

For the growing and ambitious profession of regulars, such constraints were unsupportable. Relief, however, came in the form of 'conservative medicine' espoused by Austin Flint, Worthington Hooker, Oliver Wendell Holmes, and the surgeon Frank Hamilton. In their pleas for therapeutic moderation these physicians hoped to remind their colleagues that unlike the postulate of law that a person is 'innocent until proven guilty,' 'a medicine . . . should always be presumed to be harmful.'[23]

Using probability theory and new statistical techniques developed in France, advocates of conservative medicine proposed a 'middle course' between heroic and nihilistic therapeutics, or, in the words of one of its proponents, between 'meddlesome interference [and] imbecile neglect.'[24] Rather than subscribing to the natural healer's absolute imperative to '*first* do no harm' or to the heroic practitioner's commitment to life at any cost, the conservative practitioner reasoned that statistical measurement could provide objective guidance in weighing the relative harms of both disease and treatment. Complemented by statistics, clinical empiricism thus offered a new moral norm and one that continues to influence practice today: 'If a remedy is dangerous, we are morally bound not to use it, unless withholding it involves a greater danger still.'[25]

The introduction of ethyl anesthesia in 1846 provided a turning point in the shift to conservative medicine. Objections to anesthesia were numerous and came from many sources. If its aim were simply to relieve suffering, some heroic practitioners believed that the risk posed by anesthesia was potentially incompatible with what they perceived to be their principal obligation, the preservation of life. Some natural healers objected to the anesthetic alleviation of pain because they saw pain as a sign of deviation from nature and thus as a just retribution for unnatural living. Conservative medicine, by contrast, took its inspiration from the reform movements of the nineteenth century and invoked the reformist interpretation of pain and suffering. British prison reform was grounded in the utilitarian conception of pain as evil and pleasure as good. Likewise, the anti-slavery movement in the United States fashioned its cause around the removal of human suffering. In medicine, these reformist sentiments translated into a general commitment to the minimization of pain, suffering, and harm and to the maximization of patient benefit. Insofar as it could add to the side of benefit, the administration of anesthesia was thus seen as a morally legitimate adjunct to therapy.

The introduction of the proportional calculus had practical as well as ethical consequences. Practically, therapeutic moderation helped to consolidate a profession sharply divided between the extremes of violent intervention and restrained subservience to nature. As we have seen, the regular profession regarded this consolidation as essential since patients were increasingly drawn to the milder remedies of sectarian practitioners. Ethically, the proportional calculus explicitly broadened the physician's obligation to encompass the prevention or avoidance of *both* naturally *and* medically-induced harms. In this way, the calculus invalidated the moral force that had been invested in the distinction between acts and omissions and used by heroic and natural healers to condemn the rival form of practice. This expanded obligation has continued to define physician responsibility and finds contemporary manifestation in the moral sanctions against *both* harms of omission, such as failure to diagnose breast cancer, *and* harms of commission, such as drug overdosage. As we will see in Chapter 4, this broadened obligation also establishes both beneficence and nonmaleficence as essential ingredients of the duty to 'do no harm.'

Despite its moderating influence, conservative medicine was not without its critics among the ranks of regular practitioners. Some alleged that the proportional calculation of benefit and harm supplanted clinical judgment and thereby reduced medical decision making to a rote technique. Those who espoused the epistemic primacy of a physician's judgment and 'bedside knowledge' rejected the implication that medical decision making should be rule governed or routinized. 'Any surgical operation,' said Charles Meigs, 'founded . . . on some cold and calculating computation of benefits possible, I regard as of doubtful propriety.'[26] The epistemological shift from clinical intuition to a quasi-statistical empiricism was regarded as morally suspect because it threatened to dehumanize the physician. As the nineteenth century progressed and as experimental, laboratory-based medicine gained ascendancy over the French-inspired clinical empiricism, the moral stakes were raised further still.

Laboratory science and scientific medicine

Before the American Civil War, the Paris Clinical School was a magnet for Americans studying medicine abroad.[27] Here, students learned the rigors of clinical observation by tracing the course of disease from the bedside to the autopsy room. By the end of the 1860s, however, many students and practitioners in the United States took their inspiration from the German science laboratories where observation was reinforced by the experimental method. New-found knowledge in physiology clarified basic mechanical processes in health and disease and in the action of various remedies. Later, the science of bacteriology established germs as a causal mechanism in infectious disease.

As we have seen, shifts in medical epistemology are accompanied by new moral norms. When laboratory science began to direct clinical practice, it presented heretofore the most significant challenge to the moral and professional identity of the American practitioner. It did so through a reductionist epistemology that emphasized the nature of disease entities rather than the concatenation of environmental, social, and constitutional factors that were traditionally held to influence health. The new epistemology also stressed the universal applicability of physiological and biochemical laws over the idiosyncrasies of individualized treatment. This resulted in a movement away from general (holistic) practice to specialized practice oriented to particular diseases, disorders, or organ systems. Finally, the new science of medicine was advanced by the use of precision instrumentation to establish norms for functional health and impairment. As much as instruments such as the stethoscope, the thermometer, and the ophthalmoscope (invented by von Helmholtz in 1850–51) extended the practitioner's diagnostic reach, they also served quite literally to distance the patient from the physician.[28] Direct sensory observation of the patient was now mediated by instruments. To the more traditional practitioner, the introduction of instrumentation presented a threat to professional discernment and, in so doing, exposed the patient to unknown risks. As the historian J. H. Warner has observed, the transformation in medical epistemology from clinical empiricism to experimentally-based therapeutics was tellingly reflected in the shift in metaphors used to describe medical practice. In the medical rhetoric of the period, the most common metaphor – that of navigation 'in which the application of general rules had to be fitted to the peculiarities of local winds and waters' – was replaced by an engineering metaphor, 'which embodied ideals of exactness and precision.'[29]

In general, the optimism that accompanied laboratory science was proportional to the pessimism that had characterized skeptical empiricism. With traditional therapeutics in disrepute, the laboratory offered hope that medicine would soon have a new foundation in what were now seen as the 'basic' sciences. The controversy that emerged in the 1870s and 1880s over the AMA Code of Ethics reveals the deep divisions engendered by this new professional trajectory.[30]

The Code controversy: science vs. ethics

As we have seen, the 1847 Code of Ethics was essential to the unification of the regular profession in the mid-nineteenth century. One way that the framers of the Code sought to achieve this goal was through the explicit exclusion of sectarian practitioners. The Code's consultation clause emphasized the intellectually and morally suspect character of the sectarian as well as the impropriety of consultation between sectarians and those who wished to identify themselves with the regular profession.

A regular medical education furnishes the only presumptive evidence of professional abilities and requirements, and ought to be the only acknowledged right of an individual to the exercise of his profession . . . [n]o one can be considered a regular practitioner or a fit associate in consultation, whose practice is based on exclusive dogma, to the rejection of the accumulated experience of the profession.[31]

The consultation prohibition, along with the prohibitions on advertising and the use of patent medicines, generated a great deal of hostility against the 1847 Code. Warner suggests, however, that the most formidable challenge came from the advocates of scientific medicine. By the 1870s, advocates of experimentally-based medicine dismissed the consultation clause and with it the authority of the Code as a whole, arguing that science alone was the appropriate arbiter in medical matters. According to the Code's principal detractors, any general distinction between sectarians and regulars was specious and arbitrary, for true science is entirely 'indifferent to Hippocrates and Hahnemann (the founder of homeopathy). The therapeutics of today rejects dogmas, and the therapeutics of the future will accept nothing that can not be demonstrated by the tests of science.'[32] The resolution of therapeutic controversy could, in other words, be accomplished by the application of the natural laws of science. Scientific determinations would thus obviate the need for any artificial code of ethics.

Defenders of the Code likewise grounded their rhetoric in an appeal to epistemological claims. Austin Flint and Alfred Stillé believed that medicine, no matter how scientific, would always depend upon clinical observation. This fact, as well as the irreducible individuality of the sick person, could never, by definition, be comprehended by a set of universal laws. Medicine, in other words, could never be an exact science. The 'inescapable uncertainty'[33] of therapeutic practice demanded the art of clinical judgment and this fact, maintained Flint and Stillé, demanded a moral code. Such a code was well served by a distinction between the regular and the irregular practitioner, for it was the regular physician who, having pledged fidelity to the Code, would be bound by its norms.

In 1903, pressure from state medical societies and continued rancor over the exclusivity of the AMA, led to a revision of the Code and the abandonment of its consultation clause. Although explanations for hostility to the consultation clause tend to center on the economic disadvantages that it imposed upon physicians,[34] many also objected to the fact that the consultation clause usurped the physician's judgment of what was in the best interests of the patient. To its adherents, the 1847 Code was the apotheosis of professional propriety. This allowed the Code's framers to make the simultaneous claims that 'in consultations the good of the patient is the sole object in view.'[35], and that only a *regular* practitioner is morally authorized to provide treatment. This was particularly irksome to the promoters of laboratory-based therapeutics who believed that scientific expertise provided the only warrant for clinical judgment. Thus, the stated objective of scientific practitioners opposing the 1847 Code was 'to preserve to each physician perfect liberty to decide with whom he shall act in order to secure the best interests of the sick ...'[36] By 1903, delegates of the AMA resolved that prohibitions on consultation were an unacceptable restraint on the physician's intellectual integrity and professional autonomy.

The Code controversy is important for an understanding of medical harm because it heralds the growing epistemic authority of science, and by association, the authority of practitioners to determine what is and what is not in the best interests of the sick. In other words, the resolution of the Code controversy signals the growing epistemic authority of medical science to define both patient benefit and harm.

As we have seen, prior to the advent of scientific medicine, the physician's effectiveness was intimately associated with his character, his propriety, and his embodiment of the system of beliefs shared by his patients. If, in other words, the early nineteenth century physician was called upon to practice his healing art, he was called in precisely because he was personally trusted. As scientific medicine gained authority throughout the last half of the nineteenth century, the patient's motivation to seek medical care stemmed not so much from the experience of trust and 'a shared nexus of belief and participation'[37] with a particular physician, but rather, from a growing faith in the authority of what was unfamiliar to the layman – expert knowledge.

The authority of scientific expertise

In the Jacksonian period before the Civil War, claims to expert knowledge and indeed to professional distinction were regarded with suspicion as antithetical to the democratic spirit. During that time, most of the licensure laws benefiting the regular profession were repealed, thus opening the doors to the unregulated medical practice and education that typified the much of the nineteenth century. By the Progressive era (1890–1920), the tumult and uncertainty that had characterized nineteenth-century medicine had been replaced by a consolidation of professional authority. As Starr describes it, this consolidation was attributable in part to the social legitimization of expertise.[38] In the first decades of the twentieth century, industrial capitalism, the growth of urban areas, and the demonstrable successes of science in the enhancement of public health created a demand for expertise and an attitude of deference to new forms of knowledge. In medicine, this shift was signaled at the turn of the century by the nearly universal reenactment of licensure laws.

By the beginning of the twentieth century, the therapeutic promise of scientific medicine had begun to be realized. A rabies inoculation had been available since 1886, and diphtheria, tetanus, and typhoid antitoxins at around the turn of the century. The discovery of the bacteriological etiology of wound infection and the introduction of surgical antisepsis and asepsis occurred in the 1860s to 1890s, and the development of Salvarsan as a treatment for syphilis in 1910. According to Rothman, the sentiment behind the granting of discretion to medical professionals (as well as to other professionals, to captains of industry, to parents and husbands) was that they should be given the latitude necessary to fulfill their benevolent designs. Thus doctors came to assert their manifestly superior knowledge over that of their patients.[39]

In addition to benefiting from the rising influence of science, the medical profession also consolidated its authority by deliberate efforts to assume regulatory control over medical education, licensure, and the patient's access to medicinal compounds. By the 1920s, professionally generated standards were the *sine qua non* of state licensure laws. Doctors licensed other doctors. The AMA, having led the fight for educational reform, was now the *de facto* accrediting agency for medical schools. Complementing the journalistic muckraking against patent medicines, the AMA established a Council on Pharmacy and Chemistry to set standards for drug manufacture and to evaluate claims of effectiveness. The AMA's *New and Nonofficial Remedies* became the authoritative source for drug information such that manufacturers who sought to circumvent its review process found themselves cut off from their markets. As knowledge of drug safety and efficacy was increasingly seen as the province of medical practitioners, doctors began to assume the important role of gatekeeper between drug manufacturers and patients. The 1938 Federal Food, Drug, and Cosmetic Act solidified the profession's role in drug regulation as it conferred upon the profession the responsibility for drug prescribing.[40] The AMA was well placed to implement – and to gain from – the reformist mood of the nation. With the prestige lent by science and the cultural embrace of institutional authority, physicians became the twentieth century's icons of social progress. At no time was this more evident than in the period surrounding World War II when medical research became a national program and priority.

In the late 1930s, the United States Congress for the first time authorized the Public Health Service to make grants to extramural researchers. This established an important precedent and helped to confer legitimacy on activities that had heretofore been conducted largely as a cottage industry. In 1941, Franklin Roosevelt created the Committee on Medical Research (CMR) for the purpose of systematically addressing the medical problems related to the war effort. It was under the auspices of the CMR that penicillin became widely available to both military and later civilian populations. Of all of the medical innovations of the period, penicillin was the most important both for its antibiotic and its sociological effects. Penicillin's effectiveness in subduing infection was the catalyst for widespread public endorsement of medical science. After the war, when the CMR's projects were transferred to the then National Institute of Health (NIH), the latter's research budget increased from $180,000 to $4 million. By 1950, the NIH consisted of five research divisions and had a total budget of $46.3 million.[41] In the post-war period, the development of the vaccine for polio – the leading cause of childhood disability and death from infectious disease – confirmed for the public and its elected representatives the essential importance of medical innovation. By 1960, Congressional appropriations for the NIH reached $400 million.

The growth of medical research quickly transformed the departmental structure of medical schools, the medical curriculum, and the necessary requirements for hospital privileges. These changes were met with hostility by private, non-academic physicians whose strictly clinical emphasis was seen as increasingly anachronistic in an era that emphasized research. The social rewards bestowed on medical research and researchers, however, yielded compensatory benefits for clinicians. The status and authority of the clinical practitioner were elevated by the social legitimization of science. Patients were eager to avail themselves of the miracles that scientific medicine had to offer and they looked to their physicians to perform them. In 1945, the first year that penicillin was widely available to the public, one out of four United States citizens had received a prescription for this antibiotic.[42] The hostility that clinicians felt about the dominance of research was also softened, Starr reports, by the economic prosperity that they enjoyed. Between 1945 and 1969, the annual increase in physician income exceeded the increase in the consumer price index by more than 3%. During this period, the average net profit from medical practice rose from $8000 to $32,000.[43]

The research community benefited as well, but in more subtle ways, from its association with the traditional doctor–patient relationship. As the war and later post-war initiatives gave priority to human subjects research, medical science was assumed to operate under the same norms of beneficence and nonmaleficence that governed the therapeutic relationship. In 1953, the NIH established its Clinical Center for the recruitment of patients into clinical research undertaken at its seven institutes. Patient brochures from the Center emphasized the familiar ethos of the traditional doctor–patient therapeutic relationship. 'Just like the family doctor,' the brochure stated, 'the physician in the Clinical Center has a professional and moral obligation to do everything possible to benefit the patient . . . The primary purpose of the Clinical Center is medical research in the interest of humanity, and this purpose is achieved at no sacrifice of benefit to the individual.'[44] On the strength of this assumption, the government left control over research in the hands of the scientific community.

In the course of the preceding half century, the medical profession had secured the prerogative of self-regulation. As we have seen, the socially-sanctioned policy of professional self-regulation depended largely on the granting of moral autonomy to individual physicians. Where patient care was concerned, personal accountability remained the norm. Now, as members of the profession began to direct human subjects research, that autonomy was extended to their new role. Just as the physician's integrity was deemed sufficient to safeguard the *patient*, so too was the integrity of the physician/researcher sufficient to safeguard individual *subjects*. As Rothman has observed, the fact that a NIH researcher was,

assuredly *not* a family physician, or that the well-being of humanity and the well-being of the patient might diverge, were issues the NIH did not confront. The clinical center set neither formal requirements to protect human subjects nor clear standards for its investigators to follow in making certain that subjects were well-informed about the research protocols. As a result, the hallmark of the investigator–subject relationship was its casualness, with disclosures of risks and benefits, side effects, and possible complications, even basic information on what procedures would be performed left completely to the discretion of the individual investigator.'[45]

According to the director of the National Heart Institute, by informing the patient/subject of potential risks, the researcher would 'unduly alarm the patient and hinder his reasonable evaluation of procedures important to his welfare.'[46] In other words, patient/subjects were not conceived capable of evaluating research risks in ways that would result in benefit to themselves or, quite possibly, to the researcher.

In 1962, Congress tightened regulations on the drug industry by authorizing the Food and Drug Administration (FDA) to test drug efficacy as well as safety. Despite the fact that the Congressional investigations on drug research revealed that patients were not always made aware of the experimental nature of their treatment, there was substantial resistance to the imposition of any disclosure requirements on investigators. The original language proposed to amend the FDA bill was that 'no such [experimental] drug may be administered to any human being in any clinical investigation, unless . . . that human being has been appropriately advised that such drug has not been determined to be safe in use for human beings.'[47] The language finally accepted in the amendment requested the Secretary of Health, Education, and Welfare to 'promulgate regulations so that investigators dispensing experimental drugs would obtain the consent of their subjects *"except when they deem it is not feasible or in their best professional judgment, contrary to the best interests of such human beings."* '[48] (our emphasis added).

The final language of the 1962 amendment expressed the conviction that in the context of research, the researcher, not the patient, would have ultimate authority to determine the acceptability of risk. This protective role was entirely consistent with the ethos of paternalism that characterized the relationship between doctor and patient. Not only was it the physician's obligation to benefit the patient and to 'do no harm', but knowledge of just what constituted benefit and harm was assumed to be available only to the physician. With this in mind it is useful to compare the paternalistic cast of the physician–patient relationship in the nineteenth and twentieth centuries.

Two varieties of paternalism

The beneficence advocated in the AMA's 1847 Code of Ethics can perhaps be characterized as a charitable paternalism – a type of *noblesse oblige* on the part of the gentleman-physician who could be counted on to ignore the indignities presented to him in the sickroom and to focus instead on the humanity of the ill person. The essence of charitable paternalism was captured in the Code's exhortation that the proper comportment of the physician toward the patient was one that united 'condescension with authority.'[49] In the eighteenth/nineteenth century sense of the term, 'condescension' was the magnanimous renunciation of superiority and the assumption of equality with someone of inferior status. The physician could best serve the patient through an attitude that was at once generous and authoritative. The Code's articulation of the duties owed by patients to physicians highlights the corresponding importance of obedience and gratitude. Because 'the members of the medical profession . . . make so many sacrifices of comfort, ease, and health, for the welfare of those who avail themselves of their services, [they] certainly have a right to expect and require, that their patients should entertain a just sense of the duties which they owe to their medical attendants.'[50] Included among these duties: 'to select . . . a medical advisor who has received a regular professional education'; 'prompt and implicit obedience to the prescriptions of his physician' and 'after his recovery . . . a just and enduring sense of the value of the services rendered him by his physician.'[51] Although subsequent AMA Codes omitted reference to patient duties, the trust that patients felt toward physicians was such that they continued to embrace charitable paternalism well into the early decades of the twentieth century. There are a number of reasons why this was so. As we have seen, during this period, the relationship was predicated on a common conception of health and disease. Because patient and physician were united rather than divided by medical knowledge, there was a degree of collaboration in the determination of the therapeutic regimen. Trust easily followed from the shared, collaborative healing process as well as from an intimate knowledge of the physician's character. As Rothman has pointed out, up until the 1930s, more than half of doctor–patient encounters still took place in patients' homes and most doctors continued to have localized practices that connected them directly to their neighbors and communities.[52] The contemporary conception of medical paternalism as 'beneficence which interferes with the liberty of [the] one whose good is to be promoted,'[53] is thus anachronistic when applied to the physician–patient relationship in the nineteenth and early twentieth centuries. Although, at the time, the new nation of the United States was fervent in its appeals to rights and liberty, these ideas had not yet come to characterize the patient's prerogative in medical decision making. This transformation in the physician–patient relationship would have to wait until the 1970s.

Like the charitable paternalism of the nineteenth century, the paternalistic ethos of twentieth century scientific medicine has evolved in tandem with a host of complex epistemological and cultural factors. Contemporary biomedicine has tended to operate on the basis of a reductionist medical epistemology that emphasizes the biological and physiological similarity of humans rather than their individual differences. Scientific epistemology has thus substantially displaced the individual patient both as an object and as a subject of medical knowledge. Whereas this epistemology has enhanced the diagnosis and treatment of disease, it has also – by it very focus on the biochemical basis of disorders – served to diminish the significance of the patient's particularity.[54] Through the lens of twentieth century biomedicine, the patient's self-report became a potential source of bias in the objective discernment and verification of disease. Further, insofar as the patient's complaints might not be recognized within the doctor's interpretive framework, 'the doctor's expertise might routinely negate the patient's understanding of his or her own disease.'[55] As Feinstein observes, 'the scientific aspects of modern clinical care are . . .

often focused more on the patient's laboratory identification as a diseased organism than on his bedside identity as a sick person.'[56]

The increasingly scientific character of twentieth-century medicine has also meant that patients and doctors no longer meet on a common ground of shared medical knowledge. Medical knowledge is unfamiliar to most patients, and, as such, typically separates rather than unites doctor and patient. The ascendancy and social legitimization of scientific medicine – reflected both in vast appropriations for biomedical research and in the authority of the medical profession – established the physician as the locus of epistemic authority and control in the clinical encounter. Finally, in the United States, the prestige and influence enjoyed by physicians in the twentieth century was only dreamed of by nineteenth-century 'regulars.'

These factors, all alien or unthinkable to the nineteenth century practitioner are today the commonplaces of American medicine. Their implications for the doctor–patient relationship have been profound: witness the priority of the term 'doctor' in the standard phrase 'doctor–patient relationship' which emphasizes the physician, and the physician's judgment as the most important pivot in the healing relationship.[57] Throughout this period, the Hippocratic Oath has remained a touchstone of medical morality. With the ascendancy of scientific medicine, the Hippocratic mandate – to 'help the sick *according to my ability and judgment,* but never with a view to injury and wrong-doing'[58] (our emphasis added) – has taken on new force. In the twentieth century, as in the nineteenth, the obligations of beneficence and nonmaleficence have been interpreted and exercised paternalistically. What distinguishes the paternalism of the twentieth century from that of the nineteenth is that the physician's charge to act 'according to my ability and judgment' has been legitimated by the power and promise of science. As Reiser has observed, the patient in nineteenth century America acted as narrator, the doctor as biographer.[59] In the twentieth century, the doctor has acted, and to some degree been invited to act, as the patient's *auto*biographer since he or she is understood to supply the relevant details of a patient's clinical narrative. In his book on doctor–patient communication, Eric Cassell relates a story that underscores this point. In the 1930s, he says, his grandmother went to see a specialist about a melanoma on her face. During the course of the visit when she asked him a question, he (reprimanded her) saying, 'I'll ask the questions here. I'll do the talking.'[60]

With respect to harm prevention, the physician's or investigator's superior knowledge was seen to heighten the responsibility for safeguarding patients and subjects. That belief that patients/subjects did not have sufficient knowledge to protect themselves was reflected in the disclosure requirements for research and treatment. Until 1966, when the FDA issued regulations requiring explicit informed consent to clinical trials, it was the investigator who judged what information was materially relevant to the research subject.[61] Likewise, until 1972, the 'professional practice standard' operated as the only legal norm for disclosure of treatment information. The 1972 case, *Canterbury* v. *Spence*, represents a landmark in informed consent law because it challenged professional control over information regarding the benefits and risks of therapy. As the *Canterbury* court expressed it: 'the patient's right of self decision shapes the boundaries of the duty to reveal.'[62]

As we will see, increasing emphasis on patient self-determination was attributable in part to mounting attention to the downsides of 'medical progress' – and in particular to iatrogenic illness. To understand both the historical as well as the ethical relationship between patient autonomy and iatrogenic illness, we return briefly to the post-war years – an era marked by the unbridled promotion of 'medical progress.'

Human subjects research: individual risk and the public good

The ethos of therapeutic paternalism was not the only factor that facilitated the hands-off policy with regard to medical research in the post-war period. The tradition of paternalism meshed well with the utilitarian conception of beneficence spawned by the exigencies of war. The research aims of medicine coincided with public policy initiatives that emphasized both the nation's interest in scientific preeminence and the betterment of humanity itself. Indeed, some of the most compelling rhetoric of the period combined the metaphors of war with scientific expansionism. The nation was 'marshaling its troops to wage war on disease' and, with penicillin and the sulfonamides, had all but 'conquered' diseases such as pneumonia and meningitis.[63] The most alluring ideal – reinforced by the specific action of Salvarsan in treating syphilis, of streptomycin for treating tuberculosis, and of penicillin – was that compounds could be created that would serve as 'magic bullets' in the pharmaceutical 'armamentarium.'

As a matter of public policy, the precedent of professional self-scrutiny seemed the most appropriate and perhaps most fruitful mechanism of accountability. Having witnessed how state control of research in Nazi Germany had stifled scientific progress before the war, government officials as well as researchers were wary of rigid external controls. The revelations at the Nuremberg Trials of the atrocities in Nazi-sponsored human subjects research served to reinforce the conviction that governmental regulation was suspect and that researchers in the United States should remain autonomous. Nazi researchers were considered to be so far beyond the moral pale and so much the tools of fascist ideology that the more mundane lessons of the German experience were overlooked. In particular, the government and the scientific community overlooked or ignored the fact that regardless of the political context in which it emerges, the utilitarian goal of social welfare – of the greatest good for the greatest number – is necessarily in tension and often deeply incompatible with the goal of individual welfare. But individual welfare was, of course, precisely the object of the traditional ethos of medicine and the stated justification for the granting of self-regulation to researchers. By continuing to emphasize their obligations of beneficence, now geared toward the good of the nation or humanity itself, medical researchers felt assured that they were fulfilling their established responsibilities. What they failed to recognize, however, was that beneficence was now being interpreted and understood broadly to apply not to the individual patient but to *patients* in the aggregate. In other words, beneficence was now being interpreted through the principle of utility which places individual good in the service of the good overall.

One of the catalysts for change in the regulation of human subjects research was the 1966 exposé by prominent Harvard anesthesiologist Henry Beecher. In his paper 'Ethics and Clinical Research'[64] Beecher described 22 examples of published research between 1948 and 1965 in which the investigators had risked the health or life of their subjects but had neither obtained their permission nor informed them of the potential dangers. In both the choice of subjects (from among devalued groups such as the terminally ill, alcoholics, retarded children, the poor, and military recruits) and the absence of disclosure even to those capable of comprehending, the cases reflected and promoted a utilitarian rationale. The unspoken assumption – born of and fostered during the urgency of war – was that the advance of medical science was a sufficient justification to override the rights and welfare of individuals. The 1966 exposé was not Beecher's first attempt to raise the issue of ethics and clinical research. In a 1959 paper on 'Experimentation in Man', Beecher had described the moral significance of the differences between doctor and researcher. The activities of healing and research are, he said, 'different in their procedures, in their aims and in their immediate ends.'[65] In the therapeutic relationship the doctor's principal duty is fidelity to the interests of an individual patient. In the relationship between researcher and subject, the doctor's role was not, in the first instance, fiduciary, but rather oriented to the production of socially beneficial knowledge. In the first case, the welfare of the patient was to be overriding. In the second, the demands of the protocol were paramount.

By the mid-1960s, human experimentation had become a volatile issue. With Beecher's exposé from within the profession and sustained media attention to particular abuses, the NIH could no longer maintain its uncritical, laissez-faire attitude toward either the theory or the practice of human subjects research. The NIH leadership recognized that the comparison between physician and researcher was rhetorically powerful but ethically flawed. Clinical research 'departs from the conventional patient–physician relationship,' they said, insofar as 'the patient's good has been substituted for by the need to develop new knowledge . . . [T]he physician is no longer in the same relationship that he is in the conventional medical setting, and indeed, may not be in a position to develop a purely or wholly objective assessment of the moral nature or the ethical nature of the act which he proposes to perform.'[66]

This insight became the premise for the Public Health Service's initiation of the Institutional Review Board (IRB) as the principal mechanism for review of federally funded research on human subjects. The mandate for IRBs was 'to address the rights and welfare of the individual, the methods used to obtain informed consent and the risks and potential benefits of the investigation.'[67]

As Rothman points out, the implementation of this new policy had its limitations. Most telling, for our purposes, is the fact that the NIH emphasized not the *consent* requirement in the IRB mandate, but the *review* requirement. In essence, the NIH saw the principle function of the IRB as the protection of human subjects, now by a *group* of professionals rather than by the lone – and interested – researcher. Although these changes did, to some degree, constrain utilitarian reasoning by affirming the individual subject as the focal point of questions regarding benefit and harm, there was little, if any, emphasis placed on informing the research subject or empowering that subject to make his or her own assessment of benefit and risk. Instead, the subject was asked to sign a consent form and was assured the right to withdraw from the study at any time. As Rothman puts it, 'the NIH leadership was unwilling to abandon altogether the notion that doctors should protect patients, and to substitute instead a thoroughgoing commitment to the idea of subjects protecting themselves . . . The goal was to ensure that harm was not done to the subjects, not to see that the subjects were given every opportunity and incentive to express their own wishes.'[68]

The consent requirements in the IRB mandate, like those in the FDA's 1962 regulations on the investigatory use of experimental drugs, were subordinated to the more familiar, paternalistic role of the investigator as protector and guardian.

The evolution of regulations on human experimentation in the 1960s was shaped in part by a struggle between two paradigms. One, the venerable paradigm of paternalism where the physician/investigator benefits and protects the patient/subject 'according to my ability and judgment.' The other, the emerging paradigm of patient autonomy which asserts the patient's right to self-determination in the medical context. These original considerations of patient consent in the 1960s, no matter how weak their implementation, heralded the patient rights movement that would gain momentum over the next decade. As we will see, growing concern over iatrogenic illness contributed to the patient rights movement and to a redefinition of the professional obligation to 'do no harm.'

Endnotes

1 The Oath. In *Hippocrates*. (Trans., WHS Jones. Loeb Classical Library.) Cambridge, MA: Harvard University Press, 1923–1988, vol. 1, p. 299.
2 Epidemics I In *Hippocrates*, vol. 1, p. 165 (see No. 1).
3 Ackerknecht EH. *Therapeutics from the Primatives to the 20th Century*. New York: Hafner Press, 1973.
4 Nutton V. Humoralism. In Bynum WF, Porter R, eds. *Companion Encyclopedia of the History of Medicine*. New York: Routledge, 1993, ch. 14 (pp. 281–91).
5 Edelstein L. The Hippocratic physician. In Tempkin O, Tempkin CL, eds. *Ancient Medicine. Selected Papers of Ludwig Edelstein*. Baltimore. The Johns Hopkins Press, 1967.
6 Risse G. Medical care. In Bynum WF, Porter R, eds. *Companion Encyclopedia of the History of Medicine*, ch. 4 (pp. 45–77).
   See also Kudlien F. Medical ethics and popular ethics in Greece and Rome. *Clio Med* 1970; 5:91–121. Kudlien argues that public suspicion and prejudice against drugs, cutting and cautery (or in other words, 'medicophobia') resulted in physicians refusing to intervene in these ways lest they incur public reproach.
7 Rosenberg CE. The therapeutic revolution. In Vogel MJ, Rosenberg CE, eds. *The Therapeutic Revolution: Essays in the Social History of Medicine* Philadelphia: University of Pennsylvania Press, 1979, p. 3.
8 Rosenberg CE, p. 5 (see No. 7).
9 Nutton V (see No. 4).
10 Butterfield LH (ed.). *Letters of Benjamin Rush*, vol. II. Princeton: American

Philosophical Association, 1951, p. 695. (Letter to JRB Rodgers, 3 October, 1793.) In December, 1799, George Washington came down with a throat infection that caused him great pain and constricted his breathing. In the 48 hours before his death, doctors blistered his throat, administered an enema, and bled him three times – the last time taking a quart of blood.
See Dowling HF. *Fighting Infection: Conquests of the Twentieth Century.* Cambridge, MA: Harvard University Press, 1977, p. 1.

11 Sullivan RB. Sanguine practices: A historical and historiographic reconsideration of heroic therapy in the age of Rush. *Bull Hist Med* 1994; 68:225.

12 Sullivan RB, p. 68 (see No. 11).

13 Sullivan RB, p. 228 (see No. 11).

14 Butterfield LH, p. 723 (letter to Mrs. Rush, 23 October, 1793), (see No. 10).

15 Ackerknecht EH. *Medicine at the Paris Hospital 1794–1848.* Baltimore: The Johns Hopkins Press, 1967.

16 Bynum WF. *Science and the Practice of Medicine in the Nineteenth Century* Cambridge: Cambridge University Press, 1994, pp.43–4.

17 Ackerknecht EH, p. 134 (see No. 15).

18 Pernick MS. *A Calculus of Suffering: Pain, Professionalism and Anesthesia in Nineteenth Century America.* New York: Columbia University Press, 1985, p. 20.

19 Rush B. Lecture XII On the Opinions and Modes of Practice of Hippocrates. In *Sixteen Introductory Lectures.* Philadelphia: Bradford and Innskeep 1811, p. 286.

20 Pernick MS, p. 20 (see No. 18).

21 Pernick MS. The calculus of suffering in nineteenth-century surgery. *Hastings Ctr Rep* 1983; 13:28.

22 Hooker W. *Physician and Patient*, p. 219. (Cited in Pernick MS. *The Calculus of Suffering*, p. 271, n.45.)

23 Holmes OW. Currents and counter-currents in medical science. Annual Address before the Massachusetts Medical Society, May 30, 1860. In *Medical Essays 1842–1882.* Boston: Houghton Mifflin, 1911, p. 202. Holmes used colorful rhetoric to emphasize this point. 'Throw out the opium,' he said 'throw out the few specifics which art did not discover, and is hardly needed to apply; throw out wine [whose] vapors produce the miracle of anesthesia, and I firmly believe that if the whole materia medica as *now used*, could be sunk to the bottom of the sea, it would be better for mankind – and all the worse for the fishes.' Although this passage is often and certainly was at the time considered a declaration of therapeutic nihilism, Holmes vigorously denounced all practices whether sectarian, nature-trusting or regular that were based on theoretical dogma or faulty inference.
See, in the same collection, Homeopathy and its kindred delusions, p. 1–102.

24 Pernick MS, p. 99 (see No. 18).

25 Pernick MS, p. 100 (see No. 18).

26 Pernick MS, p. 122 (see No. 18).

27 Ackerknecht EH, (see No. 15).

28 Reiser SJ. The science of diagnosis: Diagnostic technology. In BynumWF, Porter R, eds. *Companion Encyclopedia of the History of Medicine*, ch. 36 (pp. 826–51).

29 Warner JH. Ideals of science and their discontents in late 19th century American medicine. *Isis* 1991; 82:454–78 (see p. 458).

30 Our discussion of the Code controversy is based on the analysis offered in Warner JH (see No. 29).
31 American Medical Association, *Code of Medical Ethics, 2nd edn.* New York: *William Wood & Company, 1868, pp. 21–22. (Cited hereafter as AMA Code, 1847).*
32 Warner JH, p. 468 (see No. 29).
33 Warner JH, p. 468 (see No. 29).
34 *See*, for example, Rothstein WG. *American Physicians in the Nineteenth Century: From Sects to Science.* Baltimore: Johns Hopkins Press, 1992, p. 314–16.
35 AMA Code, 1847, p. 21 (see No. 31).
36 Report of the Association for Preventing the Re-enactment in the State of New York of the Present Code of Ethics of the American Medical Association. Quoted in Warner JH, p. 472 (see No. 29).
37 Rosenberg CE, p. 21 (see No. 7).
38 Starr P. *The Social Transformation of American Medicine.* New York: Basic Books, 1982.
39 Rothman DM. *Strangers at the Bedside: A History of How Law and Bioethics Transformed Medical Decision-Making.* New York: Basic Books, 1991, p. 99.
40 Temin P. *Taking Your Medicine: Drug Regulation in the United States.* Cambridge, MA: Harvard University Press, 1980.
41 Starr P, pp. 340–2 (see No. 38).
42 Beaty HN, Petersdorf RG. Iatrogenic factors in infectious disease. *Ann Intern Med* 1966; 65:641–55.
43 Starr P, p. 354 (see No. 38).
44 Cited in Rothman DM, p. 55 (see No. 39).
45 Rothman DM, p. 55 (see No. 39).
46 Cited in Rothman DM, p. 55 (see No. 39).
47 Rothman DM, p. 64 (see No. 39).
48 Rothman DM, p. 66–7 (see No. 39).
49 AMA Code, 1847, p. 4 (see No. 31).
50 AMA Code, 1847, p. 8 (see No. 31).
51 AMA Code, 1847, pp. 8–14 (see No. 39).
52 Rothman DM, p. 112 (see No. 31).
53 Buchanan AE. Philosophical foundations of beneficence. In E.E. Shelp, ed. *Beneficence in Health Care.* Dordrecht: D. Reidel, 1982, p. 50.
54 See Reiser SJ. The era of the patient: Using the experience of illness in shaping the missions of health care. *JAMA* 1993; 269:1012–17.
55 Nicolson M. The art of diagnosis: Medicine and the five senses. In Bynum WF, Porter R, eds. *Companion Encyclopedia of the History of Medicine*, ch. 35, p. (819).
56 Feinstein A. *Clinical Judgment.* Baltimore: Williams and Wilkins, 1967, p. 36.
57 Medical ethicists, notably, Robert Veatch, have offered the term 'patient–physician relationship' as a more appropriate designation that emphasizes the patient's prerogative in the clinical encounter. In 1996 the *Journal of the American Medical Association* adopted this term to launch a new section that re-emphasizes patient-centered care as the moral core of medicine.
See Glass RM. The patient–physician relationship: *JAMA* focuses on the center of medicine. *JAMA* 1996; 275:147–8.

Laine C, Davidoff F. Patient-centered medicine: A professional evolution. *JAMA* 1996; 275:152–6.

58 The Oath. In *Hippocrates*, vol. 1, p. 299 (see No. 1).

59 Reiser SJ. The science of diagnosis: Diagnostic technology. In WF Bynum and R Porter, eds. *Companion Encyclopedia of the History of Medicine*, ch. 36, p. 829

60 Cassell EJ. *Talking with Patients*, Vol. 1: *The Theory of Doctor–Patient Communication*. Cambridge, MA: MIT Press, 1985; cited in Laine C, Davidoff F (see No. 57).

61 Curran WJ. Governmental regulation of the use of human subjects in medical research: The approach of two federal agencies. *Daedalus* 1969; 98:542–94.

62 *Canterbury* v. *Spence* No. 22099 US Ct of Appeals, DC Circuit, May 19, 1972. 464 Fed Rep 2d 772.

63 Bush V. *Science, The Endless Frontier: A Report to the President on a Program for Postwar Scientific Research*. Washington, D.C., National Science Foundation, 1960 (First pub. 1945), p. 49.

64 Beecher HK. Ethics and clinical research. *N Engl J Med* 1966; 274:1354–60. The most comprehensive analysis of Beecher's impact on the regulation of research is found in Rothman DM, ch. 4 (see No. 39). We rely on Rothman's analysis in what follows.

65 Rothman DM, p. 82 (see No. 39).

66 Cited in Rothman DM, p. 89 (see No. 39).

67 Rothman DM, p. 89 (see No. 39).

68 Rothman DM, p. 92 (see No. 39).

3

Medical harms and patients' rights: the democratization of medical morality

According to the Oxford English Dictionary, the term 'iatrogenic' was introduced in 1924 in Bleuler's *Textbook of Psychiatry*.[1] An iatrogenic disease was one having a primarily psychological manifestation brought on by a physician's diagnosis. To be sure, the remarks of the physician were implicated in this definition, but the suggestibility of the patient was also regarded as a factor in the development of the illness. In his description of the natural history of a specifically iatrogenic neurosis, Bleuler explains that 'the physician solemnly diagnoses "enlargement of the heart," whereupon the patient is frightened and breaks down until the X-ray photograph resorted to by another physician relieves him of his nightmare.'[2] Although it is not surprising to find psychiatric literature attributing a psychological etiology to ill health, the prevailing medical epistemology of the late nineteenth century also helps to explain this early conceptualization of iatrogenic illness. In the holistic interpretation of illness (and health) dominant throughout the nineteenth century and central to the early history of psychiatry, communication between doctor and patient was conceived as one among the many factors that could alter the patient's experience of well-being. Indeed, the AMA's (American Medical Association) 1847 Code highlights the potential risks of this verbal exchange in its observation that 'the life of a sick person can be shortened not only by the acts, but also by the words or the manner of a physician. It is, therefore, a sacred duty . . . to avoid all things which have a tendency to discourage the patient and to depress his spirits.'[3] This sentiment was echoed as well by Francis Peabody in his 1927 treatise 'The care of the patient,' in which he says 'You will find that physicians, by ill-considered statements, are responsible for many a wrecked life, and you will discover that it is much easier to make a diagnosis than it is to unmake it.'[4]

As medical science shifted its attention to disease specificity and confirmed the legitimacy of this approach with biological specifics such as penicillin, the etiology of *iatrogenic* illness was correspondingly reconceived.[5] It was no longer exclusively identified with doctor–patient communication but rather, increasingly with the utilization of new diagnostic and therapeutic agents. In the post World War II period, the phrase iatrogenic illness gained a broader application informed both by this scientific epistemology and by the exaltation of medical progress.

In the post-war years, the sense of optimism and urgency that infused medical research extended to the therapeutic relationship. Pharmacological and surgical treatments used in military populations quickly diffused into clinical practice. As of 1953 in the United States, 140,000 medicines were listed for sale, 75% of which had been introduced in the preceding ten years.[6] Between 1929 and 1969, consumer expenditures for prescription drugs rose more than 25-fold from $190 million to $5.3 billion.[7] In 1945 alone, the first year that it was widely available to the public, one out of four United States citizens had received a prescription for penicillin.[8] The broad endorsement of scientific expansionism was reiterated in federal support for hospital construction. With funding from the 1946 Hill-Burton Act, the ratio of hospital beds to population increased to roughly 4.5 per 1000. During this period, the population also achieved unprecedented access to hospital and physician care through the growth of medical benefits plans such as Blue Cross and Blue Shield. By the end of 1954, 60% of the population had some kind of hospitalization insurance and 50% had insurance for surgical care.[9] 'Progress' through scientific achievement was the rallying cry of the era.

In this chapter, we discuss the evolution of the concept of iatrogenic illness in the post World War II period. We examine the post-war utilitarian justification for iatrogenic harms and its replacement in the 1960s and 1970s by a more critical conception responsive to the emerging call for patient rights. We also discuss the impact of the authoritative right of patient self-determination on medical ethics and physician accountability.

The price of progress

In the 1950s, publications by David Barr and Robert Moser brought attention to the phenomenon of iatrogenic illness and exemplified the widespread confidence in medicine characteristic of the period. In his 1956 article on the 'Hazards of modern diagnosis and therapy,' Barr described the harms associated with medicine as 'the price we must pay for modern management of disease.'[10] In other words, the complexities of modern medicine entailed unavoidable costs that had to be borne if the commitment to therapeutic advance was to be maintained. As such, Barr's conceptualization of the problem implicitly endorsed the ultimate utility of medical innovations despite his observation that they induced life threatening or fatal reactions in one out of 20 hospitalized patients.

During the same year, Robert Moser identified iatrogenic illnesses as diseases resulting from the development of potent new therapeutic agents and improved surgical procedures. Iatrogenic illnesses were, in his words, 'diseases of medical progress.'[11] In what would become the foundation for his 1959 book-length treatment of the subject, Moser detailed a variety of illnesses resulting from medical therapy. He dubbed one conspicuous phenomenon 'antibiotic abandon.' Following its introduction, penicillin soon became a panacea, dispensed for everything from infection, to fever, to colds, to general prevention of illness. Administered to nearly 80% of the population by the 1950s, penicillin had even found its way into folk culture in the form of a children's skipping song:

Mother, mother, I am ill!
Call the doctor from over the hill!
In came the doctor, in came the nurse,
In came the lady with the alligator purse.
Penicillin, said the doctor,
Penicillin, said the nurse,
Penicillin, said the lady with the alligator purse.[12]

By 1957, a nationwide survey had shown that penicillin was responsible for 80% of life threatening drug reactions in general hospitals and that in 50% to 90% of cases antibiotics were administered without any clear indications.[13] As evidenced by its prominent placement as the first chapter in every edition of Moser's book, it was the antibiotic experience that catalyzed the study of iatrogenic harm.[14]

Common to these early discussions and emblematic of the perception of iatrogenic complications in the 1950s was the notion that they were the sequelae of *sound* and *sanctioned* medical practices. Notwithstanding his awareness of profligate prescribing, Moser defined 'diseases of medical progress' as 'diseases that would not have occurred if sound therapeutic procedure had not been employed.'[15] Similarly, in Barr's unsystematic investigation, the term 'iatrogenic disease' refers to the 'unfortunate sequelae and accidents attributable to sanctioned and well-intentioned diagnosis and therapy.'[16]

The articles by Barr and Moser were signal contributions to the literature on iatrogenic harm. They were also products of their time. Their
purpose was not to challenge the social mandate of medicine or to question
the quality of medical care but rather to highlight some of the inevitable
risks associated with new drugs and techniques. These authors and others
who published texts in the 1960s[17] explicitly rejected the philosophy of
'therapeutic nihilism,' which was one of the nineteenth-century's rejoin-
ders to medically induced harm. Instead, their investigations of iatrogenic
illness reflected a firm confidence in medicine and its practitioners despite
the documented extent of complications. Like nineteenth century advocates of conservative medicine, these authors of the 1950s and 1960s called
for a more judicious, 'rational therapeutics' guided by the physician's
understanding of risk and benefit.[18] As we will see, however, it was not
until the 1970s with the doctrine of informed consent that the patient
would gain authority in determining the relevance and the acceptability of
risk. In the 1950s and 1960s, the determination of medical benefit, risk, and
harm was still the exclusive prerogative of physicians.

One notable exception to the utilitarian sentiment among post-war
investigations of medical harm was the 1953 paper by Henry Beecher and
Donald Todd on deaths associated with anesthesia and surgery.[19] As we
have seen, Beecher became known for his challenges to uncritical acceptance of the medical *status quo*. The paper on anesthesia and surgical deaths
was but the first salvo in the career of this medical maverick. Beecher and
Todd's paper presented findings from a prospective study of almost
600,000 anesthesia procedures administered over five years in ten university hospitals. In addition to identifying a higher risk of mortality associated with curare (the use of which doubled over the period of the study),
Beecher and Todd found that the overall death rate from anesthesia was
1:1560. As they pointed out, this exceeded by almost two and one half
times the death rate from polio in the United States during the same
period. They concluded that, 'Anesthesia might be likened to a disease
which afflicts 8,000,000 persons in the United States each year. More than
twice as many citizens out of the total population of the country die from
anesthesia as die from poliomyelitis. Deaths from anesthesia are certainly
a matter for public health concern.'[20]

This inquiry by Beecher and Todd can be distinguished from those by
Barr and Moser in a number of ways that help to explain why it was not
readily embraced as the model for investigation of iatrogenic complications. On the most mundane level, the Beecher study did not identify itself
with 'iatrogenic illness' *per se*, which three years later would emerge as an

interesting new disease classification. Secondly, when the phrase 'iatrogenic illness' gained currency, it referred specifically to complications arising from new therapies – with the implication that medical progress had some inevitable though unfortunate costs. Beecher and Todd, by contrast, emphasized their dismay at the turmoil that persisted in the profession of anesthesia *even after* its 100-year history. True, part of the turmoil was attributable to the introduction of new agents but this did not excuse the fact that the profession lacked a program for assessing the safety and effectiveness of the compounds that it used. Finally, although the Beecher and Todd study did lead to reform in anesthesia practice, it did not become a standard bearer for medical self-examination because it struck a discordant note in an otherwise harmonious paean to medical progress. Like Codman's early efforts to study and publicize patient outcomes, Beecher and Todd's emphasis on therapeutic evaluation and the quality of care, was ahead of its time.

The first explicit and systematic prospective study of iatrogenic complications was conducted by Elihu Schimmel at the Yale University medical service in 1960 and 1961.[21] Although this study was conventional in limiting its focus to noxious responses resulting from 'acceptable diagnostic or therapeutic measures,' it broadened its scope to include *all* untoward reactions, regardless of severity. Like Barr, Schimmel found that life threatening or fatal reactions occurred in almost 5% of patients. He also found, however, that one out of every 12 (8.3%) patients experienced a moderately severe complication requiring extra treatment or extra hospital days. This broader definition revealed iatrogenic illness as a significantly larger and more complicated phenomenon.

Patient's rights and medical harm

The decade of the 1960s was a period of enormous social change in America. The civil rights movement and the second wave of feminism emphasized the rights of traditionally disenfranchised citizens as a basis for an authentic participatory democracy. Social disillusionment focused on the institutions of government for their support of racial and gender inequality and for the social and human costs of the Vietnam war. Disillusionment spread to other institutions as well, institutions whose benevolent reputations were increasingly seen to mask narrow self-interest. Trust in discretionary authority gave way to movements for the empowerment of the individual. As we have seen, public concern about the conflicting interests of medical researchers was already leading to regulations aimed at safeguarding individual subjects and granting them some decisional control in the research context.

The perception of medical harm in the *therapeutic* context – otherwise known as iatrogenic illness – was also called into question during this period. By the mid-1960s, the conservative definition of iatrogenic harm – as the negative sequelae of *sound and sanctioned* treatment – had begun to be replaced by a definition that included complications resulting from faulty or contraindicated care. For the first time in the professional literature on the subject, investigators expanded the scope of their inquiries to include the negative sequelae of errors, omissions, and miscommunications. Studies of iatrogenic illness from the 1950s had been intended to alert the medical community to the 'hidden and general dangers' of medicine.[22] The newer and more comprehensive investigations took this danger for granted and went further to explore the scope of medical harm and its specific solutions.

One of these studies was conducted by William Reichel[23] and included adverse reactions related to medications and procedures as well as to medical and nursing errors. The Reichel study, which focused on elderly hospitalized patients, found that almost 30% experienced an untoward reaction resulting from their care. In a 1967 study of the frequency and severity of adverse reactions during hospitalization, Ogilvie and Ruedy defined an iatrogenic complication as '*any* undesired or unintended consequence of the care of the patient';[24] they found complications occurring in almost one-quarter of medical service patients. Nine percent of these were life-threatening, fatal, or unresolved at the time of discharge.

In a twist on the military metaphors that had infused the post-war rhetoric of medical progress, Seckler and Spritzer observed in 1966 that 'the explosive advance in our knowledge and capabilities in medicine does not differ from any other explosion; individuals exposed to it are liable to be harmed.'[25] Citing Schimmel's findings that 20% of hospitalized patients experienced deleterious effects as a result of their care, the authors extended their analogy. These statistics would seem to suggest, they said, 'that the individuals closest to the center of the explosion are most vulnerable to be most frequently and seriously injured.'[26] Seckler and Spritzer were among the first in the professional literature to question whether the good derived by humankind from advances in medical science justified harm to particular patients – that is, whether the utilitarian rationale for medical harm was still valid. 'Very few people,' they said, 'would care to challenge the fact that our present day knowledge and capabilities in medicine have been productive of more good for humankind than harm. Can we, however, fully justify doing more harm to our patients simply because we can now do more good?"[27]

In the 1970s, doctors were not the only ones asking this question. Concerns about medically induced illness were increasingly voiced by health care consumers and their elected officials. As medical harm, like so many other issues of the period, began to be viewed through the lens of individual rights, the autonomy that had, since the late nineteenth century, been cultivated and enjoyed by the medical profession, increasingly came under the control of more public and democratically forged institutions. In addition, the ethos of personal accountability and self-scrutiny that had defined the profession of medicine no longer seemed adequate to the complexities of institutionalized health care delivery or to the multifaceted risks to which patients were increasingly exposed. Thus the decades of the 1960s and 1970s were marked by the imposition of new forms of accountability upon the medical profession. On the one hand, the practice of medicine was subject to greater oversight by public and regulatory bodies that stimulated and enforced the call for a more rational therapeutics. On the other hand, professional paternalism was increasingly challenged by the publicly and politically-forged ethos of patient self-determination. In Part III, we discuss how nosocomial infection, adverse drug reactions, and unnecessary surgery became the focus of formal oversight during this period. We examine how monitoring and prevention and control strategies as well as outcomes data contribute to new standards of technical performance that form the basis of both accountability and quality improvement efforts in these areas.

In the remainder of this chapter we describe how the articulation of a substantive right of patient self-determination in both law and medical ethics influenced professional accountability by shifting the locus of decisional authority from doctor to patient. We examine the most dramatic manifestation of this shift in the emergence of the doctrine of informed consent. In Part II, we build upon this discussion, arguing that ethical norms are the fundamental mechanisms of accountability in health care.

Informed consent: shifting the locus of authority

As we saw in Chapter 2, informed consent to *research* became the focus of administrative regulations in the 1960s. Both the DHEW (now the Department of Health and Human Services) and the FDA instituted policies imposing disclosure and consent requirements on human subjects researchers. Informed consent to *treatment*, by contrast, evolved in case law.

It was the 1957 decision in *Salgo* v. *Leland Stanford Jr.*[28] that introduced the phrase 'informed consent.' The case involved a patient who suffered paralysis of the legs after undergoing a transthoracic aortography. This now obsolete diagnostic technique involved a puncture to the aorta through the back in order to inject radio-opaque dye. The patient, Martin Salgo, sued his doctors arguing that they were negligent both in their performance of the technique and in their failure to warn him of the risk of paralysis. What is significant about the *Salgo* decision is that, for the first time, the court imposed upon physicians an 'affirmative duty of disclosure.'[29] Although earlier courts – most notably the New York court in *Schloendorff* v. *Society of New York Hospitals* (1914) – had emphasized the patient's prior consent as a requirement for medical intervention, they had not specifically commented on the type or scope of information that would be needed to legitimate the patient's consent. The *Salgo* court, by contrast, ruled that the patient had a right to full disclosure of the nature, benefits, and risks of a procedure as well as alternatives to it. In other words, in decision-making regarding medical treatment and its associated risks (and benefits), the patient's informed choice should play a guiding role.

What is striking about the *Salgo* decision is that it draws on two very different types of justification to support its argument.[30] The first is a justification grounded in the physician's fiduciary duty and supported by the principles of beneficence and nonmaleficence. The second justification featured in the *Salgo* case is grounded in the patient's right to self-determination. In the precedent-setting *Schloendorff* case, Judge Cardozo famously argued that 'every human being of adult years and sound mind has a right to determine what shall be done with his own body; and a surgeon who performs an operation without his patient's consent commits an assault for which he is liable in damages.'[31] *Salgo* extended the principle of patient self-determination beyond consent (the focus of *Schloendorff*) to the disclosure of information.

A number of noteworthy distinctions can be made between these two justifications. Interpreted under the principles of beneficence and nonmaleficence as an element of due care, the management of information is relevant insofar as it has the potential to enhance or undermine the success of treatment. In the first two-thirds of the nineteenth century, malpractice judgments indicate that courts often deliberated about the issue of non-disclosure or deception insofar as it had, by undermining the patient's involvement, undermined the patient's health.[32] By contrast, we have seen that the original conceptualization of 'iatrogenic illness' in the early twentieth century emphasized the *pathogenic* potential of disclosure. Indeed as the physician's expertise came increasingly to be seen as the arbiter of sound therapeutics, the potential benefits of disclosure – that is, of patient involvement in decision making – came to be overshadowed by its potential for harm. Thus the therapeutic privilege emerged as a justification for withholding information. Therapeutic privilege is supported by a paternalistic argument that the doctor's duty of nonmaleficence justifies denying the patient the information and opportunity to give consent. Pivotal to this argument is that the information itself might exacerbate the patient's condition.[33] The *Salgo* court made use of this justification in its assertion that 'the physician has . . . discretion [to withhold alarming information from the patient] consistent, of course, with the full disclosure of facts necessary to an informed consent.'[34] The force of the therapeutic justification for disclosure (in this case, its potentially negative effect on clinical outcome) seems to have blinded the court to the potential contradiction between the physician discretion it allows and the 'full disclosure' it requires. As Faden and Beauchamp have observed, however, the fact 'that there can be a divergence between the interests and goals of patients and those of physicians is a fundamental premise of informed consent itself.'[35]

In contrast to the therapeutic or 'due care' justification for informed consent (which we discuss in more detail in Chapter 5), the justification grounded in patient self-determination is premised on the intrinsic value of patient autonomy. Such a justification makes no reference to the outcomes afforded by patient choice and information but rather holds these things to be good in themselves. Within this framework, lies, silences, or evasions intended to benefit the patient are failures to respect the patient's rational agency. On this view, paternalistic deception is morally suspect precisely because it undermines the patient's ability and opportunity to decide for him or herself. On the due care justification for informed consent, physician deception could be justified by therapeutic outcome. On an autonomy-based justification, failure to obtain consent is sufficient grounds for an action even if the subsequent outcome was unanimously agreed to be beneficial. Katz has observed that this justificatory tension at the heart of the *Salgo* decision represents 'Anglo-American law's conflicting vision of human beings as autonomous persons and its deference to paternalism.'[36] Katz may be right in his assessment, but the tension seems to go deeper than a conflicting vision in the law. The tension between protection and self-determination – between the principles of nonmaleficence and beneficence on the one hand and autonomy on the other – is also at the heart of contemporary clinical ethics and of the patient's expectations of medical providers. As discussed in Chapter 6, this tension also raises an important question about the current conceptualization of iatrogenic harm, namely the extent to which the values of the patient will influence determinations regarding not only risk, but also occurrent harm. As we will see, to the extent that we recognize the concept of harm to be informed by the values of providers and individual patients, the tension between these principles will, in the clinical setting, give way to a negotiated understanding of benefit and harm.

In the 1960s and 1970s, the tensions in the *Salgo* case were displayed in two judicial standards of disclosure for informed consent. In the *Salgo* case and many that followed it, the courts held that the degree of disclosure made to patients was essentially a question for medical judgment. This 'professional standard of disclosure' followed naturally from the rules of recovery in negligence cases generally wherein 'reasonable professional judgment' provided the basis for assessment of the appropriateness of care and the level of skill of a provider.[37] In 1972, the professional practice standard of disclosure was called into question in a number of cases, including the landmark *Canterbury* v. *Spence*.[38] In *Canterbury*, the patient had a laminectomy to relieve severe back pain. After the surgery, the patient fell out of his bed and some hours later suffered major paralysis. The patient had not been informed prior to surgery of the risk of paralysis and the appeals court judged that this failure to disclose constituted negligence on the part of the provider. The court asserted that the duty to disclose risks and alternatives was founded on the duty of due care, that is, on the physician's duty as a fiduciary entrusted to promote the patient's health interests. Where the court broke new ground, however, was in the determination that disclosure should be made according to a standard of what a 'reasonable patient' would want to know about treatment, *not* according to standards of professional judgment.

The context in which the duty of risk-disclosure arises is invariably the occasion for decision as to whether a particular treatment procedure is to be undertaken. To the physician, whose training enables a self-satisfying evaluation, the answer may seem clear, *but it is the prerogative of the patient, not the physician to determine for himself the direction in which his interests seem to lie.* To enable the patient to chart his course understandably, some familiarity with the therapeutic alternatives and their hazards becomes essential.[39] [Our emphasis added.]

In its pioneering endorsement of a patient-centered standard of disclosure, the *Canterbury* court was echoing a cultural shift toward the recognition of patient values as authoritative in medical decision making. This shift was also reflected in a number statements published during the early 1970s that emphasized the rights of patients. In 1969, the Joint

Commission on Accreditation of Hospitals (JCAH) was asked by the National Welfare Rights Organization (NWRO) to include in its 1970 *Accreditation Manual* a statement addressing the concerns of patients. The NWRO was a group that advocated for the poor by urging charitable institutions to adopt a rights orientation. Recognizing disparities between hospital care for the poor and the nonpoor, the NWRO offered a list of 26 recommendations to the JCAH for its 1970 *Standards Manual*. Among those included in the Joint Commission's 1970 preamble was the statement that 'the patient has the right to receive . . . adequate information concerning the nature and extent of his medical problem, the planned course of treatment and prognosis.'[40] The JCAH preamble was the basis for the most influential document of the period, the American Hospital Association's (AHA) *A Patient's Bill of Rights*. In this statement, the AHA affirmed that 'the patient has the right to obtain from his physician complete current information regarding his diagnosis, treatment and prognosis in terms the patient can reasonably be expected to understand.'[41]

If we take a closer look at these documents, we find that, despite their groundbreaking endorsement of patient rights in the context of medical decision making, they remain well within the ethical tradition that emphasized the primacy of beneficence and nonmaleficence. Just as the courts had consistently relied on a therapeutic justification for informed consent, so too did these statements of institutional policy advance the notion of respect for the rights of the patient as 'an integral part of the healing process.'[42] Indeed, these documents also underscored the necessity for physician discretion in the communication of information not deemed 'medically advisable.' In contrast to Faden and Beauchamp who suggest that these documents, when applied to medical decision-making, 'literally invit[ed] the replacement of the beneficence model with the autonomy model,'[43] we believe that they rather reveal the persistent tension between these two paradigms.[44] The effect of the 'Patient's Bill of Rights' and the JCAH preamble, however, eclipsed their still quite conservative intent and rationale. This was due, in part, to the language of patient rights adopted in these documents, a language with a bracingly revolutionary potential in this era of other politically charged rights movements. To affirm patient rights was to identify a source of medical obligations outside of the professionally-generated canons of conduct. Indeed, after the publication of the AHA document, governmental bodies began adopting legally binding bills of patient rights.[45]

Now that an important moral norm governing medicine had been identified in the domain of public policy, the professional monopoly on medical ethics was over. Physician discretion did not properly extend to evaluative questions outside the purview of medical expertise. This fact was made manifest in the 1976 New Jersey Supreme Court decision in the case of Karen Ann Quinlan. In April 1975, Quinlan (22 years old) was brought into the emergency room in a coma from which she never emerged. After several months, her parents sought to have her removed from the respirator so that she could die a natural death. The hospital and the physicians argued against withdrawal of treatment on the grounds of the State's interest in preserving human life and upholding the ethical integrity of the medical profession. They argued that 'removal of the respirator was not supported by accepted medical practice' and that 'no court . . . should require a physician to act in derogation of [the] sacred and time-honored [Hippocratic] oath.'[46] The judges in the Superior Court substantively agreed, they said, by noting that 'our society has chosen to entrust to the medical profession the responsibility for determining when death occurs and what treatment shall be administered to the living.'[47] In its subsequent decision in favor of the Quinlans, the New Jersey Supreme Court asserted that medical practice 'must, in the ultimate, be responsive not only to the concepts of medicine but to the common moral judgment of the community at large.'[48] As Appelbaum et al. observe with regard to the Quinlan decision,

physicians had heretofore considered the physician–patient relationship by beginning from the patient's submission to the physician's professional beneficence. The law enlarged that perspective by viewing the relationship within the wider social framework, emphasizing instead that patients voluntarily initiate the relationship and have the right to define its boundaries to achieve their own ends. The goals sought by patient and physician were generally the same; but when they differed, the law was capable of demonstrating to medicine the validity of autonomy concerns.[49]

It was during this period that biomedical ethics was born as an interdisciplinary field bringing together philosophers, theologians, lawyers, and medical historians. The dominant strain of biomedical ethics in the United States has grown out of the liberal political tradition's articulation of the rights of individuals. The traditional obligations of beneficence and nonmaleficence have now been joined by principles of autonomy and justice.

Medical nemesis: the paradox of 'progress'

In the 1970s, the issues of autonomy and medical harm intersected not only in deliberations concerning medical malpractice, the disclosure of risk, and the right to refuse treatment; they were also underscored in Ivan Illich's landmark book *Medical Nemesis: The Expropriation of Health*.[50] As we have seen, in one of the first professional expressions of caution regarding the harmful effects of medical progress, Seckler and Spritzer observed in 1966 that 'very few people would care to challenge the fact that our present day knowledge and capabilities in medicine have been productive of more good for humankind than harm.'[51] Ten years later, in *Medical Nemesis*, Illich challenged the fundamental premise of medical 'progress,' arguing that institutionalized medicine was overwhelmingly pathogenic and actively 'sickening.' Not only did a large percentage of patients experience unnecessary harms at the hands of health care providers but, with the over-medicalization of society, they also increasingly relinquished control of their health to institutions. Cultural iatrogenesis is 'the ultimate evil of medical *progress,*'[52] he said. 'It occurs when people accept health management designed on the engineering model ...[that translates] human survival from the performance of organisms into the result of technical manipulation.'[53] In its most pernicious form, medical iatrogenesis, Illich argued, paralyzes autonomous action by destroying the potential of people to deal with their human weakness, vulnerability, and uniqueness in a personal and self-directed way.[54] Like Prometheus and Sisyphus, who were condemned by Nemesis to a self-defeating and captive existence, the medical industry and those of us who naïvely subject ourselves to its machinations have created a self-reinforcing iatrogenic loop where remedies themselves become pathogenic. Health, argued Illich, does not come by way of passivity and dependence but by way of freedom.

What is striking about Illich's radical critique of iatrogenic illness is that it is grounded in a vision of autonomy as a substantive good – as the essence of humanity and human well-being. Because Illich emphasizes self-care outside of the physician–patient dyad, he does not link his critique with the legal and ethical principle of patient self-determination. It is clear, however that in his view, autonomy is integral to individual human health. By extension, to deprive persons of their autonomy is to harm them by directly and indirectly depriving them of their health.

Conclusion

The spirit of individual sacrifice that defined the United States in war-time persisted into the post-war 1950s. During this time, the acknowledged harms associated with medical care were seen through a lens that subordinated concerns about individual welfare to the net good afforded by medical advancement. The definition of iatrogenic illness as 'diseases of medical progress' reflected this utilitarian sentiment. At the same time, the medical profession – as the quintessential embodiment of scientific achievement – gained unprecedented authority and prestige. By the 1950s, the moral and professional authority of the physician was decisively linked to scientific knowledge. This expertise conferred upon physicians the prerogative in all decisions concerning medical care. In the 1960s and 1970s, this prerogative was challenged by new forms of professional accountability to patients, to governmental bodies, and to formal institutional oversight. The medical profession strongly resisted the notion that moral norms governing medicine should come from outside the canons of professional practice. When asked, for example, if an interdisciplinary governmental committee should be convened to deliberate about the ethical issues in organ transplantation, heart transplant surgeon Christiaan Barnard argued that doctors (not the public) were the only ones qualified to respond to questions regarding patient need, resource allocation, and the definition of death. To suggest otherwise, he said, was not only an insult to doctors but a threat to progress.[55] These same sentiments were echoed in the *Quinlan* case and in debates over the wisdom and propriety of patient involvement in decision-making through informed consent. Confident in the authority conferred by scientific expertise, doctors saw it as their moral duty to act for the good of the patient as they understood it. Any rule perceived to divert the physician from discharging this duty would threaten the ethical integrity of the medical profession. In the 1970s professional control was called into question as the interests and values of patients and physicians were seen to diverge. As medical sociologist Paul Starr has observed, the emphasis on patient rights in both law and ethics 'challenged the distribution of power and expertise' in medicine.[56]

Finally, just as the harms associated with heroic practice gave rise to therapeutic skepticism in the eighteenth and nineteenth centuries, so, too, did the harms of twentieth century technological and bureaucratic medicine. One response common to both eras was the call for patients to forgo altogether the ministrations of physicians and to take greater responsibility for their health. Nineteenth-century reformers such as Elizabeth Cady Stanton made the link between health and individual liberty, urging (especially female) patients to 'take the liberty of being their own physician.'[57] In the 1970s, social critic Ivan Illich renewed this call, arguing that freedom from the pathogenic culture of technological medicine was the only way to avoid medical iatrogenesis and to achieve health.

Therapeutic skepticism and medical consumerism represent two critical responses to medical harm and to practitioner accountability. In Part III, we explore the corresponding responses of assessment and regulation. In Part II, however, we turn from a descriptive to a prescriptive account, offering ethical and conceptual analyses of medical harm that encompass norms of beneficence, nonmaleficence, and respect for patient autonomy.

Endnotes

1 A Supplement to the Oxford English Dictionary, vol. II. Oxford: Clarendon Press, 1976, p. 225.
2 Bleuler E. *Textbook of Psychiatry* (Trans., by A. A. Brill). New York: Macmillan, 1924, p. 502.
3 AMA Code, 1847, p. 6 (for full reference see Chapter 2, No. 5).
4 Peabody FW. The care of the patient. *JAMA* 1927; 88:877–82.
5 A parallel phenomenon is noted by Pernick in the late nineteenth century shift from a malpractice to a battery theory of liability for medical consent. Pernick maintains that the battery theory (which holds the doctor liable for failure to disclose information regardless of the outcome of the medical treatment) was adopted precisely at the time when the transmission of information and the patient's participation in the therapeutic encounter were dismissed as having any important causal influence on health and sickness. See Pernick MS. The patient's role in medical decision-making: A social history of informed consent in medical therapy. In President's Commission for the Study of Ethical Problems in Medicine and Biomedical and Behavioral Research. *Making Health Care Decisions*, vol. 3. Washington, DC: USGPO, 1982, p. 30.
6 Barr DP. Hazards of modern diagnosis and therapy – the price we pay. *JAMA* 1956; 159:1452–6.
7 Temin P. *Taking Your Medicine: Drug Regulation in the United States.* Cambridge, MA: Harvard University Press, 1980, p. 4.
8 Beaty HN, Petersdorf RG. Iatrogenic factors in infectious disease. *Ann Intern Med* 1966; 65:641–55.
9 Starr P. *The Social Transformation of American Medicine*. New York: Basic Books, 1982, p. 313.
10 Barr DP (see No. 6).
11 Moser RH. Diseases of medical progress. *N Engl J Med* 1956; 255:606–14.
12 Meyler L. *Side Effects of Drugs.* Amsterdam: Elsevier, 1952, p. vi.
13 Beaty HN, Petersdorf RG (see No. 8).
14 Whorton JC. 'Antibiotic abandon': The resurgence of therapeutic rationalism. In Parascondola J, ed. *The History of Antibiotics: A Symposium.* Madison, WI: American Institute of the History of Pharmacy, 1980, pp. 125–35.
15 Moser RH, p. 606 (see No. 11).
16 Barr DP, p. 1452 (see No. 6).
17 For example, 'Because of the delicate nature of the subject, it is imperative at the outset to state unequivocally what this book is definitely not about. It is not intended to support or encourage any concept of therapeutic nihilism' Spain DM. *The Complications of Modern Medical Practice: A Treatise on Iatrogenic Diseases.* New York: Grune and Stratton, 1963, p. xv.

18 See, for example, the editorial statement inaugurating the journal *Clinical Pharmacology and Therapeutics* in 1960. The journal 'will provide the perceptive practitioner with up-to-date information of the type he needs and seeks . . . [by concentrating] on "*the effects of drugs in man*, their proper and enduring evaluation, their actions and their therapeutic and toxic effects".' Modell W. Editorial *Clin Pharm Ther* 1960; 1(1):1–2.

19 Beecher HK, Todd DP. A study of the deaths associated with anesthesia and surgery. *Ann Surg* 1954; 140:1–34.

20 Beecher HK, Todd DP, p. 28 (see No. 19).

21 Schimmel EM. The hazards of hospitalization. *Ann Intern Med* 1964; 60:100–10.

22 Barr DP (see No. 6).

23 Reichel W. Complications in the care of five hundred elderly hospitalized patients. *J Am Geriatr Soc* 1965; 13:973–81.

24 Ogilvie RI, Ruedy J. Adverse reactions during hospitalization. *Canad Med Ass J* 1967; 97:1445–50.

25 Seckler SG, Spritzer RC. Disseminated disease of medical progress. *Arch Intern Med* 1966; 117:447–50.

26 Seckler SG, Spritzer RC (see No. 25).

27 Seckler SG, Spritzer RC, p. 449 (see No. 25).

28 *Salgo* v. *Leland Stanford Jr. University Board of Trustees*, 317 P.2d 170 (Cal Ct App 1957).

29 Appelbaum PS, Lidz CW, Meisel A. *Informed Consent: Legal Theory and Clinical Practice*. New York: Oxford, 1986.

30 These two types of justification for informed consent are discussed in Faden RR, Beauchamp TL. *A History and Theory of Informed Consent*. New York: Oxford University Press, 1986.

31 *Schloendorff* v. *Society of New York Hospitals*. 211 N.Y. 125, 105 N.E. 92 (1914).

32 Pernick MS. The patient's role in medical decision-making: A social history of informed consent in medical therapy. In President's Commission for the Study of Ethical Problems in Medicine and Biomedical and Behavioral Research. *Making Health Care Decisions*, vol. 3. Washington, DC: USGPO, 1982, p. 1–35.

33 Another more expansive premise in arguments for therapeutic privilege is that the physician has a duty to protect the patient against him/herself, that is, against potentially harmful choices that she/he might make. This premise finds support in the Hippocratic injunction to 'keep the sick from harm and injustice.'
    See Childress J. *Who Should Decide?: Paternalism in Health Care*. New York: Oxford, 1982, p. 36. The court in *Canterbury* v. *Spence* argued against this assumption saying that the therapeutic privilege 'does not accept the paternalistic notion that the physician may remain silent simply because the divulgence might prompt the patient to forego therapy the physician feels the patient really needs.' Such a notion, the court points out 'might devour the disclosure rule itself.' *Canterbury* v. *Spence* No. 22099 US Ct of Appeals, DC Circuit, May 19, 1972. 464 Fed Rep 2d 789.

34 *Salgo* v. *Leland Stanford Jr. University Board of Trustees*, 317 P.2d 170 (Cal Ct App 1957).

35 Faden RR, Beauchamp TL, p. 135 (see No. 30).

36 Katz J. Informed consent – A fairy tale? In Walters L, Beauchamp TL, ed.

Contemporary Issues in Bioethics, 2nd edn. Belmont, CA: Wadsworth, 1982, p. 192.

37 Appelbaum PS, Lidz CW, Meisel A, p. 41 (see No. 29).

38 *Canterbury* v. *Spence* No. 22099 US Ct of Appeals, DC Circuit, May 19, 1972. 464 Fed Rep 2d 772.

39 *Canterbury* v. *Spence*, p. 781.

40 Joint Commission on the Accreditation of Hospitals. *Standards Manual*. Oakbrook Terrace, IL: JCAH, 1970.

41 A Patient's Bill of Rights. Chicago: American Hospital Association, 1973. Reprinted in Reich WT, ed. *The Encyclopedia of Bioethics*, vol. V. New York: Simon and Schuster/Macmillan, 1995, p. 2619.

42 A Patient's Bill of Rights (see No. 41).

43 Faden RR, Beauchamp TL, p. 95 (see No. 30).

44 In fact the professional practice standard is still the dominant rule in informed consent law despite an ideological shift toward patient autonomy. See Faden RR, Beauchamp TL, p. 31 (see No. 30).

45 Veatch RM. *A Theory of Medical Ethics*. New York: Basic Books, 1981, p. 47.

46 *In the Matter of Karen Quinlan: The Complete Briefs, Oral Arguments, and Opinions in the Superior Court of New Jersey* (vol. I) and in the *New Jersey Supreme Court*, vol. II. Arlington, VA: University Publications of America, 1976, p. 144–5.

47 *In the Matter of Karen Quinlan*, vol. II, p. 144 (see No. 46).

48 *In the Matter of Karen Quinlan*, vol. II, p. 308 (see No. 46).

49 Appelbaum PS, Lidz CW, Meisel A, pp. 142–3 (see No. 29).

50 Illich I. *Medical Nemesis: The Expropriation of Health*. New York: Pantheon Books; 1976.

51 Seckler SG, Spritzer RC, p. 449 (see No. 25).

52 Illich I, p. 34 (see No. 50).

53 Illich I, p. 34 (see No. 50).

54 Illich I, p. 32–3 (see No. 50).

55 Rothman DM. *Strangers at the Bedside: A History of How Law and Bioethics Transformed Medical Decision-Making*. New York: Basic Books, 1991, p. 173.

56 Starr P, p. 389 (see No. 9).

57 Pernick MS, p. 27 (see No. 5).

PART II

4

The moral basis of medicine: why 'do no harm'?

The literature on iatrogenic illness is replete with references to the Hippocratic injunction against harming patients. The cardinal tenet, of medicine, says R. L. Kane is *primum non nocere*.[1] R. P. Ferguson observes that, 'The sense of nonmaleficence goes back to the oath of Hippocrates and is, of course, encapsulated in our quintessential maxim: first do no harm.'[2] In a study on the 'frequency and morbidity of invasive procedures', Schroeder, et al. advise that, 'The stricture that physicians 'first, do not harm' mandates scrupulous avoidance of procedures in which possible results do not justify risks involved.'[3] Walco et al., in a recent paper on 'The ethics of pain control in infants and children' state that 'The fundamental principle of responsible medical care is . . . do no harm.'[4] Despite its almost universal endorsement, we have seen that the obligation to do no harm has been interpreted relative to historical circumstance and the value commitments of individuals and institutions. In the nineteenth and early twentieth centuries we saw the obligation strained by the professionalization of medicine. In many ways, the physician's loyalty was divided between preventing harm to the profession and preventing harm to the patient. This tension was induced and exacerbated by key institutions – medical schools, hospitals, and the American Medical Association (AMA). Also during this period, the grounding of medical epistemology in experimental science served to divert attention from the patient's particularity to the more general manifestations of disease. 'Do no harm' was now interpreted relative to the more 'objective' criteria of medical science.

The expansion of human subjects research and medical science in the 1940s and 1950s also called into question the physician's allegiance to the Hippocratic maxim. By their failure to clarify and distinguish between their competing obligations as healer and researcher, doctors often exposed unwitting patients to risk and to measurable harm. Again, institutional interests fostered this blurring of roles. The United States government, committed to marshaling its scientific resources for the war effort, and later for the goal of scientific preeminence, allowed individual researchers almost total autonomy. With the commitment to scientific progress that defined the post-war period, the obligations of beneficence and nonmaleficence were increasingly interpreted within a utilitarian framework that linked these duties to populations rather than individuals. As in public health generally, this commitment to the health of the United States citizenry and, indeed, of humanity supplied the implicit justification for many medical harms to individuals.

In the 1960s and 1970s, one response to the tradition of physician paternalism and growing reports of iatrogenic harm was the emergence of the field of medical ethics and with it the demand for a more patient-centered medical ethos. During this period, the traditional obligations to benefit the patient and to do no harm were joined by a new moral norm – patient self-determination – drawn from the tradition of Enlightenment liberalism. The endorsement of patient autonomy in both law and medical ethics was an affirmation of patients' rights to participate in decision-making regarding their medical care and, specifically, to make informed choices about the risks entailed by that care. It was also a call for greater accountability on the part of health professionals to moral norms at the heart of democratic society.[5] No longer would the more traditional and paternalistically-interpreted norms of beneficence and nonmaleficence satisfy the demands of accountability. Rather, they would be met only by the inclusion of the patient's perspective in medical decision making. The profession's traditional commitment to the patient was no longer seen as a sufficient safeguard against harm. Nor was it believed to be authoritative in determining benefit.

In recent years, changes in health care financing in the United States have given prominence to the interests of insurer/provider organizations such as health maintenance organizations (HMOs) and other organizations that employ physicians and provide insurance coverage to patients. These interests are largely financial and may involve profit-taking as well as economic efficiency. Increasingly, the job of cost-control is being assigned to physicians and authority for treatment decisions is shifting from patients and their doctors, to benefits administrators. Alongside these changes in health care financing and delivery, there is a new model of medical ethics that locates the normative basis of medicine in the demands of the free market. Thus, while the values of the marketplace increasingly drive the health care system, they are also championed as the legitimate basis for medical ethics.

In the face of these momentous transformations in health care, an account of iatrogenic illness that intends to make plausible moral claims about the centrality of the obligation to 'do no harm' cannot simply assert the authority of the principles of nonmaleficence and beneficence. Neither can it appeal to ancient Hippocratic origins as a sufficient justification. Such an account must offer an argument about the moral basis of medicine and the source of the obligation to avoid and prevent harm to patients. If we want to have moral norms we must justify them with moral arguments. Otherwise, the imperatives that guide the practice of health care professionals will be drawn from the marketplace or from law or legislation.[6] This chapter examines a number of philosophical accounts of the source of the obligation to 'do no harm' and argues that this obligation is best sustained by a fiduciary model of the healing relationship.

Common morality and prima facie principles

Up until the 1970s, the Hippocratic Corpus was seen to be the source of medical morality in the West. Where the Corpus was silent or held to be anachronistic, new norms (for example, regarding consultation) were fashioned by the established profession. Rather than make use of philosophical argumentation or justification, the nineteenth and early to mid-twentieth century versions of Hippocratic ethics relied almost exclusively on the justificatory force of traditional and professional authority. This was entirely consistent with the image of the autonomous, authoritative – and authoritarian – physician. The physician's prerogative governed the technical as well as the moral domains, in other words, both the domains of practice and ethical policy.

The patients' rights movement in the 1970s identified a source of medical obligations *outside* of the professionally-generated canons of conduct. Medical ethicists soon provided philosophical frameworks for this emerging ethos. One of the most influential of these philosophical treatments of medical morality has been *The Principles of Biomedical Ethics* first published in 1979 by Tom Beauchamp and James Childress.[7] We discuss their philosophical perspective on a duty to 'do no harm.'

Now in its fourth edition, *The Principles of Biomedical Ethics* is premised on the authority and practical value of common sense moral beliefs. Emphasizing the general acceptance of the norms of autonomy, beneficence, nonmaleficence, and justice, Beauchamp and Childress argue that these principles reflect a social consensus not enjoyed by any contested moral theory. These principles, therefore, as established features of the moral point of view, provide the framework for what they call a 'common morality ethics.' Because of their general endorsement, these four principles are, according to Beauchamp and Childress best understood to be prima facie binding with no assigned priority or ranking. To say that autonomy, beneficence, nonmaleficence, and justice are prima facie binding obligations is to say that each is a *de facto* obligation whose violation is wrong unless it is justified by another prima facie duty.[8] For example, although surgeons and surgical nurses have a binding obligation of nonmaleficence, that is, to avoid harming a patient, that obligation can be justifiably overridden by the principles of beneficence and autonomy. The violation of nonmaleficence may be justified, on the one hand for example, by the anticipated benefits of the surgery to which the patient consented. If, on the other hand, the patient requests a surgical intervention whose anticipated harms (e.g. because of the patient's advanced age or other risk factors) are disproportionate to anticipated benefit, the doctor may feel that the performance of the surgery would be an unjustifiable violation of nonmaleficence. It is at this point of tension between obligations (to respect patient autonomy and the patient's conception of benefit vs. nonmaleficence) that the parties would need to engage in a process of deliberation whereby the competing principles could be specified and balanced to account for the particular context. The patient might, for example, want to have the surgery in the context of a research protocol. Beneficence in this case would encompass benefits to others through the advancement of scientific knowledge. On the basis of the patient's more robust notion of benefit (assuming that the patient makes a competent decision to enter the protocol), the duty to avoid harm might be outweighed. Another example touches on the sort of harm that comes to mind when we think of iatrogenic illness. Here, we might say that nurses are required by the principles of nonmaleficence and beneficence to prevent decubitus ulcers in bedridden patients. As Beauchamp and Childress point out, in health care, these principles are specified through standards of due care. In order to determine whether the actions that contributed to the patient's development of bed sores were justified we would need to determine: (1) whether the risk of the decubitus ulcers was justified by the anticipated benefits of the patient's stay in bed and (2) whether the nurse(s) abided by standards of due care in efforts to prevent the decubitus ulcers.

Rather than ranking the principles in any fixed order, Beauchamp and

Childress offer a procedure of 'specification' and 'balancing' as the means by which conflicts among principles are resolved. Specification involves the explication and adaptation of principles relative to the particular situation at hand. Balancing involves practical deliberation about how competing principles should be weighed. Both methods are used in combination to provide a coherent account of a moral problem and, if the problem has not been 'dissolved' by specification, a justification of its resolution one way or another.

We need not examine these procedures in detail but point out simply that they represent a view that we share regarding the importance of practical judgment in cases that involve uncertainty in the dynamic between general rules and particular situations. Unlike an absolutizing procedure that resolves complexity in favor of a single principle (such as the paternalistic prioritization of a 'doctor-knows-best' beneficence or the libertarian prioritization of respect for autonomy), practical judgment involving specification and balancing assumes that decisional complexities cannot be satisfactorily resolved by the rigid application of rules. Neither moral nor medical problems are, in other words, solved at the level of theory. They are resolved by individuals deliberating together about the values that they bring to the particular context of decision making.

What are the implications of Beauchamp and Childress' approach for the obligation to 'do no harm'? It is clear that in this account, the obligations of nonmaleficence and beneficence are inescapable. Even in cases where they are justifiably overridden by other prima facie principles, they do not 'disappear or evaporate . . . they leave "moral traces" which should be reflected in the agent's attitudes and actions.'[9] The moral obligation to do no harm can be justifiably overridden but it can never be erased.

In their account, Beauchamp and Childress offer some useful conceptual distinctions in their discussion of the norms of beneficence and nonmaleficence. These distinctions will provide a framework for our explication of the notion of due care in Chapter 5 and, for the moral evaluation of medical harm in Chapter 6.

Beauchamp and Childress rightly point out that as action guides, nonmaleficence and beneficence are overlapping and continuous principles. At times, we can prevent harm to someone (e.g. a patient who is bleeding profusely from an injury site), only by actively benefiting them (applying a tourniquet). Despite the continuity between these obligations, Beauchamp and Childress offer an important conceptual distinction between them. Whereas nonmaleficence specifically involves forbearance (refraining from action), beneficence involves positive actions.[10] Thus, we can say that under the obligation of nonmaleficence,

(1) one ought not to inflict evil or harm;
(2) one ought not to impose unnecessary or unreasonable risks of harm.[11]

Under the obligation of beneficence,

(1) one ought to prevent evil or harm;
(2) one ought to remove evil or harm;
(3) one ought to do or promote good.

This distinction is useful for a number of reasons. First, it provides a more fine-grained account of the traditional maxim to 'do no harm' by linking this maxim to obligations of *both* nonmaleficence *and* beneficence.[12] In this way, the distinction is able to provide grounds for the moral evaluation of both harms of commission (under the principle of nonmaleficence) and harms of omission (under the principle of beneficence). Secondly, it provides the conceptual resources to deal with the fact that certain medically- or surgically-induced harms may be justified in light of the benefits that they furnish. In other words, the aim of achieving a desired net benefit or a net reduction of harms may justifiably and without contradiction involve harming. Sometimes you must do harm to avoid or prevent harm.

The *Principles of Biomedical Ethics* sustains an obligation to do no harm by appealing to the 'common morality.' What this account does not provide, however, is an explanation of *why* common morality *does* support the centrality of these obligations in health care.[13] At a time when health care in the United States is increasingly viewed within a market model, to be constrained only by those regulations governing all commercial enterprises, it seems essential to explain *why* it is that society places special obligations on health care providers. It is precisely this question that motivates the work of Edmund Pellegrino. According to Pellegrino, the norms governing clinical activity are grounded in the fiduciary nature of the healing relationship.[14]

The fiduciary nature of the healing relationship

In his work, Pellegrino describes the nature of the healing relationship as a concatenation of three elements: 'the fact of illness, the act of profession, and the act of medicine.'[15] First and foremost, the healing relationship is distinguished by the vulnerability of the ill patient. This is what Pellegrino calls 'the fact of illness.' Illness disrupts our self-perception and thus our relationship to the world and to our future in it. Whereas we ordinarily take for granted the consonance between our bodies and our selves, in illness, 'the body stands opposite to the self . . . it intrudes on our existence rather than enhancing and enriching it.'[16] Instead of being the vehicle of our chosen modes of self-expression, the body (or mind) becomes an obstacle to that self-expression. Pellegrino describes the experience of illness as 'an ontological assault.'[17] It is characterized by a sense of disruption, by anxiety, uncertainty, and often fear and pain that together force us to place ourselves under the power of another person – the health professional. The vulnerability that we experience as a result of illness is thus compounded by the fact that the possibility of benefit depends on our willingness to reveal our bodies, our personal lives, and personal histories to another. We must entrust to the health professional those things about which we care most deeply.

The fact of illness calls medicine and health professionals into existence and gives rise to what Pellegrino calls 'the act of profession.' This is the second constitutive element of the healing relationship. The act of profession is quite literally the 'declaration,' – the 'profession,' – that the physician or other health care provider makes when he or she offers services to the patient. By offering oneself as a physician, an individual ' "declares aloud" that he has special knowledge or skills, that he can heal, or help and that he will do so in the patient's interest.'[18] The relationship formed by the one in need and the one who promises to heal or help is thus characterized by inequality. The physician has precisely the knowledge, skill, and resources that the patient lacks. For this reason, the model of contract, which is premised on the equality of the participants, does not adequately describe the relationship. By holding oneself out as someone who can heal or help, the physician announces her/his good will and thus invites the trust of the patient. By virtue of a physician's public 'profession,' a context for trust pre-exists and in fact invites the establishment of a particular physician–patient relationship.

Given the inequality between them, the physician's pledge to act in the patient's interest is necessarily a pledge that he or she will not exploit the patient's vulnerability, and will also help in positive ways to diminish that vulnerability as much as possible. It is here that the notion of patient autonomy becomes a crucial element in Pellegrino's account. Our willingness to become patients and to depend on the physician's resources is an acknowledgment that our valued autonomy is limited by the circumstances of illness. Thus, it is only by enhancing and encouraging the patient's diminished autonomy that, according to Pellegrino, the physician can genuinely serve the patient's interests.[19] Only in this way can the physician dignify the experience of illness as it is perceived and endured by someone in particular.

The third feature of the medical relationship, the act of medicine, is 'the vehicle of authenticity and the bridge which joins the need of the one seeking help with the promise of the one professing to help.'[20] It is the end at which the physician–patient relationship aims – the telos of the clinical encounter. The act of medicine is built upon the diagnostic and therapeutic questions 'what is wrong?' and 'what can be done?' The information gleaned in addressing these questions must then be particularized into a recommendation for this patient. The act of medicine is thus the response to the subsequent prudential question: 'what should be done?' As Pellegrino describes it, the act of medicine, that which constitutes *medicine qua medicine,* is 'a right and good healing action taken in the interests of a particular patient.'[21] The healing action is right, in the sense that it is technically, scientifically, and logically sound and in conformity with the patient's need. The healing action is good in the sense that it accords with the goals and values of the patient in the achievement of healing or wholeness. According to Pellegrino, these features distinguish medicine as a morally unique activity.

We find in the ontology of the healing relationship, perhaps, the broadest meaning of the maxim to 'do no harm': the enterprise of healing is a moral enterprise oriented to patient well-being.[22] In this sense, the maxim 'do no harm' constitutes a broad warning against the abuse of authority and expertise possessed by the healer. More positively, it summons practitioners to be faithful to the trust that they have invited.

In their book, *For the Patient's Good*, Pellegrino and Thomasma argue that these three features of the healing relationship establish the healer's essential role as that of a fiduciary.[23] When a physician offers her/his services to a patient, she/he is professing that she can be trusted to act in the interests of the patient. This act of profession is not simply an 'institutional fact'[24] or a promise that is subject to revision. Rather, it derives its force from the 'fact of illness.' Medicine exists because people become ill; the physician is a physician only given the fact that ill people become patients. In addition, the dependency relation fostered by the physician's 'act of profession' gives moral weight to the promise.[25]

In the law, a fiduciary typically has specialized knowledge, expertise and access to resources. In addition, the fiduciary is a 'person entrusted with power or property to be used for the benefit of another and legally held to the highest standards of conduct.'[26] Because the fiduciary relationship is based on dependence, reliance, discretionary authority and trust, the fiduciary's activity is regulated with regard to conflicts of interest and other potential threats to the welfare of the fiducie.[27] In describing the fiduciary relationship Justice Cardozo (who wrote the celebrated opinion in *Schloendorff* v. *Society of New York Hospitals* mentioned in the last chapter) held that,

> many forms of conduct permissible in a workaday world for those acting at arm's length, are forbidden to those bound by fiduciary ties. A trustee is held to something stricter than the morals of the marketplace.[28]

According to Pellegrino and Thomasma, the health care provider's duty to do no harm is grounded neither in the authority of the Hippocratic tradition nor simply in the 'common morality' but, rather, in the fiduciary nature of the healing relationship. To abandon medical ethics to the marketplace would be to abandon the meaning of illness and the trust on which healing is based.

Libertarian theory: medical ethics for the free-market

In sharp contrast to Beauchamp and Childress's assumption that the common morality sustains an obligation to do no harm, Engelhardt's libertarian theory of health care ethics is based on the assumption that in our pluralistic society there are *no* commonly shared values or commonly shared views of the good. As a result, any secular ethics that aspires to universal application must eschew *content* (a theoretical commitment to any sort of substantive good) in favor of agreed upon moral *procedures* grounded in mutual respect and permission. As a libertarian, therefore, Engelhardt believes that moral authority can only be located in *actual* agreements between persons, that is, actual agreements between autonomous individuals.[29] Unless they are based on actual consent, broad 'contentful' principles or policies (such as the principle to provide help to those in need) risk being coercive. Coercion or force is incompatible with secular ethics because individual freedom alone is 'the condition for the possibility of fashioning a secular moral world.'[30]

Already one can begin to see the consonance between this libertarian argument and the model of free market consumerism. Individual choice activates and sets the boundaries for transactions between persons. What are the implications of such a theory for medical ethics and the moral assessment of medical harm? To answer these questions we need to understand first what Engelhardt means by the term 'person.'

According to Engelhardt, persons are 'the constituting sources of the moral world.'[31] That is to say, morality is logically possible only because there exist beings who (1) are self conscious (for only self-conscious beings are able to engage in moral discourse), (2) are rational (for irrationality could not support a coherent view of morality), and (3) have a minimal moral sense, that is, some 'understanding of the notion of worthiness of blame and praise.'[32] Given these defining conditions, the only beings who, strictly speaking, 'count' in moral or medical moral decisions are those who meet the criteria of personhood. Infants, young children, and mentally retarded or brain impaired children or adults do not meet these criteria and are not, therefore, necessary for the possibility of morality. According to Engelhardt,

Fetuses, infants, the profoundly mentally retarded and the hopelessly comatose provide examples of human nonpersons. They are members of the human species but do not in and of themselves have standing in the secular moral community.[33]

Another implication of this pivotal concept for Engelhardt's theory is that medicine is regarded not as the agent of the sick and vulnerable, but as 'the agent of persons.'[34]

Medicine is the agent of persons. It is engaged on their behalf. It is restrained by obligations to respect the wishes of persons and directed by the [freely chosen] goal of doing good to persons.[35]

In Engelhardt's theory, therefore, the defining characteristics of personhood establish the moral boundaries of medicine. Health care providers have no obligations to the sick *per se*, but only to persons who contract with providers for particular goods. It is up to persons, strictly speaking, to decide whether or not the interests of those who cannot engage in such contracts (children, the incompetent) will be considered in the arena of health care.[36]

In this libertarian theory of medical morality, the absence of common values and the prohibition against force together entail a rejection of the classical and common sense notion that healing is the good sought by medicine or that health care providers necessarily have any positive obligations to patients. Instead of orienting the focus of medical ethics toward a particular value such as healing, Engelhardt's theory must and does reject the possibility that healing is itself morally significant except insofar as it is mutually agreed upon as desirable. Deprived of the notion of healing as a unifying feature of all 'health care' enterprises, Engelhardt's analysis must identify another moral center for medicine and for medical ethics. That center, is, as we have seen, permission or mutual respect. As Engelhardt has observed, the common thread that relates different health professions is not healing as a desired goal – but, a 'common set of puzzles.' [37]

I will not use the term *health care* in the narrow sense (i.e. the preservation or promotion of health) . . . Instead I will favor the broad sense of health care that includes a collection of somewhat competing professions (e.g., doctors of medicine, doctors of osteopathy, nurses, dentists, occupational therapists, physician assistants, clinical psychologists) with differing but overlapping interests, who face *a common set of puzzles regarding the rights and obligations of professionals, patients and societies concerning health care.*[38] [Our emphasis added.]

Thus, for Engelhardt, health care is not necessarily a morally distinctive enterprise, rather, it is the locus of certain perplexities involving free individuals. 'That which creates the substance of [the provider-patient] relationship also fashions its limits: the free choices of individual men and women.'[39]

At this point we can begin to discern the implications of such a theory for a prohibition against harm. It is clear that in Engelhardt's libertarian theory, the coherence of morality itself demands that doctor and patient abide by the principle of permission (mutual respect, non-interference, forbearance, respect for autonomy). Unlike the principle of permission, which is 'constitutive,'[40] 'the principle of beneficence,' Engelhardt claims, 'is not required for the very coherence of the moral world.'[41] The participants in particular medical relationships may act to benefit a patient only if the goods sought have been determined by mutual agreement. There is no *duty* of beneficence in a secular morality: it is a 'moral ideal' rather than a moral obligation; beneficent acts are 'meritorious' rather than required.[42]

Just as there are no canonical 'goods' in a secular pluralist society, so there are no canonical harms. A secular pluralist morality, therefore, requires that any content to the concept of harm be provided by individuals. As far as refraining from harming is concerned, Engelhardt regards 'harm' from two perspectives: first, the perspective of the one who acts (let us say doctor or nurse RX); secondly, the perspective of the one acted upon (let us say patient P). From the perspective of P (the one acted upon), RX (the one acting) has an obligation *not* to do to P what P believes to be harmful. This obligation finds its justification not in a principle of non-maleficence, but rather in the more fundamental principle of permission, which Engelhardt states as follows: 'do not do unto others that which they would not have done unto them, and do for them that which one has contracted to do.'[43]

When 'harm' is looked at from the perspective of RX, however, the principle of nonmaleficence takes on a novel meaning. According to

Engelhardt, the principle of nonmaleficence is a special application of the principle of beneficence.[44] Under this principle, RX is not obliged to provide to P a service that RX finds harmful, namely, in violation of the principle of beneficence. The moral force of nonmaleficence, then, is that RX not be required to do anything that RX, in the context of RX's own belief system, believes to be harmful to P. Thus, it is clear that nonmaleficence here is simply another version of the principle of permission. A doctor cannot, for example, be forced to remove a vital organ from a healthy patient if the doctor finds such an act morally repugnant. There is no moral sanction against such assistance, however, if both patient and physician agree. In other words, any obligation to avoid harm as well as the substance of that obligation must be established by mutual agreement.

Within these theoretical constraints, there would be no such thing as iatrogenic 'harm' *per se*, only iatrogenic effects whose beneficial or harmful character would be determined by individual patients and others. An iatrogenic effect determined by the patient to be harmful would be morally significant not because it was a harm *per se* (since there are no objective harms on this account) but rather because it involved the violation of the autonomy of the patient. The most egregious violation would be the failure to obtain consent for an intervention. Other violations would include breach of contract, including the failure to keep a promise or to abide by an agreement. These are first and foremost violations of mutual respect. Again, whether these violations result in 'harms' (for example to the patient's body) will depend on the patient's explicit identification of effects as harmful.

Clearly, such a theory which gives absolute priority to the principle of permission or autonomy places great demands on the patient (who is a person) to be able to anticipate and judge the meaning and consequences of various interventions. Likewise, if authority for all interventions is to be justified by permission alone, then patients and providers would need to anticipate in adequate detail all of the subtleties involved in the continuous series of judgments and acts that comprise medical care.[45] According to Engelhardt, however, 'the principle of permission does not require that individuals be informed, only that they be given the opportunity to inform themselves.'[46] It is, in other words, the responsibility of the patient who contracts with this doctor/nurse/technician to know what the doctor/nurse/technician stands for and what the doctor/nurse/technician will provide. In this way, Engelhardt's view is consistent with the provision of medical services as a free-market transaction – governed by agreements between buyer and seller and by the prudential principle of *caveat emptor* or 'let the buyer beware'. In addition, in this highly rationalistic view of persons as autonomous choosers, the vulnerability of the sick patient and his or her often diminished capacity for deliberation during illness, are not necessarily germane. Similarly, this view of persons/autonomous choosers as the source of any moral authority for a medical intervention means that doctors have no *de facto* obligations to those who cannot 'give permission' (children, the incompetent or unconscious) unless their interests are represented by a 'person' in the strict sense.

In this libertarian theory, persons may, of course, choose to convey trust to individual or institutional providers; in other words they may forego serial permissions and allow discretionary authority to those who provide them services. But why would they? Because, according to Engelhardt either they don't value their autonomy, or because they share a common view of the good with the providers in whom they accordingly invest trust. In this theory, Engelhardt allows for the possibility that trust and substantive obligations of beneficence/nonmaleficence might be established within the bounds of what he calls 'communities'. A community is a group that is formed on the basis of shared values. It may be based on religious values such as Roman Catholicism or doctrines of the Jehovah's Witnesses or it might equally consist of agreements made between a health care plan and its subscribers. It is here that Engelhardt envisions a role for substantive rather than simply procedural morality. Of course any concrete conception of benefit and harm embraced by the community and definitive of it would have to be agreed upon by its members (who are persons). Engelhardt reminds us that, 'No one may independently or unilaterally fashion the concrete character of health care . . . for the character of health care is to be created' by autonomous individuals.[47]

Thus, on Engelhardt's view, when one speaks of professional–patient relationships, one might be speaking of two communities: the community of those who choose to affiliate with something called a 'profession' and endorse its norms; and a broader and overlapping community of professionals and patients who come together on the basis of a common view of the good to seek and provide health care. This need not, however, be the case. An unwilling doctor is not, according to Engelhardt, *required* to affiliate with a 'profession' – for this would be coercive. Of course, as we saw in our discussion of the consolidation of the profession in the nineteenth century, individual doctors may find it difficult if not impossible to practice unless they commit themselves to certain professional norms. In Engelhardt's theory, any amount of leverage or 'peaceable manipulation' is permissible as long as it does not make rational choice impossible.[48]

Doctors who want to practice may thus find it expedient or prudent to agree to abide by certain standards lest they forfeit opportunities for practice. Such standards may certainly have as their aim the advancement of the patient's health interests. They may also, however, legitimately have as their aim maximal short-term profit, or cost-savings. The patient who is affiliated with this community ostensibly shares the values (and standards) that govern health care. If it turns out that the patient no longer endorses these values, she may 'opt out' by affiliating with a community that more accurately reflects her beliefs.

In the last decade, health care financing and delivery in the United States have shifted largely from fee-for-service arrangements to some form of managed care. In the process, the locus of health care decision-making has shifted from the doctor–patient relationship to managed care administrators and employer groups. Now, 'the contract that carries primacy is often the one between the employer and the managed care organization, not the implicit contract between physician and patient.'[49] As individuals (who may also be patients) come to exercise less control over the substance of employer-sponsored health plans and the choice of specific treatment options, we must ask about the implications of this development for Engelhardt's concept of community.

In any free market transaction, consumers are at liberty to 'exit' or opt out of arrangements with which they are dissatisfied. In health care, third parties have become the primary consumers. Every time employers switch to more economical health plans or physician networks, they are exercising the 'exit' option. When the exit option becomes the primary mechanism for expressing dissatisfaction, accountability is said to be 'mediated by the marketplace.'[50] In Engelhardt's view, this type of accountability is most appropriate in a peaceable secular, pluralist society because it involves the least coercion and the greatest amount of consent.[51]

Although Engelhardt puts forward the notion that patients and providers could come together within the context of a community of shared values, the realities of health care coverage militate against such an ideal. Most of us who have access to health care, gain that access through the insurance plans of our employers. Most people cannot afford to 'opt' out of the employer's plan and purchase their own coverage. In addition, about one-half of insured employees have no choice among alternative plans.[52] Because employees rarely have a voice in selecting the plan with whom their employers contract, they do not have any say about the character or quality of care purchased and may not be able to continue seeing their own doctor. Of course, on a libertarian scheme, employees may exit their current jobs and choose to work for companies that provides better 'benefits' but this is contingent not only on their ability to find other employment but on the new employer's commitment to the type of coverage that the prospective employee found appealing. The ideal of patients being able to freely choose the health care community that reflects their values seems unrealistic in light of the current structure of health care financing and delivery. This may only be underscored as health care institutions and medical knowledge are increasingly seen as proprietary.

We can now recapitulate the implications of Engelhardt's theory for an obligation to do no harm. First and foremost, in this libertarian construal of morality, harm to others is prohibited by the principle of permission. One may not do to another that to which the other has not consented. Neither individual nor institutional health care providers have any *special* obligation to avoid harm to patients. What obligations they do have stem from the basic requirements of mutual respect, including both consent and promise keeping. Because patient or community permission defines the positive obligations of health practitioners, practitioners cannot be held accountable for failure to provide care or services that are not agreed upon by the relevant agents. Without an operative and substantive obligation of beneficence, there can be no sanctions against what we would ordinarily understand to be blameworthy omissions. In a libertarian theory, the only blameworthy omissions are those that involve breach of contract.

The idea of an 'objective' conception of harm is, on this view, rejected, for just as there are no canonical goods in a secular, pluralist society, neither are there any canonical harms. Whatever benefits a patient hopes to gain, whatever harms she/he hopes to avoid, must be articulated and determined by contract. Providers may, but are not required to, abide by standards of competence or care, but they must make clear to the patient what they can and will provide. Patients (who are persons) and providers may join together to form communities that embrace particular views of the good. Membership in such a community may imply that consent is given for interventions that advance the good and that consent is withheld for interventions that cause preponderant harm. Although it is possible to imagine doctors, nurses, and patients sharing a commitment to patient welfare – since this has been the traditional presumption in health care – the shift of decisional authority from the doctor–patient relationship to health plan administrators has, in fact, created and heightened conflicts in the physician's loyalty to this goal.

Do no harm: fiduciary or contractual obligation?

The fiduciary and contract models represent powerful and competing visions of the provider–patient relationship. Each articulates a conception of the provider's moral obligations to the patient. As we saw in Beauchamp and Childress's analysis of the principles of beneficence and nonmaleficence, the duty to do no harm involves not simply the negative obligation of forbearance (one ought not to inflict evil or harm) *but also* and more importantly, the positive obligation to benefit (one ought to prevent and remove harm). Thus, the duty to do no harm unequivocally imposes a positive obligation on health care providers. On the market model offered by Engelhardt, however, positive obligations emerge only from contractual agreements. Thus, the duty to do no harm becomes, on this view, a truncated imperative of generic non-interference. Harm is only morally problematic because it violates the principle of permission.

Such a vision is most compatible with an unregulated or minimally regulated free-market model of health care. As this model comes to the fore, it will be challenged to account for the ways in which medicine does not mirror market or commercial contracting. It will be challenged to account for the significance of illness and the disparity of power between provider and patient. And it will be challenged to account for the fact that in decision-making regarding both their health care and their health care coverage, patients rarely have the knowledge or access to information that is available to 'consumers' of other goods or services.

At the opposite end of the spectrum we find the fiduciary model espoused by Pellegrino and Thomasma.[53] Here the vulnerability and dependence of the patient, the disproportionate power possessed by the health care provider and the provider's offer to help, unequivocally impose upon providers the obligation to act in the interests of the patient and to hold the patient's good 'in trust.' The physician has a *de facto* duty of beneficence, therefore, that pre-exists the articulation of specific goods by the individual patient. It is on this basis that we have moral expectations of physicians that go beyond the limited specificity achievable by contract. In addition, the duty to act in the patient's interests explains not only why we have legitimate moral expectations that our unchosen relationships with providers (for example, in an emergency situation) will serve our health interests but also why we hold providers accountable for harms of omission.

Although the fiduciary model continues to be the dominant model in both medical ethics and law, it is increasingly strained by a changing health care system in which physicians are held accountable to interests other than those of the patient. As physicians become more accountable to corporate agents and, in particular, accountable for their financial performance, the fiduciary model will press them to express their obligations of beneficence and nonmaleficence in active advocacy for the interests of patients.[54] The fiduciary model will also be challenged to address the conditions under which the interests of the patient may be justifiably weighed against the legitimate interests of others.[55]

Following Pellegrino and Thomasma, it is our view that the obligation to do no harm is grounded in the fiduciary nature of the healing relationship. We believe that the peculiar vulnerability of the patient and the trust invited by the health care provider together explain why health care providers, unlike shopkeepers, have positive obligations of beneficence toward those whom they serve. We also believe that as health care comes to be increasingly reinterpreted in the language of the marketplace – as 'patients' become 'customers,' 'subscribers,' or 'covered lives'[56] we risk losing sight of the fact that patients are not just the 'consumers' of health care, we are its direct object. The harms associated with medical care are considerable. On the market model, harm is only morally repugnant when and if it reflects a breach of contract between autonomous persons. Otherwise it is simply unfortunate. On the fiduciary model, iatrogenic harm is morally repugnant precisely because as patients we have legitimate moral expectations that medicine will serve our good.

Endnotes

1 Kane RL. Iatrogenesis: Just what the doctor ordered. *J Community Health* 1980; 5:149–58.
2 Ferguson RP. Iatrogenesis: The hidden and general dangers. *Hosp Prac* 1989; 24:89–94.
3 Schroeder SA, Marton KI, Strom BL. Frequency and Morbidity of invasive procedures: A report of a pilot study from two teaching hospitals. *Arch Intern Med* 1978; 138:1809–11.
4 Walco GA, Cassidy RC, Schecter NL. Pain, hurt, and harm: The ethics of pain control in infants and children. *New Engl J Med* 1994; 331:541–4.
5 Veatch R. *A Theory of Medical Ethics.* New York: Basic Books, 1981.
6 Rich S. Managed care, once an elixir, goes under the legislative knife: Cost-cutting feared harmful to patients. *Washington Post* September 25, 1996, p. A1.
7 Beauchamp TL, Childress JF. *Principles of Biomedical Ethics.* New York: Oxford University Press, 1979.
8 Beauchamp TL, Childress JF. *Principles of Biomedical Ethics*, 4th edn. New York: Oxford University Press, 1994, p. 33.
9 Beauchamp TL, Childress JF, p. 105 (see No. 8). Because the specification

and balancing of obligation involves intersubjective deliberation and also, at times, subordination of important values, much will depend on the character of the agents in deliberating well and in acknowledging what is lost and gained in our moral choices. In this way, health care ethics must also go beyond principles to an assessment of moral character.

10 Beauchamp TL, Childress JF, p. 192 (see No. 8).

11 We have added this form of nonmaleficence (the imposition of unreasonable risk) to Beauchamp and Childress's schema. Such a specification is appropriate to the medical context since, in medical decision making, the physician has an essential role in the calculation of risk. This prohibition is adjusted and further specified in the process of informed consent.

12 As we have seen, if the healer only had a negative obligation, that is, to refrain from direct harm, then the moral demands would be no different than the noninterference owed by and to members of society generally. The healer's obligation to do no harm, however, encompasses positive duties as well. This is one way in which the healing relationship is morally distinctive.

13 Similarly, Robert Veatch argues that a society establishing principles of morality by contract, would support the idea of role-specific duties for health care providers. Veatch does not, however, explain *why* such duties would be regarded as necessary. See Veatch R (see No. 5).

14 The following discussion is drawn from:
Sharpe VA. *How the Liberal Ideal Fails as a Foundation for Medical Ethics or Medical Ethics 'In a Different Voice'* (Dissertation)] Georgetown University, Washington, DC, 1991.
Sharpe VA. Justice and Care: The implications of the Kohlberg-Gilligan debate for medical ethics. *Theoretical Medicine* 1992; 13:295–318.

15 Pellegrino ED. Toward a reconstruction of medical morality: The primacy of the act of profession and the fact of illness. *J Med Phil* 1979; 4:32–55.

16 Pellegrino ED (see No. 15).

17 Pellegrino ED (see No. 15).

18 Pellegrino ED, p. 46 (see No. 15).

19 This conception of benefit is captured in Pellegrino and Thomasma's notion of beneficence-in-trust. On this account, the concept of beneficence, or doing the patient's good, cannot be collapsed into the concept of paternalism because paternalism is precisely the *interference* with the liberty of the one whose good is to be promoted.

20 Pellegrino ED, p. 47 (see No. 15).

21 Pellegrino ED (see No. 15).

22 Jonsen AR. Do no harm: Axiom of medical ethics. In Spicker S, Engelhardt HT, Jr, eds. *Philosophical Medical Ethics: Its Nature and Significance.* Dordrecht: Kluwer, 1977, pp. 27–41.

23 Pellegrino ED, Thomasma DC. *For the Patient's Good: The Restoration of Beneficence in Health Care.* New York: Oxford, 1988, ch. 2–4.

24 Searle J. How to derive 'ought' from 'is'. *Phil Review* 1964; 73:43–58.

25 See Goodin R. *Protecting the Vulnerable.* Chicago: University of Chicago Press, 1985, p.44: 'Promises usually carry special obligations but only because other people are relying upon you to discharge them.'

26 Rodwin MA. Strains in the fiduciary metaphor: Divided physician loyalties and obligations in a changing health care system. *Am J Law and Med* 1995; 21:241–2.

27 Rodwin MA, has coined the term 'fiducie' to refer to the person whose good

is held in trust by the fiduciary (see No. 26).

28 *Meinhard* v. *Salmon*. 164 N.E. 545, 546 (N.Y. 1928) cited in Rodwin, p. 244 (see No. 26).

29 Engelhardt HT, Jr. *The Foundations of Bioethics*, 2nd edn. New York: Oxford, 1996, p. 73.

30 Engelhardt HT, p. 97 (n. 87) (see No. 29).

31 Engelhardt HT, p. 183 (n. 19), (see No. 29).

32 Engelhardt HT, p. 139 (see No. 29).

33 Engelhardt HT, (see No. 29).

34 For a critique of Engelhardt's notion of personhood see Sharpe VA. *How the Liberal Ideal Fails as a Foundation for Medical Ethics* (see No. 14).

35 Engelhardt HT, p. 276 (see No. 29).

36 If, indeed, one can speak of interests at all in the absence of any common conception of the good.

37 Engelhardt HT, p. 8 (see No. 29).

38 Engelhardt HT, Jr. *The Foundations of Bioethics*. New York: Oxford, 1986, p. 8.

39 Engelhardt HT, p. 289 (see No. 29).

40 Engelhardt HT, p. 107 (see No. 29).

41 Engelhardt HT, p. 105 (see No. 29).

42 Engelhardt HT, pp. 106–7 (see No. 29).

43 Engelhardt HT, p. 123 (see No. 29).

44 Engelhardt HT, p. 114 (see No. 29).

45 Pellegrino ED, Thomasma DC, p. 110 (see No. 23).

46 Engelhardt HT, p. 320 (see No. 29).

47 Engelhardt HT, p. 320 (see No. 29).

48 Engelhardt HT, p. 308 (see No. 29).

49 American College of Obstetricians and Gynecologists Committee on Ethics. Policy Statement No. 170. *Physician Responsibility Under Managed Care: Patient Advocacy in a Changing Health Care Environment.* Washington, DC: ACOG, 1996.

50 Emanuel EJ, Emanuel LL. What is accountability in health care? *Ann Intern Med* 1996; 124:229 39.

51 Engelhardt HT, p. 171 (see No. 29).

52 Starr P. Look who's talking health care reform now. *New York Times Magazine* September 3, 1995.

53 The contrast between these two models is manifested in corresponding 'codes of ethics' recently offered by Engelhardt and Pellegrino.
See Engelhardt HT, Rie MA. Morality for the medical-industrial complex: A code of ethics for the mass marketing of health care. *N Engl J Med* 1988; 319:1086–89.
Crawshaw R, Rogers DE, Pellegrino ED, et al. Patient–physician covenant. *JAMA* 1995; 273:1553.

54 AMA Council on Ethical and Judicial Affairs. Ethical issues in managed care. *JAMA* 1995; 273(4):330–35.

55 We take up this question in Chapter 5.

56 Annas G. Reframing the debate on health care reform by replacing our metaphors. *N Engl J Med* 1995; 332:774–7.

5

Due care as a specification of the duty to 'do no harm'

In practice, the obligation to do no harm has traditionally been articulated in the doctrine of 'due care'; the notion that patients are due or owed a certain standard of care by health care providers. According to Beauchamp and Childress, these requirements follow from the imposition of risk. In the treatment of the patient, standards of due care 'can be met only if the goals sought justify the risks that must be imposed to achieve the goals.'[1] Historically, the standards governing practice have been determined largely by the medical profession. They have also been mandated by governmental regulation.

In recent years, third-party payers attempting to get more value for their health care expenditures, have begun to place greater emphasis on knowing what works, using what works, and doing well what works in the delivery of care.[2] In so doing, these economic agents have emerged as a new and powerful source of standards oriented not only to the quality of medical and nursing care but also to its cost. As more explicit attention is given to quality and cost in health care, we will need to determine whether and to what degree new efforts at standardization are coincident not simply with greater efficiency and economy but, more importantly, with the duty to do no harm. In this chapter, we argue that the shift to more evidence-based standards in medicine is a promising one to the extent that it is guided primarily by moral, rather than financial considerations. We emphasize this point in our discussion of due care in the establishment of standards themselves. We then discuss the demands of due care in the selection of treatment, in provider–patient communication and in the delivery of care.

Establishment of standards

The authentication of due care begins with the establishment of the standards that will guide medical and nursing practice. There are two important dimensions to due care in the establishment of professional standards: the evidentiary basis of the standards and the objective that the standards are designed to meet.

As safeguards against risk to patients, practice standards depend, first and foremost, on the availability of valid and reliable evidence regarding the risks and benefits of treatment alternatives. Valid and reliable evidence, in other words, is the basis for valid and reliable standards. Until recently, standards of practice emanated almost exclusively from the profession through professional journals and societies. The formulation of standards was largely unsystematic and rarely based on rigorous evidence regarding outcomes.[3] From the late nineteenth century to the 1970s, the locality rule in medical malpractice reflected and supported the concept that standards were and should be largely decentralized in formation and application.[4] Recent work in health services research has suggested that there is indeed, wide geographic variation in the use of procedures and services.[5] However, rather than supporting the idea that medical practice does and should operate according to local standards, geographic variation studies have led to widespread acknowledgment of the need for more universal standardization[6] and, to this end, a more substantial evidentiary basis for medical practice.[7] This conviction has given rise to a number of strategies for the explicit determination of indications for the appropriate use of medical and surgical services.[8] It may not be too strong a suggestion, however, that in some cases, the notion of due care is itself undermined by the absence of an adequate evidentiary basis for medical practice.[9]

Richard Smith, the editor of the *British Medical Journal,* has recently argued that the use of medical interventions that are not supported by sound evidence of benefit and risk represents a breach of contract. 'Patients,' he says, 'assume that the doctors know that the treatment they are using is beneficial. That the doctors themselves may not understand that the evidence for the treatments they are using is weak or non-existent seems to me to explain but not to excuse the breach.'[10] In essence, Smith is acknowledging that the duty of due care is violated when – because of inferior or insufficient evidence – unwitting patients are exposed to unknown therapeutic risks. Smith places the moral burden for this breach on physicians themselves. By performing procedures whose risks and potential benefits are largely unknown, physicians violate their obligations of nonmaleficence and fidelity to the patient.

Although we endorse the claim that physicians are morally responsible in such circumstances, we contend that their responsibility lies principally in the demands of informed consent: in knowing and in communicating to patients the quality of the evidence supporting treatment options. Thus, we do not believe that individual physicians can be held accountable for standards themselves, which may be either dubious or unsettled. The burden of accountability for due care must extend, therefore, to those who promulgate professional practice standards. Because the *proliferation* of practice standards may cause as much uncertainty and confusion as the *absence* of established guidelines, legislation – or in other words, a new and more explicit 'contract' as Smith might say – may be required to establish the authoritative source for these standards. It has recently been proposed, for example, that a National Medical Standards Board could act to oversee the determination, dissemination and monitoring of standards.[11] The determination of standards brings us to the second dimension alluded to above: the objective to be met by the standards.

As we have pointed out, due care 'can be met only if the goals sought justify the risks that must be imposed to achieve the goals.' In this era of health care cost-containment, standards are being promulgated not only by licensing boards and specialty societies but also by third-party payers. In light of the increased attention to the cost of health care, there is valid concern that cost containment will increasingly overshadow patient welfare as the primary objective of insurer-generated standards.[12] These concerns focus on economic motivations in both the formulation and the establishment of guidelines.

In the formulation of guidelines, economic motivations may result in poorly designed studies that either limit the study population or the breadth of outcomes studied as a basis for standards. As Morreim points out, economically motivated protocols may ignore qualitative outcomes because they are more difficult and more expensive to measure. 'Studies of cancer therapies, for instance, often examine such easily measured factors as mortality or tumor shrinkage, to the exclusion of such important matters as quality of survival.'[13] Further, guidelines based on a limited study population (of young males, for example) may subsequently be applied to a population including females or the elderly who may be ill-served by the generalizations gleaned from the research protocol.[14]

Even if they are based on painstaking and careful research, clinical standards may pit patient welfare against economic concerns. As debates about the authoritative source of practice standards continue, it will be useful to keep in mind the distinction between cost-benefit and cost-effectiveness analysis. Cost-benefit analysis is a decision-making tool based on the ratio between the revenues (direct or indirect) of a product or program and its associated monetary costs. A ratio favoring net gain justifies costs. In this calculus, relevant considerations are measured in monetary terms and economic efficiency has intrinsic value. Cost-benefit analysis takes no interest in the nature of the product or program at issue, but only in the ratio between the economic gain and loss entailed in its production. Cost-effectiveness analysis, by contrast, identifies the least costly means for achieving a goal valued on moral or cultural grounds – a goal expressive of interests not 'priced' by the markets.[15] In the context of practice standards, cost-effectiveness analysis allows that such non-economic interests as health and harm prevention are valued for their own sake as policy objectives. Economic efficiency is valued, therefore, only as a means to the achievement of these intrinsic goods.[16]

At the policy level, the question at stake in the promulgation of practice standards, then, must be whether and to what extent economic efficiency may justify certain risks to patients. Correlatively, we must ask what level of anticipated benefit justifies the cost associated with a particular standard of care. This question has recently come to the fore in debates regarding post-partum discharge policies[17] and is at the heart of future deliberations regarding the cost and quality of health care in our country. Although we cannot address these important issues here, we would point out that an answer to these questions regarding the relative weight of cost, risk, and benefit may depend on the economic interests at stake; on whether, for example, economic efficiency serves the interests of shareholders in the achievement of profit or the interests of justice in the distribution of limited funds for health care.

We have argued that patient benefit and forbearance from the imposition of unnecessary risk are goals integral to the moral identity of medicine. When economic efficiency supplants patient welfare as the principal goal for the development of practice standards, the resulting standards are morally suspect. Indeed, given their departure from the traditional object of practice, we may appropriately call them 'efficiency guidelines' or 'resource rules' rather than 'standards of care.'

To argue that the development of standards should be motivated by and oriented to the goal of patient welfare does not in any way resolve the problems attendant upon their implementation in a particular case. Standards are, by their very nature, indifferent to individual circumstances.

Whether they be rules of law, ethical principles, or scientifically-based practice standards, they are general principles of judgment. Although their generality and abstractness make them broadly applicable, these features also, of necessity, may prevent them from explaining or addressing the uniqueness of the individual case. Tensions between the general and the particular are evident at every level of a study of medical harm. They are manifest in 'idiosyncratic' or 'allergic' drug reactions; in general and individual conceptions of harm and benefit; in clinical judgment whereby a broad body of knowledge is brought to bear in 'a right and good healing action for the particular patient.'[18] The idiosyncratic drug reaction reminds us that particular patients cannot be wholly subsumed under general laws and that clinical medicine is marked by uncertainty and unexpected occurrences, negative as well as positive.[19] General and individual conceptions of harm and benefit remind us, as we will see in our next chapter, that our concepts must be capable of specification. The moral demands of a right and good healing action for a particular patient – that is, the moral demands of beneficence, nonmaleficence and respect for patient self-determination – remind us that in clinical medicine, the 'particular' in question is not just a particular body but an individual patient with moral and legal rights and protections.[20] These imperatives compel us to further specify due care in the selection of treatment, provider–patient communication and, the delivery of care.

Selection of treatment

Due care in the selection of treatment involves the identification of strategies that will minimize risk and maximize benefit to the patient. Accordingly, due care, requires the physician's knowledge and comprehension of the available evidence and standards, and his or her ability to tailor these assessments to the unique circumstances and needs of the individual patient. This involves the physician's diligence in keeping up with the professional literature and guidelines, as well as his or her competence in assessing the literature and in conveying to the patient the relative risks, benefits, and costs of various forms of treatment.

As treatment decisions increasingly come under the control of the purchasers of health care through utilization review, pre-admission certification and diagnostic-related group (DRG) coordination, treatment options may be limited or constrained in ways that expose patients to greater risk or deprive them of some beneficial services. Plans may place restrictions on the physician's freedom to prescribe medications and diagnostic tests. They may dictate the length of hospital stay, and many aspects of the general treatment plan. Morreim has argued that in the selection of treatment, physicians can no longer be held accountable to a standard of care that requires them to utilize expensive technological resources. Such a standard, she argues, is based on the erroneous assumption that physicians have control over these resources when, in fact, they are owned and increasingly controlled by government, business, and insurers. To say either from a legal or a moral point of view that the physician is *required* to take X-rays or to 'keep the patient in the hospital as long as is medically necessary regardless of insurers' reimbursement decisions . . . [is to] place the physician in the impossible predicament of being required to deliver resources that he no longer controls – and in the case of law, of being exposed to potential liability for failing to do the impossible.'[21] On the assumption that physicians owe to their patients only what is theirs to give, Morreim advocates for a divided standard of due care. On the one hand, physicians would be held to a Standard of Medical Expertise (SME). This element of due care would retain the traditional mandate that physicians owe the same standard of knowledge, skill, and diligence to each patient. On the other hand, the Standard of Resource Use (SRU) would govern the physician in his or her utilization of material and fiscal resources. Because patients will have varying economic, legal, and moral entitlements to these proprietary resources (through, for example, in the United States, their contracts with managed care organizations or their eligibility for social programs such as Medicaid), physicians' obligations regarding resource use will vary according to patient entitlement. Under the SRU, physicians will not be obligated to 'deliver resources *per se*, but to work conscientiously within a resource nexus.'[22] The physician's chief resource duty, according to Morreim, will be economic advocacy both immediately for individual patients and more remotely for all patients in order to improve resource policies – presumably by rendering them more equitable. With the interests of economic agents increasingly influencing the use of services and resources, the physician's fiduciary duty is no longer limited, Morreim says, to the avoidance of 'vulgar exploitation of vulnerable patients in order to line his pockets with a little extra gold.'[23] Fidelity now involves a more active advocacy on behalf of the patient's interests.

Morreim's proposal is a provocative one. It acknowledges that the prerogatives of medical decision-making, while once in the hands of physicians, now rest to a large degree with the economic agents of health care. Accordingly it suggests that accountability for resource use must not be borne by physicians alone but also by these economic agents. Like Morreim, we will not attempt to resolve the enormously complex question of justice in access to and in the distribution of health care. We can only point to some of the contours of this complexity by focusing on the enhanced obligations of physician to patient.

Whether under a traditional fiduciary model or under a model such as Morreim's that divides the standard of care, due care in the selection of treatment will continue to require that factors which impose identifiable risk must be disclosed to the patient. These include clinical as well as economic and administrative determinants. Because the meaning of risk, benefit, and burden is intimately connected with the patient's own conception of a desired quality of life, due care in the selection of treatment requires open communication and collaboration with the patient to determine the treatment plan. This is one of the moral foundations of informed consent and one which is jeopardized by institutional policies that forbid physicians to discuss services that are not covered by the patient's plan.[24] Such policies undermine the physician's fidelity to the patient. Moreover, such policies point to a fundamental public policy question confronting the United States today – what is the scope and what are the boundaries of the *institutional* provider's obligation of due care in the selection and provision of treatment? Beyond informing patients of coverage exclusions, what, for example, is the scope of the managed care plan's obligation to serve the interests of individual patients? This question is central to debates in the United States about how health care should be structured and financed. Although we cannot address this important question here, we can say that when the goals and values of institutional providers conflict with the physician's fiduciary duty, due care requires that the physician act as an advocate on behalf of the patient's health interests.

Increasingly, physicians are encouraged to practice according to clinical pathways or practice guidelines. As we mentioned above, guidelines or standards are general principles of judgment. As such, they may not address the unique needs of the individual patient. If the health interests of the patient are to guide decision-making, then there must be some flexibility in the specification of these standards. This is just as true in the tailoring of lengths of hospital stay as in the tailoring of medication dosages. The question of how much flexibility will be allowed in the application of standards is, of course, a question of the amount of control that institutional providers will exert over the judgment of physician and patient. To meet the needs of the individual patient, the physician's advocacy may involve appeals to the utilization reviewers for additional hospital days or to a managed care plan's medical director for a more expensive but more efficacious antibiotic. Advocacy should above all be based on therapeutic goals. The only morally legitimate form of cost control that the physician should undertake in the care of the individual patient is that of providing rational medicine; the wise use of tests and treatment.[25] Considerations regarding the amount of benefit or potential incremental benefit which a particular patient may be due in circumstances of scarcity, raise important questions about the cost-worthiness of different outcomes and ultimately about distributive justice. Above all, these distributive questions must be addressed at the level of policy within institutions, states, and at the national level. Stewardship of resources is a common responsibility and one that cannot be borne or discharged by physicians alone.

Provider–patient communication and the decision-making process

In the previous sections, we have alluded to the importance of provider–patient communication in meeting the obligation of due care. In health care, the demands of communication are reflected most prominently in the doctrine of informed consent. As we discussed in Chapter 3, there are two moral justifications central to the doctrine of informed consent. The first is the 'therapeutic' or 'due care' justification that emphasizes informed consent as a way of preventing patient harm and promoting patient benefit. Informed consent supports these goals by emphasizing that the patient's own conceptions of benefit and burden and the patient's own evaluation of risk are central to determinations regarding the right course of treatment. The second justification for informed consent is the patient's right of self-decision, a right that is articulated in both law and contemporary medical ethics and that establishes the patient's moral authority in medical decision-making. To exclude the patient from the decision-making process is to undermine the patient's moral agency and thereby to 'wrong' him. As Faden and Beauchamp observe, in the justification based on beneficence and nonmaleficence, 'autonomous choice is valued extrinsically for the sake of health or welfare.' In the latter, it is valued 'intrinsically, for its own sake.'[26] In the present discussion of informed consent, we emphasize the first of these two moral justifications; that is, informed consent as an aspect of due care.[27]

The moral requirements of due care in provider–patient communication are linked to the purposes that communication serves in serving the patient's welfare. As a means of establishing and sustaining a relationship based in trust, due care in communication requires a number of moral skills or virtues on the part of the provider: attentiveness (listening, not interrupting); responsiveness (responding to patients' questions and concerns with clear, jargon-free language); patience (a willingness to work through difficult and confusing choices with the patient); respectfulness (taking seriously the patient's concerns and choices); and empathy (imaginatively identifying with the patient's vulnerability in illness). These skills or virtues are required in all health care professionals who directly provide patient care.

As a means of providing information, due care in communication requires honesty and integrity on the part of the practitioner. Substantively, this will translate into disclosure not only of clinical risks, benefits, costs, and uncertainties but also of any economic and administrative constraints that may increase patient risk. As we saw in Chapter 3, in the law of informed consent, due care is expressed in standards of disclosure. Whereas disclosure according to the 'professional' standard, for example, may meet the legal obligation of due care, this standard might not lead to disclosure of risks that an individual patient considers pertinent. This is yet another manifestation of the inevitable tension between the general and the particular. As Beauchamp and Childress observe, although legal standards of disclosure may 'be appropriate for the needs of the courts or even for some institutional policies . . . they should serve only to initiate the communication process necessary for good decision-making.'[28] In other words, from the point of view of beneficence and nonmaleficence, effective communication between providers and patients is never restricted to the minimal requirements of the law.

As a means of arriving at an appropriate and individualized plan of care, due care in communication requires a method of determining the patient's decision-making capacity and comprehension of information and options. It also requires the provider's honesty in making a professional recommendation and his or her openness to the patient's conception of the appropriate course. This openness does not mean abandoning the patient to make his or her own decision. It means collaborating openly with the patient to determine the operative goals of care and the therapeutic strategies most suited to the achievement of these goals. Institutional policies that restrain the physician from disclosing services not covered in a plan are at odds with the provider's fiduciary obligation of due care. If beneficial resources and services are denied to the patient as a matter of institutional policy, this must be made clear to patients.[29]

The due care justification for informed consent requires us to revisit the question of the potentially harmful effects of disclosure itself. In Chapter 3, we noted that in the nineteenth century, attention to medically induced illness frequently emphasized the risks associated with information and the manner in which it was transmitted to the patient. The minimization of these risks was offered as a paternalistic justification for the physician's withholding of information regarding the seriousness of the patient's disease or of the risks associated with treatment. A corollary justification for nondisclosure consisted in the concern that if risks were made known, the patient might forego needed care. In the twentieth century, these concerns have manifested themselves in the doctrine of therapeutic privilege which asserts an exception to the requirements of informed consent. Understood broadly, therapeutic privilege permits nondisclosure of any information that the physician believes will have an adverse effect on the patient's physical, psychological, or emotional well-being. Understood narrowly, it permits nondisclosure of information that might either foreclose a rational decision or render the patient incompetent.[30]

A number of important considerations must be factored into the assessment of justifications for nondisclosure. As empirical claims, the physician's beliefs about the harm to be avoided or the benefit to be gained by nondisclosure are subject to fallibility and uncertainty. The physician may be wrong about the patient's ability to tolerate the information and may ultimately be wrong about the predicted outcome. As evaluative claims these justifications are highly paternalistic in their exclusion of the patient's perspective from the evaluation of risk. The inevitability of predictive uncertainty and the strong possibility that the patients' values and interests may diverge from those of the physician are powerful arguments against any presumption that physicians can automatically know what is best for patients. In addition, any attempt to avoid harm by nondisclosure must consider the very real prospect that the patient may be harmed by choices made on the basis of what is, in fact, incomplete information. Practitioners who appeal to nonmaleficence as a justification for nondisclosure should not ignore the fact that this ostensibly altruistic motivation may mask more self-serving aims, namely to avoid interactions that are difficult, uncomfortable, or time consuming. Therapeutic privilege can be easily abused.

If we accept the premise that communication between doctor and patient can effect patient well-being – a key premise in arguments for therapeutic nondisclosure – then it is illegitimate to consider risks alone. One cannot, in other words, restrict one's attention to the *pathogenic* potential of disclosure. One must also consider the benefits to the patient afforded by honest communication and the benefits that are lost through deception. Honest and open communication can strengthen the trust relationship between provider and patient. It can provide patients with the information that they need to make decisions not only regarding their health care but other aspects of their lives. In addition, research increasingly indicates that a process of communication and decision-making that encourages patient involvement will be empowering to the patient and may lead to improved health outcomes.[31] Finally, honesty and openness are ways of respecting patient autonomy, the basis of responsible moral agency. In the face of these considerations, a 'therapeutic' justification for nondisclosure may be difficult to support.

From another perspective, however, a due care justification for nondisclosure may be authoritative. This perspective is informed by ethnographic studies that highlight the variation in cultural attitudes towards truthtelling in medicine. A study of the perspective of a Native American tribe, the Navajo, on the disclosure of negative information, for example, points out that in the traditional Navajo worldview, language does not just describe but, indeed, *shapes* reality and controls events. Thus, 'discussing the potential complications of diabetes with a newly diagnosed Navajo patient may, in the view of the traditional patient, result in the occurrence of such complications.'[32] Within this cultural context, both nonmaleficence and respect for the patient's autonomy not only *justify* but *require* nondisclosure.

In light of the diversity in cultural and individual beliefs, it is inappropriate to make any absolute judgments about the harmfulness of medical information. The reality of different cultural perspectives, however, provides an important lesson for both clinician and patient. The lesson for clinicians is that to honor the obligations of beneficence, nonmaleficence, and respect for patient autonomy, they 'must get to know their patients well enough to discern when, and if, those patients wish to contravene the mores of prevailing medical culture. This requires a degree of familiarity and sensitivity increasingly difficult to come by but morally inescapable for every physician who practices in today's morally and culturally diverse world ...'[33] The lesson for patients is that we should, as much as possible, make our values known to providers and should seek to understand their compatibility with the values of the provider.

Delivery of care

The obligation of due care extends, finally, to the processes by which clinical decisions are implemented – in other words, to the matter of how care is delivered to patients.

The delivery of health care encompasses complex and overlapping processes often involving a diversity of providers within various institutional structures. The obligations of beneficence and nonmaleficence thus extend to all providers who work together in in-patient and out-patient care: the physicians who direct and coordinate care; the unit secretaries who transcribe medication orders; the nurses who administer medicines and oversee the patient's daily needs; the technicians who are responsible for laboratory testing; the support staff who handle patient charts and reports; the pharmacists who dispense prescription orders; and the orderlies who transport patients to locations within the hospital setting. At or between any of these points in the delivery of care, delayed or neglected actions, technical or judgmental errors, or communication failures may result in serious adverse consequences for the patient. In addition, quality failures may be the result of poor system design or management decisions such as unrealistic work loads, over-scheduling, inadequate training,[34] or economic policies that jeopardize patient interests. Leape has recently reported that potentially preventable error and poor system design are, in fact, the cause of most iatrogenic injuries.[35]

Due care in the delivery of health services requires effective communication and cooperation among providers so that the patient's care is provided in a continuous and coordinated fashion. It also involves practical and organizational strategies to eliminate system-related sources of risk in the processes of care. An institutional commitment to providing technical and policy support is essential to these efforts. This will involve sophisticated analyses of the processes of care[36], mechanisms such as provider benchmarking and feedback on adverse events, computerized surveillance of adverse drug reactions[37], medication error review[38], and nosocomial infection control.[39] We believe that the implementation of Continuous Quality Improvement (CQI) strategies holds promise as an approach to the identification and prevention of harmful quality failures in the delivery of care.[40] In our next chapter, we discuss CQI as the basis for a new model of quality and accountability in health care.

Endnotes

1 Beauchamp TL and Childress JF. *Principles of Biomedical Ethics*, 4th edn. New York: Oxford, 1994, p. 194.
2 Berwick DM. Health services research and quality of care. *Med Care* 1989; 27(8):763–71.
3 Office of Technology Assessment. *Assessing the Efficacy and Safety of Medical Technologies*. Washington DC: U. S. Government Printing Office, 1978.

Wennberg JE, Bunker JP, Barnes B. The need for assessing the outcome of common medical practices. *Ann Rev Publ Health* 1980; 1:277–95.
Eddy DM. Clinical policies and the quality of clinical practice. *N Engl J Med* 1982; 307:343–7.

4 Waltz JR. The rise and gradual fall of the locality rule in medical malpractice litigation. *De Paul Law Review* 1969; 18:406–20.

5 Wennberg JE, Barnes BA, Zubkoff M. Professional uncertainty and the problem of supplier induced demand. *Soc Sci Med* 1982; 16: 811–24.
Siu AL, Sonnenberg FA, Manning WG, et al. Inappropriate use of hospitals in a randomized trial of health insurance plans. *N Engl J Med* 1986; 315:1259–66.

6 The idea of national standards of care has analogously been endorsed in recent case law: 'each physician has a duty to use his or her knowledge [to] treat . . . each patient, with such reasonable diligence, skill, competence, and prudence as are practiced by minimally competent physicians in the same specialty or general field of practice throughout the United States, who have available to them the same general facilities, services, equipment and options.' *Hall* v. *Hilburn* 466 So 2d 856, 873 (Miss, 1985).

7 Chassin MR. Standards of care in medicine. *Inquiry* 1988; 25(4):437–53. As we will see in Chapter 10, just what constitutes 'evidence' or adequate evidence is the subject of considerable debate.

8 This is the mandate for outcomes assessment by the US Agency for Health Care Policy and Research and the Cochrane Collaboration. It has also been the catalyst for pioneering research by the RAND Corporation, the Institute of Medicine, the US Task Force on Preventive Medicine, and for McMaster University's Evidence-Based Medicine Working Group.
See Marwick C. Federal agency focuses on outcomes research. *JAMA* 1993; 270:164–5.
Chalmers I. The Cochrane collaboration: preparing, maintaining, and disseminating systematic reviews of the effects of health care. *Ann NY Acad Sci* 1993; 703:156–65.

9 Schoenbaum SC. Toward fewer procedures and better outcomes. *JAMA* 1993; 269:794–6.

10 Smith R. The ethics of ignorance. *J Med Ethics* 1992; 18:117–8,134 (p. 118).

11 Leape LL. Translating medical science into medical practice: Do we need a National Medical Standards Board? *JAMA* 1995; 273(19):1534–7.

12 Gray BH. *The Profit Motive and Patient Care: The Changing Accountability of Doctors and Hospitals*. Cambridge, MA: Harvard University Press, 1991, ch. 11.

13 Morreim EH. *Balancing Act: The New Medical Ethics of Medicine's New Economics*. Washington, DC: Georgetown University Press, 1995, p. 53.

14 Healy B. Women's health, public welfare. *JAMA* 1991; 226(4):566–8.
National Women's Health Resource Center, *Forging a Women's Health Research Agenda*. Washington, DC: National Women's Health Resource Center, 1991.

15 Sagoff M. *The Economy of the Earth*. New York: Cambridge University Press, 1988, p. 38.

16 For a more detailed discussion of cost-benefit and cost-effectiveness see Beauchamp TL and Childress JF, pp. 293–318 (see No. 1).

17 Rich S. Managed care, once an elixer, goes under legislative knife: cost-cutting feared harmful to patients. *Washington Post* September 25, 1996,

p. A1.

18 Pellegrino ED. Toward a reconstruction of medical morality: The primacy of the act of profession and the fact of Illness.' *J Med Phil* 1979; 4: 47.
See also Davis FD. *Phronesis and the Physician: A Defense of the Practical Paradigm of Clinical Rationality.* (Doctoral dissertation.) Georgetown University, Washington, DC, April, 1996.

19 See Gorovitz S, MacIntyre A. Toward a theory of medical fallibility. *J Med Phil* 1976; 1:51–71. These authors argue that the ideal of scientific rationalism is flawed because *knowledge* is not just of universals (laws, rules) but of particulars as well. Epistemologically this is important for understanding medical error (and thus harmful error) because, according to Gorovitz & MacIntyre, there is a certain degree of error built into our understanding of particulars (in this case, patients). This gives rise to a 'necessary fallibility' in clinical medicine.

20 These are some of the considerations that, in fact, prompt the distinction between 'standards' and 'guidelines'. Whereas a standard, implies specific requirements to which one must conform, a guideline provides a guide or general indication for a course of action. The term 'practice guideline' allows that there is flexibility in application.

21 Morreim EH, p. 88 (see No. 13).

22 Morreim EH, p. 88 (see No. 13).

23 Morreim EH, p. 63 (see No. 13).

24 Morain C. Looking for more controls on managed care in California. *A M News* 1995, May 8; 5:6.
Pear R. Doctors say HMOs limit what they can tell patients. *New York Times* December 21, 1995, p. A1, B13.
Pear R. The tricky business of keeping doctors quiet. *New York Times* September 22, 1996, p. E7.

25 Pellegrino ED. Managed care and managed competition: Some ethical reflections. *Calyx* 1994; 4:1–5.

26 Faden RR, Beauchamp TL. *A History and Theory of Informed Consent.* New York: Oxford University Press, 1986, p. 14.

27 The relationship between harms and wrongs is an interesting one that deserves more attention than we can give it here. Some harms, such as battery, may also be wrongs (to the extent that they violate the patient's autonomy). More interestingly, wrongs may also be harmful in the sense that they disempower the patient and undermine the patient's autonomy, which, like physical and cognitive functioning, can be seen as instrumental to patient welfare. As we noted in Chapter 3, this is the fundamental premise of Ivan Illich's *Medical Nemesis.* Autonomy is essential to human well-being and the general and particular ways in which it is undermined by medicine constitute iatrogenic harms.

28 Beauchamp TL and Childress JF, p. 150 (see No. 1).

29 Mechanic D. Trust and informed consent to rationing. *Milbank Q* 1994; 72:217–23.

30 Faden RR, Beauchamp TL, pp. 37–8 (see No. 26).

31 Greenfield S, Kaplan S, Ware JE Jr. Expanding patient involvement in care: Effects on patient outcomes. *Ann Intern Med* 1985; 102:520–8.
Greenfield S, Kaplan SH, Ware JE, Jr, et al. Patients' participation in medical care: effects on blood sugar control and quality of life in diabetes. *J Gen Intern Med* 1988; 3:448–57.

32 Carrese JA, Rhodes LA. Western bioethics on the Navajo reservation. *JAMA* 1995; 274:826–9.
33 Pellegrino ED. Is truth telling to the patient a cultural artifact? *JAMA* 1992; 268:1734–5.
34 Dearden CH, Rutherford WH. The resuscitation of the severely injured in the accident and emergency department – a medical audit. *Injury* 1985; 16:249–52.
35 Leape LL. Error in medicine. *JAMA* 1994; 272(23):1851–57.
36 Wenzel RP, Pfaller, MA. Infection control: The premier quality assessment program in United States hospitals. *Am J Med* 1991; 91(Supp. 3B): 27S–31S.
37 Classen DC, Pestotnik SL, Evans RS, Burke JP. Computerized surveillance of adverse drug events in hospital patients. *JAMA* 1991; 266(20):2847–51.
38 Allan EL, Barker KN. Fundamentals of medication error research. *Am J Hosp Pharm* 1990; 47(3):555–71.
39 Haley RW, Culver DH, et al. The efficacy of infection surveillance and control programs in preventing nosocomial infections in US hospitals. *Am J Epidemiol* 1985; 121:182–205.
40 Berwick DM. Continuous improvement as an ideal in health care. *N Engl J Med* 1989; 320(1):53–6.

6

Conceptual and ethical dimensions of medical harm

Thus far in our discussion of the moral basis of the injunction against patient harm, we have left the concept of harm largely unspecified. We have not, in other words, explained what counts as a harm to be avoided in the clinical context or what sort of effects are to be considered harmful. In this chapter we examine the values that inform the concept of harm in patient care. Building on our analysis of the moral basis of medicine in the previous chapter, we argue that a more patient-centered ethos will regard the individual patient's values as central not only to determinations of benefit and risk but also to occurrent harm. On the basis of these observations, we provide a framework for the moral evaluation of medical harm and the imposition of risk. We consider conditions under which iatrogenic harm or the imposition of risk may be justified and conditions under which they may be excused. Our discussion of potential excusing conditions for iatrogenic harm makes reference to recent empirical work on the complex etiology of medical mistakes and quality failures. We argue that a model of collective agency and accountability may provide a more fruitful basis for iatrogenic harm prevention than do traditional models of individual agency and accountability.

The concept of 'iatrogenic illness'

As we saw in Chapter 3, the term 'iatrogenic illness' originated in early twentieth century psychiatric writings and referred to neurotic manifestations induced by a physician's diagnosis. The harm in question was an identifiable illness produced by the words of an incautious physician to a suggestible patient. By the 1950s and 1960s, iatrogenic illness was no longer exclusively identified with doctor–patient communication, but rather, with the effects of new diagnostic and therapeutic agents. Iatrogenic illness was now understood to encompass those complications, diseases, disorders, and toxic reactions that resulted from 'sound and sanctioned' medical practice. During this period, iatrogenic harms were understood to be unfortunate but unavoidable 'diseases of medical progress.' By the early 1970s, definitions of iatrogenic illness were extended to include harms associated with faulty and contraindicated care. It was during the period of the 1960s and 1970s that adverse drug reactions and nosocomial infection were formally classified as particular types of iatrogenic complication. Today the study of iatrogenic adverse effects has been undertaken in almost every specialty and in relation to particular procedures, products, and treatment combinations.[1]

Although the concept of iatrogenic illness has undergone a considerable evolution in the medical literature, the harms in question have continued to be defined as 'complications', 'diseases', 'disorders', 'injuries', 'adverse events,' or 'illnesses.' Although these terms have rarely been further specified, they tend to reflect a narrowly clinical interpretation of harm that excludes non-clinical or non-disease-specific outcomes that the patient may consider harmful. This assumption is made explicit in an early definition of adverse drug reaction (ADR) which was conceived by Cluff et al., as 'any response to a drug that was unintended and undesired *by the physician* who prescribed it.'[2] Although this approach is very practical from the standpoint of detection and prevention of certain medically induced complications, from a moral standpoint, it is limited in its failure to acknowledge the essential relevance of the patient's self-report in interpreting the harmful effects of care.

Thus, there are both practical and ethical challenges in conceptualizing iatrogenic harm. The concept must be general enough to be workable and yet must account for the patient's own subjective assessment of the setbacks associated with treatment. Analogous challenges, of course, surround the concepts of 'benefit' and 'risk' in patient care. As we saw in Chapter 3, one of the most significant contributions of contemporary medical ethics has been to place the values and preferences of the patient at the center of medical decision-making. In this chapter, we extend this more patient-centered model to include the shared determination not only of risk and benefit but also of occurrent harm. Before we address the practical and ethical questions concerning the *scope* of the concept of harm in patient care, it will be useful to lay out the fairly straightforward elements of a definition of iatrogenic harm: those involving its *source* and its *object*.

Conceptualizing iatrogenic (comiogenic) harm: its source, object, and scope

Source

It is generally held that what distinguishes a harm as specifically 'iatrogenic' is that it would not have happened but for a person's exposure to the health care setting and/or health care providers. Taken in its literal sense, however, the term 'iatrogenic' means 'originating with the physician' (*iatros*). This narrow conception of the source of medical harm is inadequate because physicians are clearly not the only providers whose acts or omissions occasion patient harm. Harms may also result from the acts or omissions of nurses, technicians, support staff, pharmacists, orderlies, device or pharmaceutical manufacturers, or, indirectly, from the acts or omissions of institutional administrators. Although the proximal cause of a harm may be a drug, a defective supply, device, or a hospital pathogen, it is providers, operating under the obligations of due care, who bear the burden of responsibility for the patient's exposure to these potentially harmful agents. From an ethical point of view, therefore, the *source* of an iatrogenic harm should be understood broadly to include all health care providers who are directly or indirectly responsible for the care of the patient. Because the root *iatros* does not adequately capture the diversity in the sources of medical harm, a new term is required. We suggest the term 'comiogenic,' which uses the same Greek root *komein* (meaning care or attendance) found in the word 'nosocomial'. A comiogenic harm or adverse effect, therefore, is one that originates with care – and, more specifically, with care of patients.[3] This coinage has the advantage not only of a linguistic association with the term nosocomial but, more importantly, it reflects the diversity in the possible sources of patient harm. From an ethical point of view, this neologism invites a broader ascription of responsibility for medical harm. From this point on, except where it is historically inaccurate, the term comiogenic will be used to refer to the harms associated with patient care.

Object

It has been proposed that an iatrogenic harm can have as its *object* either patients, care giving institutions, or particular communities.[4] This seems to cast the net too broadly. Although it is undeniable that the negative results of medical care (just as medicine's positive results) may have an effect on third parties, including the patient's family, community, or health care institution, it is the patient him or herself who is the direct object of medical harms.[5] If a country falls into disarray after its leader dies of a surgical mishap, we do not properly say that the nation was 'harmed by medical care.' Rather, we recognize that there are other negative consequences that may flow from a medically induced death.

This having been said, it is worth noting that it is often precisely these secondary effects that motivate concern about the phenomenon of comiogenic illness. For instance, the two largest studies of iatrogenic adverse effects – The California Medical Feasibility Study and the Harvard Medical Practice Study – were initiated to address concerns about the economic impact of these occurrences on health care insurers. Likewise, as we will see in Chapter 9, attention to unnecessary surgery has come primarily from private or governmental insurers who focus on the aggregate economic costs of the phenomenon rather than on its direct affect on patients. Thus framed, the issue of unnecessary surgery is properly understood as one of 'surgical overuse' rather than one of harm to patients.

As discussed in Chapter 4, in its broadest sense, 'do no harm' is a general injunction that medical skills should be used to minimize patient risk and harm. In keeping with this principle, therefore, we would identify the patient as the direct object of comiogenic harm and as the prime beneficiary of moral and practical safeguards against it. An investigation of the ethical dimensions of comiogenic harm, in other words, will focus on the harmful effects of medical care (broadly defined to include nursing and dental care) to *individual patients*, not on its indirect effects on resource utilization or cost-containment efforts. By making this distinction and identifying the patient as the proper object of comiogenic harm and the principal beneficiary of safeguards against it, we also establish a standpoint from which to evaluate the legitimacy of policies that may subordinate the health interests of the patient to the achievement of such goals as cost-efficiency.

Finally, by emphasizing the *patient* as the object of comiogenic harm, we intend to distinguish this type of harm from the harm that may befall human research subjects. As we saw in Chapter 3, despite early impressions to the contrary, the aims of therapy and research are different and potentially divergent. In the case of the individual who knowingly and willingly enters a research protocol that has no therapeutic component, the conceptual distinction between the two types of harm is straightforward. The research subject has not initiated contact with the researcher (who may be a physician) in order to seek care but, typically, in order to earn money or to make a contribution to medical knowledge. The *non-therapeutic* research subject consents to an activity and its associated risks without any expectation that this activity will serve the patient's health interests or that the researcher will place the patient's interests uppermost. Correlatively, the explicit goal of the researcher is the achievement of knowledge rather than patient benefit. As a result, the researcher's activities are not governed by a duty of due care or by any fiduciary obligation to the research subject. Although an injury to a non-therapeutic research subject may be harmful, we do not properly call it 'comiogenic' because the harm is not at variance with an established duty to promote the good of the research subject.

The case of injuries associated with *therapeutic* research is somewhat different. In therapeutic research the physician plays a dual role as healer and investigator.[6] In each role, the physician is committed to certain values. As healer, the physician is committed to the value of patient benefit and the avoidance of patient harms. As investigator, the physician is committed to scientific knowledge and the rigor of the research protocol. At almost any point in the clinical experiment, these values can come into conflict. When a study design requires randomization or blinding, the physician is necessarily in ignorance of the patient's therapeutic regimen and will have difficulty interpreting the patient's clinical course. Further, if the patient seems to be in danger under the constraints of the protocol, the physician as scientist would be reluctant to discontinue the experiment until the patient's decline had been statistically associated with the treatment itself. As the patient's fiduciary, however, the physician would be required to abandon the research goals in favor of the patient's health. In the context of therapeutic research, the physician's fiduciary role remains paramount and as such, any harm to the patient, although potentially the result of a research design or a rigid adherence to the protocol, is properly speaking 'comiogenic'. Although the potential for conflict of this sort does not categorically rule out therapeutic research, the imposition of risk in such cases as well as the occurrence of harm will require special justifications and explanations. Loss of knowledge can rarely provide a sufficient justification for harm to the patient.

Scope

In common usage, a *harm* is some sort of damage, impairment or injury. When something is said to be 'harmful', it is understood to have caused or to have the potential to cause damage or impairment. To say that someone 'has been harmed' is to say that they have undergone, experienced, or been subjected to some sort of injury or setback. Implicit in all of these notions is some positive or normative conception of proper functioning, well-being or interests – the concept of harm, in other words, is understood only with reference to some positive conception of value. A harm undermines something in which we have some stake or about which we care. Because the concept of harm is fundamentally evaluative, it makes sense that an attempt to understand comiogenic harm must begin by identifying the sources of value that give meaning to the concept of harm in patient care. Given its evaluative nature, the historical appropriation of the concept by the medical profession represents both an ethical and an epistemological blunder. The presumption that physicians have unilateral authority to determine harm and benefit assumes either that these are simply factual determinations or that physicians have a monopoly on values. The first assumption is an epistemological error, the second is the basis of paternalism. Below we examine the evaluation of harm from the clinical point of view and from the point of view of the individual patient.

Clinical evaluation of harm: adverse outcomes assessment

From the clinical point of view, there is a normal or healthy state of the human organism. This state can be empirically assessed by a set of identifiable physical signs, or by such objective measures as temperature, blood gas levels, cardiac output, or thyroid function levels. The clinical values that the practitioner brings to the healing encounter are those inculcated through clinical education, training, and practice. They provide the basis for evaluating particular states as healthy or diseased, and for evaluating particular effects as beneficial or harmful. In clinical practice and research, these assumptions find expression in particular outcomes measures.

Mortality and morbidity continue to be focal outcomes in clinical care, but the experience of chronic conditions, age-related functional disorders, and impairments to mobility have increasingly advanced quality of life as the main goal that motivates patients to seek care. As a result, over the last few decades, outcomes assessment has begun to include not only mortality, morbidity, and such 'paraclinical' outcomes[7] as laboratory values, radiographic, and cytology results, but also health outcomes related to the quality of life associated with illness and treatment. A great deal of work has been done in this area and is reflected in such clinimetric and psychometric indices as the Sickness Impact Profile (SIP), the Activities of Daily Living Index (ADL) the Spitzer Quality of Life Index and the Medical Outcomes Study (MOS) Short Form.[8]

Although there remain important and unresolved methodological issues in the assessment of health-related quality of life, there is a general consensus that health status should include markers for: physical functioning (pain, energy levels, mobility, sexual function, sleep quality); cognitive functioning (memory, concentration, perception, reasoning); social and role functioning (communication, job performance, independence); emotional well-being (affective responses, suffering, anxiety, vitality), as well as biological and physiological markers.[9]

This broadened notion of outcomes is indicative of a major shift that is occurring in our social conception of the function of medical care – a shift from medicine as a disease-oriented to a health-oriented enterprise. Whereas narrow physiological indicators are intended only to capture information regarding disease or some notion of '(ab)normal' function, health status measures are intended to capture information on the *impact* of disease, illness, and treatment on a patient's life and goals.[10] This shift in perspective invites a broader conceptualization of comiogenic harm as well as new tools for its identification and assessment.[11] As clinically discernible or measurable phenomena, comiogenic adverse effects should be understood to include not only abnormal biological and physiological markers and patient mortality but also impairments to health status. This conceptualization of adverse outcomes will yield a more comprehensive picture of the risks and harms associated with clinical care.

As a practical matter, in reconceiving harm in broader terms reflective of health status, one positive step forward would be to change the current MEDLINE classification from 'iatrogenic *disease*' to 'comiogenic *harm*.' As a subset, the classification, 'comiogenic adverse effect' not only would accommodate a broad spectrum of disease- and health-related outcomes but would also be amenable to scaling by degrees of severity. In turn, this subcategory could accommodate classifications such as 'adverse drug event' and 'nosocomial infection' that are current in the literature.

The patient's evaluation of harm

The patient comes to the clinical encounter not as an instance of clinical norms but as a unique individual with a particular history, constellation of relationships and values, desired life plan, and moral point of view. Although the patient and practitioner may have a common interest in the integrity and normal functioning of the body, and in the absence of pain, suffering, and disfigurement, they interpret and often weigh these interests differently. In our discussion of informed consent in Chapter 3, we saw that with the ascendancy of the principle of patient autonomy, contemporary medical ethics has placed the patient's values at the center of decision-making regarding medical benefits and risks. Consistency requires the same shift with regard to the conceptualization of harm and harmful outcomes. The epistemological justification for this shift is that the concepts of harm and benefit are evaluative and that their meaning depends on an understanding of the values that inform them.[12] A more patient-centered ethic will underscore the provider's obligation to inform the patient of potential adverse outcomes and to solicit and take seriously the patient's self-report regarding unacceptable risks. In addition, such an ethic requires providers to be responsive to the patient's subjective experience of the downsides of care.

At the conceptual level, a patient-centered ethos focuses not only on clinically determined adverse events but on the patient's 'illness experience' as such. Recent work in the philosophy of medicine usefully distinguishes the concepts of illness and disease.[13] Illness is the human experience of the sufferings and unwelcome symptoms associated with embodiment. By contrast, classifications of disease are interpretive tools that help to explain illness in terms of theories of disorder.[14] Seen within this framework, the phrase comiogenic *illness* would specifically refer to the patient's lived experience of the negative effects of care and treatment. Unlike a comiogenic *adverse effect*, comiogenic *illness* would refer to an experience whose significance is expressed through the patient's personal narrative rather than through any application of scales, checklists, or measures. A patient's suffering in illness can be exacerbated not only by treatment that is painful or debilitating but also by providers who are insensitive, unresponsive, or hurried. It can be exacerbated not only by nosocomial infection but also by the dehumanizing experience of intensive care. To place the patient's well-being and the avoidance of patient harm at the moral center of health care means that each encounter with a patient is a moral opportunity, not simply to avoid comiogenic adverse effects, but to mitigate the suffering, anxiety, and powerlessness of patients who are vulnerable to the vicissitudes of the healing process.

The distinction between the clinical evaluation and the individual patient's evaluation of harm roughly parallels the distinction made in the law of informed consent. There, we find a distinction between a 'reasonable person' and a 'subjective' standard of disclosure. As the classification of clinical outcomes has expanded beyond morbidity and mortality to include health-related quality of life, the medical profession is moving more towards a 'reasonable person' account of harm and benefit. Thus, although the 'professional' rather than the 'reasonable person' standard of disclosure is still the dominant rule in informed consent law,[15] the professional conception of outcomes increasingly coincides with a more common sense, functional understanding of benefit and harm. Our identification of comiogenic *illness* as the illness experience of the individual patient is comparable in some ways to the subjective standard of disclosure. In both cases, it is the individual patient who has interpretive authority.

While our broad conceptualization of comiogenic harm as inclusive of the patient's subjective experience might appear to heighten the provider's obligations of beneficence, nonmaleficence, and respect for patient self-determination, we believe that it simply elucidates these fundamental obligations in an area that has previously been obscure. Indeed, a conceptualization embracing both 'objective' and 'subjective' accounts of harm is already implicit in many of the prevention and control strategies for adverse drug reactions and adverse surgical outcomes, as well as in the motivation for much of the care provided by nurses, social workers and psychologists. The importance of the patient's conception of outcomes is reflected also in patient satisfaction surveys and in explicit efforts to make care more patient-centered. As the Picker/Commonwealth Program for Patient-Centered Care reminds us, health care quality can be described in two dimensions: one has to do with technical excellence, the other, with the patient's experience of care.[16] The claim that the individual patient's values give meaning to the concept of harm does not represent a dramatic shift or place a heavier moral burden on providers. It simply underscores the moral demands of individualized care.

Moral evaluation of comiogenic harm and provider accountability

Our analysis of the duty to do no harm revealed that the health care provider has an obligation: (1) not to inflict harm or to impose unreasonable risks of harm on patients, (2) to prevent harm to and to remove harm from patients, and (3) to promote the patient's good. As we saw in Chapter 4, the 'do no harm' principle is not absolute, but is conditioned by various factors. These conditions help us to assess responsibility and blame for harmful actions and outcomes. In what follows, we differentiate between justification and excuse as key aspects of the framework of provider accountability. We also examine some of the practical and moral challenges that accompany the evaluation of harmful mistakes.

Justifiability and excusability

For harmful acts or outcomes to be defensible, they must be either justifiable or excusable.[17] Ordinarily, justificatory appeals are made with reference to harm-causing or risk-imposing *actions or non-actions*. By contrast, when we speak of excuse or excusing conditions, we generally do so with reference to harmful *outcomes*. Further, in offering a *justification* for a harm-causing action or the imposition of risk, an agent admits responsibility for the action but argues that it was right, sensible, or permissible on the basis of some countervailing claim.[18] With regard to patient harm, a justification implies that the principle of nonmaleficence or beneficence is overridden. An excuse, by contrast, implies that harm occurred despite a commitment to these principles.

Justification

In clinical care, there are two principal justifying conditions for harm-causing actions and the imposition of risk. The first is consent by the informed, competent patient (or valid surrogate). The second is that the anticipated harm is necessary to achieve patient benefit and is proportionately less harmful than the condition for which the patient sought care. The moral justifiability of harm-causing action may be understood, in other words, relative to the countervailing prima facie obligations of beneficence and nonmaleficence (due care) and respect for patient self-determination.[19]

In Chapter 4 we argued that the duty to do no harm is grounded in the fiduciary nature of the healing relationship. We also observed that the fiduciary obligation of the provider is strained when the provider is held accountable to interests other than those of the patient. In previous chapters, we have identified a history of tension in the physician's responsibility to patient welfare. Now, with the significant and dramatic changes in the delivery and financing of health care, we must address the conditions under which the provider's obligations to others may justify actions that either impose substantial risk upon, or cause harm to, the patient. As Morreim has argued, in the new ethics of medicine's new economics, 'the physician's obligations to the patient . . . must be weighed against the legitimate competing claims of other patients, of payers [and] of society as a whole.'[20] In what follows we examine the scope and legitimacy of competing claims on the physician's loyalty. We look specifically at circumstances where the physician's obligation to the patient conflicts with the physician's obligations to other patients, to the public health, to research and education, and to employers and third party payers who require physicians to act as financial gatekeepers.

Duties to a physician's other patients

In terms of justifying harm or risk to the patient, the least complicated competing claim is that of another patient for whom the physician has simultaneous responsibility. A triage situation, for example, may justify a harmful omission to one patient in order to prevent greater harm to another whose situation is more dire. In such a situation, helping one patient at the expense of another presents no challenge to the fiduciary model *per se* but requires that the principles of beneficence and nonmaleficence be interpreted within the constraints of distributive justice. In a triage situation, the scarce resources of time and expertise necessitate a specification of those principles in view of the relative needs of the patients.

Public health interests of society

A more complicated matter involves conflict between the caregiver's obligation to the individual patient and to the public health. Physicians for example, have a duty to report cases of venereal disease and some infectious diseases including AIDS. Infection control nurses, likewise have an obligation to place notices on the hospital door or labels in the chart of a patient with positive HIV or hepatitis B (HBV) status. Typically, these examples center on the justifiability of violating the patient's autonomy, privacy or confidentiality. In other words, in the first instance, the conflict does not center on the justifiability of violating the obligation to 'do no harm'. Nevertheless, it seems fair to say that violating someone's confidentiality or privacy, if not harmful in itself (insofar as it may, for example, be detrimental to emotional well-being), at least has the potential to cause secondary harms to the person whose confidentiality is violated. Reporting an AIDS case to public health authorities or by highlighting that information within the hospital, may result in job or insurance discrimination that then deprives the person of access to needed care. As Beauchamp and Childress point out, 'in a sufficiently just political system there is a moral obligation to obey the law, but this obligation too is prima facie.'[21] They go on to argue that, just as moral justifications may be offered to override a duty of nonmaleficence, so too may they be offered to override legal duties, such as notification that may result in inadequate treatment for a patient. When obligations conflict in this way, a satisfactory justification for a breach of confidentiality will depend on the following considerations:[22]

(1) It should be clear that there is a high probability of harm to a third party or third parties.
(2) It should be clear that the potential harm is a serious one.

(3) It should be clear that the action taken (e.g. the disclosure of confidential information) can be used to prevent harm to a third party.

These considerations must be weighed against the following factors:

(4) There are personal risks to the individual whose autonomy is limited or violated.
(5) Loss of trust resulting from the action may reduce the health provider's ability to help the individual patient and may deter others from seeking care.
(6) There may be other social costs (such as a loss of trust in health care providers) associated with this violation of individual liberty.

The same considerations should guide deliberation in cases where the physician must impose risk or harm upon the patient in order to protect an identifiable third party. An example is the tension between the physician's obligation to the patient and the duty to warn someone to whom the patient presents a threat.

Medical research and education

In Chapter 2 we discussed the potential conflicts posed by a physician's dual role as clinician and researcher. A similar tension characterizes the physician's dual role as clinician and educator. In both cases, the obligation to serve the well-being of the individual patient may be in conflict with other aims. While it is true that the clinician-researcher can at times be motivated primarily by self-interest, particularly an interest in advancing career or reputation, these personal interests do not provide a sufficient justification for patient harm. Indeed, the regulation of human subjects research through Institutional Review Boards is an acknowledgment that, among other things, patients (and other human subjects) should be protected against the self-interest of the researcher.

The question of justification is more complicated when the conflict is between obligations to serve the interests of individual patients and the interests of humanity or society. Such conflicts are common when physicians are engaged in research or education *and* patient care. In the context of therapeutic research, the goal of the research protocol to serve future patients with an improved therapeutic regimen, may be at odds with the obligation to prevent harm to the individual patient. In the context of clinical education, educational objectives that, for example, cause delay in the patient's transfer from the emergency room to the intensive care unit may place the patient at risk.

In general, justifications for human subjects research and the use of patients to achieve educational objectives are based on an appeal to the principle of utility. Aggregate benefits to society are believed to justify risk and indeed harm to a particular individual. As we saw in Chapter 3, a similar utilitarian rationale informed the post-war characterization of iatrogenic illness as 'the price we must pay for the modern management of disease.' In essence, the period exemplified the utilitarian presumption of research, but on a grand scale. If the underlying assumption of human subjects research is that medicine is a social good for which some individual sacrifice is required, then the assumption in the 1940s and 1950s was that medical *progress* was itself such a social good. The spirit of individual sacrifice and collective mobilization characteristic of the war years provided the implicit justification for medical harm and produced the perception of these harms as 'diseases of medical progress.' The 1957 AMA 'Principles of medical ethics' reflected this utilitarian spirit in its pronouncement that, 'The principal objective of the medical profession, is to render service to humanity ...'[23]

With the rise of the patient's rights movement in the 1960s and 1970s, the validity of the utilitarian justification for patient harm was called into question. Since that time, the legal and moral requirements of informed consent have become necessary justifying conditions for medical research. Other steps, such as the exclusion of the clinician from particular forms of human subjects research, have been taken to reduce the potential for conflict between the physician-investigator's duty to the patient and the interest in obtaining knowledge through a rigorous research protocol. When comiogenic harms occur in the context of therapeutic research, their justification will depend not only on the validity of the informed consent process but also on the physician's ability to demonstrate that the harm was not the result of any disregard for the patient's needs in order to sustain the goals of research.

Although informed consent has become a necessary condition for human subjects research, it has not played as prominent a role in justifying the imposition of risk to achieve educational objectives. One reason is the presumption that there is adequate supervision of physicians-in-training such that educational objectives pose no additional risk. Of course, this presumption is not always realistic. Hospital staffing policies may, for example, discourage adequate oversight.[24] In addition, an uncritical acceptance of educational goals combined with assumptions about the adequacy of supervision may prevent teaching institutions and educators from continuously and critically assessing teaching strategies so that the risk of patient harm is reduced. Where teaching is combined with patient care, educational objectives can easily seem paramount.

From a public policy standpoint, medical education will continue to be an important social good. As such, it might be argued that, as individuals who benefit from medical advancements, we have a collective duty to give back to the system by making ourselves available so that this good may be sustained. This is a version of the principle of reciprocity. Just as physicians and nurses are indebted to the society and individual patients who have made their education possible, so too are individual patients indebted as the beneficiaries of teaching exercises performed on previous patients.[25]

From the point of view of institutional and individual providers who have a fiduciary obligation, every effort must be made to examine how educational goals may be achieved with minimal risk to patients. An institution's general openness to informing patients of their role in physician and nurse education may be proportional to its confidence in its supervision, staffing, and work-load policies. From the point of view of the individual student, who, for example, is performing a first venipuncture, informing the patient of one's status, and requesting permission to perform the intervention, shows respect for the patient and for the importance and integrity of the educational process.

Employers and third-party payers

Physicians play a pivotal role in the economics of health care. It has been estimated that 75% of health care expenditures in the United States are tied to decision-making by physicians through their power to prescribe and through their recommendation of services to patients.[26] As a result, efforts to control health care costs focus on strategies to modify physician behavior. In managed care, these strategies may include such financial incentives as bonuses to physicians who discharge patients earlier, or who limit referrals for tests or specialty care. Strategies may also involve penalties centered around economic performance. If physicians do not contribute to the achievement of the economic goals of their employer or of a plan with which they are affiliated, they may risk being fired or dropped from the plan. In essence, these strategies operate by placing the self-interest of the physician in contest with the interests of the patient, particularly the patient whose care requires a greater than average amount of time or money.

Without question, the traditional fee-for-service reimbursement system may also pit the physician's interests against those of the patient. Because they stand to gain financially for each billable service, physicians are encouraged to do more rather than less in a fee-for-service scheme. Such incentives clearly have the potential to increase the likelihood of comiogenic harm through unnecessary services and the compounding of risk. However, under these incentives, physicians confront only themselves as obstacles to the patient's genuine needs. The situation in managed care is substantially different. As Pellegrino has pointed out,

> when fee-for-service conflicts occur, they are the physician's direct responsibility. The physician is free to resolve the conflict in the patient's favor. Overutilization for private gain is a moral defect for which the physician is clearly responsible. In managed care, the physician is not responsible for generating the conflict but *is* responsible, nonetheless, for its resolution. Furthermore, the measure of freedom allowed in effecting a resolution is much narrower than in a fee-for-service situation.[27]

Even if a physician resists the appeal of managed care to her self-interest, for example, by refusing bonuses or forgoing a percentage of salary that might have been available to a physician for economizing on care, it is still the case that physicians who contract to work in managed care systems assume some obligation to promote the interests of the system. Inevitably these interests include cost control. In managed care, in other words, physicians may be obliged, as a condition of their employment, to promote financial interests that compromise their fiduciary role. In Chapter 5 we discussed economic advocacy – that is, patient advocacy with regard to economic constraints – as an extension of the physician's obligation of due care. In what follows, we look more closely at the duty of advocacy in the context of conflicting obligations to patients and employers.

The physician's role as economic advocate has at least two dimensions. First, advocacy requires physician disclosure of all potentially beneficial treatment options and the economic obstacles that the patient may face in obtaining them. Secondly, advocacy requires that physicians contest the denial of beneficial treatments and services. We agree with Gray and others that the obligation to appeal administrative constraints on care 'increases with the seriousness and certainty of harm to the patient's well-being.'[28] The obligation is heightened further still if the plan's exclusion of services has not been justified by plan administrators. Unless the patient's interests are to be systematically subordinated to cost-control objectives, the economic agent must justify denials of care. Of course, these justifications and, likewise, effective patient advocacy depend on the availability of sufficient information regarding the potential clinical benefits and harms of possible interventions. As we discuss in Chapter 10, medicine suffers from a dearth

of outcomes data. Often there is little solid scientific evidence to support –
or to reject – clinical recommendations. With regard to the prevention of
comiogenic harm and the minimization of risk, such data are, however,
essential. Outcomes research will continue to be one of the key requirements in the evolving, evidence-based practice of medicine.

As we saw in Chapter 2, the nineteenth century debate about the
legitimacy of clinical intervention centered largely on the propriety of
competing therapeutic maxims – the heroic rallying cry of 'better something doubtful than nothing,' versus the more skeptical one of 'better
nothing than something doubtful.' Both of these maxims represented a
particular epistemological commitment on the part of the physicians who
championed them. With the evolution of medical ethics in the twentieth
century, the prerogative for decision-making has shifted increasingly from
physician to patient; questions regarding the acceptability of risk are no
longer regarded as a strictly clinical determination but rather, as a function
of the values that both clinician and patient bring to the decision-making
process. As economic agents have become more involved in health care
determinations, they have brought yet another set of values to the decision-making process – values potentially in conflict with the patient's
health interests. When conflicts between the interests of patients and of
third party payers arise, it is the responsibility of health care organizations
to establish fair procedures for their resolution.

In Chapter 4 we argued that beneficence, nonmaleficence, respect for
patient autonomy, and justice are presumptive obligations governing
health care providers. The presumptive nature of these obligations allows
that they may be justifiably overridden only by a countervailing prima
facie claim. Because abandonment of one's role as patient advocate may
supersede as many as three fundamental principles governing patient care
(beneficence, nonmaleficence, respect for patient autonomy), the warrant
must be considerable. The physician should not, in other words, abandon
the duty of advocacy readily, for if the physician, as the patient's only
identified fiduciary, does not advocate for the patient, who will? Indeed as
Wolf has pointed out, the physician's identification of mitigating circumstances may be a managed care or a utilization review organization's only
source of information regarding needed exceptions.[29] Given this, we would
argue against contractual agreements that place physicians in the role of
financial gatekeeper for their corporate employer. Such an obligation may
not only directly conflict with the physician's duty to the patient but may
also deprive managed care or other health care employers of an important
resource for information regarding clinical appropriateness.

In the late nineteenth and early twentieth centuries, physicians played a crucial role in contributing to the financial viability of hospitals. The physician's appointment to the hospital guaranteed a steady supply of patients from his private practice. In return, the hospital provided physicians with an array of clinical opportunities and a measure of prestige. An additional result of this symbiosis was a reluctance on the part of hospitals to evaluate physician performance in anything but financial terms. Ernest Codman's pioneering work in hospital quality was, in large measure, an effort to reform standards of accountability. According to Codman, hospital quality and efficiency should be assessed in *therapeutic* rather than in *fiscal* terms. As such, the performance of physicians and nurses, and the success of the institution's administrative and educational functions should be evaluated on the basis of patient benefit, rather than institutional revenues. Despite all of the contemporary pressures to focus on financial constraints and opportunities, we reemphasize Codman's admonition and the moral demands of the fiduciary relationship. Only by examining how well or poorly patients fare can we know if medicine is doing more harm than good. From the point of view of comiogenic harm prevention, *this* is the 'bottom line.'

Justice in the distribution of health care resources

In her book *Balancing Act: The New Medical Ethics of Medicine's New Economics,*[30] Morreim argues that the fact of fiscal scarcity places limits on the physician's traditional obligation of fidelity to the patient. We disagree that scarcity itself is a *sufficient* justification for compromising this obligation, for determinations of scarcity are always relative to predefined goals. At the very least, such determinations always depend on the prioritizing of allocations and this prioritization may be based on values that are deeply at odds with the responsibilities of physicians and the goals of health care. For example, resources may be deemed scarce relative to a projected profit margin for a health care plan or they may be deemed scarce relative to a publicly established global budget for health care. In addition, an acceptance of the fact of fiscal scarcity does not in any way *require* that the responsibility for cost containment should fall to physicians. This is an easy but invalid inference drawn from the influence that the physician has in treatment determinations.

Although we do not believe that scarcity *itself* warrants the physician's abandonment of the obligations of advocacy, we do believe that considered strategies devised to achieve just distribution of scarce fiscal resources may legitimately be weighed against the physician's duty as advocate and, by extension, against his or her obligations of nonmaleficence and beneficence. In the United States, the demand for transplantable organs is greater than the supply. Rather than placing the burden of organ allocation on individual physicians, we have established policies for justice in the distribution of these scarce resources. The transplant physician's obligation to a patient who is a potential organ recipient is, thus, constrained by a distributive policy based on the principle of justice. Similar distributive policies can govern the allocation of scarce fiscal resources and, indeed, do in Medicaid and other state-sponsored health insurance plans. In order to decrease the likelihood that any particular interests are systematically advanced or denied, such policies should be the result of an open, public, deliberative process. Certainly in the development of public policy, the physician, like any other citizen has a responsibility to contribute to a just and rational scheme of distribution.

Placing the burden of fiscal accountability on the physician at the bedside effectively side-steps the question of justice and circumvents the public policy process that can lay open the priorities at the heart of health care rationing schemes.

Excuse

As we said above, in offering a *justification*, the agent of harm admits responsibility for the harm but argues that the actions or omissions that led to it were right, sensible, or permissible on the basis of some countervailing demand or obligation. In offering an *excuse*, however, the alleged agent of harm denies responsibility (and thus moral agency) for an admittedly unfortunate outcome and argues that the outcome was the result of – and, therefore, should be excused by – certain features of the situation.[31] Whereas a justification makes appeal to some compelling reason for overriding principles of nonmaleficence and beneficence, in offering an excuse, one maintains the priority of the principles of nonmaleficence and beneficence but rejects personal responsibility for their violation.

Excusing conditions for comiogenic harm might involve innocent ignorance, duress, lack of sufficient resources, the current inability to prevent the occurrence of the harm, and good-faith error.

Innocent ignorance

Among harms excused by innocent ignorance would be those that are unpredictable and that follow from the best medical knowledge and skill. A harmful ADR may result, for example, from the unforseeable influence of patient co-morbidity or sensitivity. Indeed allergic or idiosyncratic reactions are responsible for approximately 10% of adverse drug events.[32] Gorovitz and MacIntyre[33] have identified this 'necessary fallibility' as the inevitable source of some patient harms – inevitable because the predictive powers of even the most astute, informed, and conscientious provider are necessarily outstripped by the enormous complexity of factors that comprise the individual case. In that clinical knowledge is always probabilistic, it is always fallible.

Another excusing condition under 'innocent ignorance' may be that the 'best medical knowledge' was, in fact, flawed. Examples include the many harms associated with now obsolete practices in the history of medicine from mercury poisoning and puerperal sepsis in the nineteenth century to blindness in premature infants caused by the recommended high levels of oxygen in incubators in the 1940s and 1950s.[34] Individual providers cannot be held accountable for the fact that general medical knowledge is incomplete. As Marcel Proust observed, 'Even the wisest of doctors are relying on scientific truths, the errors of which will be recognized within a few years time.'[35]

Of course, although individual physicians may legitimately claim innocent ignorance when medical standards are found to be flawed, this only raises the more pressing question of responsibility and accountability for standards themselves. As we argued in Chapter 5, the authentication of due care begins with the establishment of standards. As the formulation and establishment of practice standards becomes more explicit and systematic in this era of cost-containment, we will see increased intensity in debates regarding evidence, cost, outcomes and, ultimately, who controls medical decision-making. At the heart of these debates will be the question of the values that should guide the practices and policies of institutional and individual health care providers. Regardless of where these debates take us, some degree of uncertainty will always accompany medical practice. As patients, we would be wise to recognize this inevitability so that our expectations of medicine do not exceed its true capabilities.

To return to the excuse of innocent ignorance, such an appeal might also be offered by a doctor, nurse, or technician, where the actual agent of harm was a defective supply, device, or drug. When we attribute causal responsibility to a defective piece of equipment we are saying not simply that the equipment *caused* the harm but that the event was somehow controllable. In such cases, we attribute blame for the harmful occurrence to those responsible for the product – the pharmaceutical company, the dispensary, the device manufacturer. An analogous claim of innocent ignorance on the part of the drug or device manufacturer is more problematic, however, and raises difficult questions regarding what constitutes a sufficient level of evidence for the marketing and/or use of drugs and devices. The Dalkon Shield, diethylstilbestrol (DES), and thalidomide are relatively recent examples of products marketed without sufficient recognition of their potential for harm. Social consensus on these matters tends to be reached in regulatory law in the United States through the Food and Drug Administration (FDA). We discuss some of these regulatory efforts in Chapter 8. Suffice it to say here that the moral evaluation of the manufacturer's excusability will depend, in part, on its subsequent actions. Serious mishaps require positive changes to address and respond to the defect. This is the assumption behind regulatory requirements for post-marking surveillance and adverse event reporting under the FDA's MEDWatch program.[36] For the patient, the lesson of such mishaps is that every drug, device and supply carries with it the risk of sometimes unknown but serious harm.

Finally, the possibility of appeal to innocent ignorance prompts us to say a word about the conditions under which ignorance would be culpable. In the case of medical harm, the blameworthiness of ignorance is related to the assumption of a professional role and its attendant duties. Medical and nursing professionals are, by virtue of their fiduciary role, required to maintain certain standards of knowledge by keeping up with the professional literature and staying abreast of developments in their areas of practice. To say that a provider 'should have known,' for example, that cardiac arrest was likely to result from the combination of terfenadine and erythromycin, or that diabetics whose care excludes food by mouth must have their insulin dose correspondingly reduced, is to say that the provider's ignorance in producing these harms was culpable. As we discuss later in this chapter, harms associated with what we have called culpable ignorance are often abetted by systems that encourage individual errors or make them difficult to detect. An exclusive emphasis on individual culpability, therefore, may not only fail to reveal all of the relevant causes of an adverse event, but may also be counterproductive in preventing such occurrences.

Duress

A second potentially excusing condition in the case of comiogenic harm is duress. This excuse might be offered by a paramedic, for example, whose triage of patients at an accident site results in harm to the patient whose care was delayed. In this case, duress is comparable to a third excusing condition – lack of sufficient resources. If, on the one hand an emergency room provider is not able to adequately sterilize a patient's wound site (because of a shortage of available supplies due to an error by the supply requisition department), that provider may legitimately plead lack of sufficient resources as an excuse for the patient's surgical wound infection. In such a case, accountability for the harm will rest on the requisitions department and the hospital administration. If, on the other hand, a surgeon proceeded with an elective, non-emergency, operation fully aware that sterilization was impossible, an 'insufficient supplies' excuse would obviously be invalid.

The physician's fidelity to the patient is increasingly challenged by institutional controls on decision-making and incentives that either penalize or reward the physician for the desired utilization of services. Hospitals or hospital management organizations may, for example, share profits with physicians who keep costs below certain targets; they may withhold a portion of the physician's annual pay as an incentive to keep costs down. They may deduct the cost of specialist care from the fee to the primary care referring physician, or they may exclude a physician from a provider network on the basis of that physician's financial performance. Given these circumstances, we must ask whether the physician's role in resultant patient harm is excused by an appeal to duress. To what extent, in other words, can a physician be excused for succumbing to pressures to implement the economic directives of a plan? The question of excuse here can be usefully distinguished from that of justification. As we saw earlier, justification for harm-causing action involves the invocation of some countervailing principle as a sanction for the action. The agent takes responsibility for the action but argues that it was necessary or permissable. When managed care plans seek cost-savings through policies that increase patient risk, they may do so through a justificatory appeal – cost efficiency demands certain sacrifices.[37] By contrast, in making an appeal to duress as an *excusing* condition under such circumstances, the physician denies responsibility and, therefore, blame for an adverse outcome, arguing that blame actually lay in a hospital policy of early discharge or utilization review. In order to determine the physician's moral complicity in such a circumstance, the assessment of the appeal to duress must take into consideration a number of factors. First, in the face of the potentially harmful directive, did the physician actively advocate for the patient's interests? Secondly, did the physician disclose to the patient the financial concerns influencing decision-making? Thirdly, what was the extremity of duress – would the physician have lost a generous bonus, a significant portion of salary, or her job by contradicting institutional policy? The significance of duress in such circumstances is reflected in the most prominent lawsuit to date concerning economically motivated denials of care. In the case of *Wickline* v. *State of California,*[38] 'the plaintiff who believed that she had been discharged from the hospital too early declined to sue her physicians, suing only the state Medicaid program that had denied funding for a longer stay. The physicians, she felt, were as much victims of the system as she was.'[39]

As fiscal scarcity becomes the rule in health care and as physicians increasingly function as financial gatekeepers, patients will inevitably be harmed as a result of denials of care. In such cases the burden will be on the physicians to demonstrate how they attempted to fulfill their fiduciary obligation to do no harm through patient advocacy and full disclosure of the financial influences upon decision-making. Although the excuse of extreme duress under such circumstances may mitigate the responsibility ascribed, it rarely exonerates. Indeed, having identified policies that jeopardize their ability to act in the interests of the patient, physicians now have the responsibility of taking active steps to change policies that compromise their fiduciary role and thereby compromise patient welfare. Unless they actively resist practices and policies that erode the commitment to patient welfare, physicians effectively become moral accomplices in the resulting harms.

Non-preventability

Another potentially excusing condition for comiogenic harm is its current non-preventability. It is axiomatic that all interventions, hospitalizations, and medications are associated with degrees of risk. In some situations, those risks will manifest themselves and the patient will experience a harmful outcome. It may be that the underlying disease made the patient more susceptible to a bad outcome or it may be that the patient was a victim of medicine's 'necessary fallibility.' Although non-preventable harms may be excusable, they are nonetheless opportunities to scrutinize the processes of care so that risks may be minimized in the future. What is judged non-preventable now may eventually become preventable with new approaches.

Harmful mistakes

A large percentage of comiogenic harms occur as a result of mistakes. The Harvard Medical Practice Study[40] found that 69% of iatrogenic adverse effects were due to potentially preventable errors. In a study of cardiac arrests at a teaching hospital, Bedell et al.[41] found that medication errors were responsible for almost 64% of preventable arrests. Of major adverse events associated with anesthesia, 70 out of 1089 were due to preventable errors involving breathing circuit disconnections, gas flow errors, and loss of gas supply.[42] Given the significance of error in the etiology of comiogenic harm, it is important to understand how mistakes might be evaluated and how they might influence our understanding of provider accountability.

A mistake is standardly defined as 'an error in action, opinion, or judgment caused by poor reasoning, carelessness [or] insufficient knowledge.'[43] Reflecting on the meanings of 'do no harm' enumerated earlier, we see that the blameworthiness or excusability of a harmful mistake depends on how it squares with the obligation of due care. Harms associated with recklessness, incompetence, or negligent incapacitation (e.g. the practitioner is inebriated) clearly violate due care and, as such, are inexcusable. Indeed, they are not genuine 'mistakes' since they do not result from error *per se* but from a disregard for standards themselves. When mistakes in reasoning, judgment, or action do involve erring from due care, however, they are genuine errors and, as such, are presumed to have occurred within a context of good faith.

Traditionally, the evaluation of medical error, both from a moral point of view and from the point of view of quality assurance, has emphasized individual agency. As Leape[44] has pointed out, this view of error is deeply embedded in the culture of medicine. Under a socialization process that emphasizes perfectibility and infallibility, mistakes are viewed as unusual, unacceptable, and indicative of flawed character. Implicit in this view of error is the belief that medical quality itself is essentially a function of the competence and integrity of individuals. This belief has often been explicitly articulated in the medical literature. In 1947, G. G. Ward asserted that 'the product of the hospital is health, and . . . we know that it is the character of the medical staff that determines the product of the hospital.'[45] In 1993, a physician-ethicist averred that 'in the end, the patient's greatest guarantee of quality of care is the physician's character.'[46] The same conviction was displayed in a recent Georgetown University hospital publication: 'The quality of your medical care depends on the quality of your doctor.'

Although few would deny that physician integrity and competence are important ingredients in the overall quality of care, the assumption that these characteristics are sufficient to guarantee quality belies the empirical evidence regarding quality failures. Physicians may strive for faultless performance, but the fact is that many of the immediate aspects of patient care are simply beyond their power to control. Recent research reveals that system failure and poor system or job design contribute significantly to harmful error by providing the conditions under which error will thrive. Although a physician may be the proximal cause of a deadly prescribing error, the underlying cause may be a dangerously heavy work-load or a poor system of drug information dissemination. A harmful error in drug dispensing may have been facilitated by a system that does not adequately control for look-alike drug packaging or sound-alike drug names.

In a recent study of in-hospital adverse drug events, Leape et al.,[47] found that system failures accounted for 78% of harmful errors. These findings strongly suggest that, from the point of view of actual practice, the principal locus of quality failure is not the individual but, rather, the design of systems, processes, and policies. These findings have been substantiated elsewhere. In a study by Dearden and Rutherford,[48] institutional staffing policies played a key role in critical care management errors. In particular, harmful errors were associated with staffing arrangements in which only inexperienced, junior doctors were on duty outside of regular office hours. Similarly, policies that require long working hours for residents or discourage or prevent adequate resident supervision may be significant catalysts of patient harm. In a study by Wu et al., house officers (interns and residents) reported that job overload played a part in 65% of their mistakes.[49] Such system failures were also implicated in the 1984 death of Libby Zion. Zion was a college freshman who died nine hours after being admitted to New York Hospital with fever and agitation. Review of her case identified both the policy of 36-hour resident shifts and the 'closed book order' – a common practice that allows only interns (in the United States those in their first year of residency training after receiving the MD degree) to write orders for patients – as factors contributing to her death.[50] Whereas a plea of debilitating fatigue may thus partially excuse a resident's mistake, in a case like Zion's, it simultaneously implicates the policymakers and, indeed, the professional culture that sustains the tradition of long working hours. From a moral point of view, the occurrence of such a harm compels a number of responses, among them that those who establish policy for medical training must determine whether or not the tradition of long working hours and specific supervision policies are consistent with the requirement of due care.[51] It may, of course, be that the upshot of policy deliberation, will ultimately conclude that the risks associated with education and training policies are justified on the basis of the principle of utility. From the point of view of individual interests, such a justification will remain problematic. As members of a society that endorses such policies and as potential patients, we must be prepared to accept the fact that these trade-offs may expose us to grave risk.

The process of patient care, especially in an institutional setting, involves coordination among an array of providers. At each junction of responsibility there is a possibility for miscommunication that may result in patient harm. Examples of communication failure include misinterpretation of handwriting on a prescription or in the patient's chart, misidentification of a patient or a patient's treatment plan, mislabeling or misfiling of patient records or lab results, communication delays and communication failures *per se* where one provider fails to give another information pertinent to the patient's history, diagnosis, or plan of care. Although miscommunications may originate as errors in individual judgment, action (or inaction), they are abetted by poor systems for follow-up and review. In a recent Florida case, errors and miscommunications combined to result in the amputation of a patient's wrong leg.[52] The misidentification of the patient's leg began with an entry error in the hospital's computer system. Because there was no system of checks against the original entry, the error was undetected and repeated on the operating room schedule and blackboard. When the surgeon entered the operating suite, the incorrect leg was already draped and sterilized. A surgical nurse realized the error only when the amputation was well underway. From the moral point of view, this diffusion of responsibility among members of a health care team means not that *no one* is responsible for harms associated with these failures, but that *everyone* – that is, everyone who had an opportunity to prevent the error – is responsible. This is the moral imperative behind quality improvement in the delivery of health care. On the assumption that errors and communication failures (and the harms associated with them) are largely preventable, quality improvement requires a concerted and systematic effort on the part of administrators and practitioners to identify and anticipate such failures, and to implement processes that make them less likely. It is this broader notion of causal agency and moral accountability that is captured in the shift from the term 'iatrogenic' – which implicates physicians alone – to the term 'comiogenic' – which implicates all health care providers who are directly or indirectly responsible for the care of the patient.

Communication failures can also occur between providers and patients. Beyond the technical requirements of disclosure in the informed consent process, patients need to understand how and when to take medications, what activities to avoid, what to expect after treatment, and, with decreasing lengths of hospital stay, what to expect after discharge from the hospital. For example, had the patient in the *Wickline* case[53] been alerted to possible complications following her discharge after surgery for an aortic obstruction, she might have been spared the loss of her leg to gangrene. As we argued in Chapter 4, adequate communication and coordination of care from original contact to follow-up is one of the demands of due care. Due care is not only an individual responsibility. It is a collective responsibility and extends to all levels of the delivery process.

In the foregoing discussion we have highlighted findings regarding the complex causal etiology of comiogenic complications. These findings have important implications for both the evaluation and prevention of comiogenic harm. In what follows we discuss these implications by distinguishing between two models of agency and accountability.

Agency, quality, and accountability

As we said above, the culture of medicine has historically championed the model of individual agency. This model manifests itself in a strongly internalized sense of duty to perform faultlessly and in very high standards of individual accountability. It also finds expression in the traditional scheme of quality management – known as quality assurance (QA) and in the fault-based compensation scheme of medical malpractice.

On the theory of QA, poor quality of care is understood to be the result of incompetent or careless individuals, or, as Berwick has described it, of 'bad apples'.[54] Quality is accordingly 'assured' by a system of standards, inspections, and penalties that mark the boundaries of acceptable conduct. 'Outliers,' those whose work fails to meet established standards, are identified by sophisticated inspection and measurement techniques, and brought into line by penalty and probation. The individual is regarded as the 'lone agent of success or failure.' Although physicians, in particular, are traditionally regarded as the primary agents of quality in medical care, the theory of 'bad apples' is deeply embedded and spares no one. Administrators look suspiciously on individual physicians, individual physicians look suspiciously on nurses, nurses look suspiciously on physicians and other nurses. The 'bad apple' is to blame and dismissal or discipline is regarded as the solution to the immediate problem and the deterrent for future lapses. The assumption that errors and poor quality are largely if not wholly the product of individual deficiencies naturally engenders an atmosphere of defensiveness and evasiveness that may even at times result in providers blaming the patient for bad outcomes.[55] Under the QA model, there is very little incentive to admit possible error because the mechanisms for addressing it are largely punitive. Because it discourages openness about error, this model may, in fact, be counterproductive in error prevention.

The model of individual agency is also at the heart of medical malpractice law. As a species of tort law, the primary function of medical malpractice is 'to determine when loss shall be shifted from one to another, and when it shall be allowed to remain where it has fallen.'[56] In medical matters, the most prominent theory of tort law is that of negligence. Under the law of negligence, liability for a harm depends on the following conditions: (1) the professional must have a duty to the harmed party; (2) the professional must breach that duty; (3) the affected party must suffer a harm; and (4) the harm must be caused by the breach. Compensation (or 'burden-shifting') depends upon the identification of an individual agent who, in failing to abide by established standards, caused patient harm.

In recent years, the call for tort reform in medicine has emphasized the promise of a no fault compensation scheme for medical injuries. One rationale for such a scheme is that by deemphasizing individual agency, it may encourage quality improvement programs that focus on the complex, system-related causes of patient harm.

As a quality management scheme, 'quality improvement' – also known as continuous quality improvement (CQI) and total quality management – is based on the premise of collective agency or a 'systems theory of causation.' A 'system' is 'an interdependent group of items, people or processes with a common purpose.'[57] The common purpose in health care is patient benefit and the avoidance of harm. Empirical data from both industry and health care, suggest that as many as 75% of errors can be traced to system deficiencies.[58] In light of this, the object of CQI is to 'determine what went wrong, rather than [to] identify who is to blame.'[59] Those working in the field of medical quality improvement identify their work as the fulfillment of Ernest Codman's plan for quality reform almost a century ago. Recall from Chapter 1 that the aim of Codman's plan for hospital standardization was to advance the ultimate 'product' of the hospital, namely, patient benefit. This was to be done through the 'end-result system,' which was based, he said, 'on the common-sense notion that every hospital should follow *every* patient it treats, long enough to determine whether or not the treatment has been successful, and then to inquire "if not, why not?" with a view to preventing similar failures in the future.'[60] Just as CQI operates on the assumption that 'every defect is a treasure,'[61] so Codman recognized that to effect improvement,

the first step is to admit and record the lack of perfection. The next step is to analyze the causes of failure and to determine whether these causes are controllable. We can then rationally set about effecting improvement by enforcing the control of those cases which we admit are controllable, and by directing study to methods of controlling those causes over which we now admit we have but little power.[62]

As of 1992, CQI was adopted in the United States as the model for quality assessment by the Joint Commission for the Accreditation of Healthcare Organizations (JCAHO) in their standards manual,[63] and for the first time in the history of the organization begun by him in 1914, Codman's portrait was hung on the walls of the JCAHO's Chicago offices.[64] In 1996, the JCAHO further acknowledged its debt to Codman by reprinting his pioneering and controversial *A Study in Hospital Efficiency*.[65] In 1916, the Joint Commissions' progenitor organization, the American College of Surgeons' Committee on Hospital Standardization had specifically omitted from its 'Minimum Standard for Hospitals' the analysis of patient outcomes and the reporting of preventable error. Eighty years later, these have become central elements in the organization's vision of quality.

Because one of the central conditions for quality improvement is the identification of errors and quality failures, it has been argued that the success of quality management programs (whether QA or CQI) depends upon the guarantee of confidentiality and immunity from punitive action.[66] Under the existing fault-based compensation system, however, confidentiality and immunity are achieved largely at the expense of the injured patient. Through the doctrine of legal privilege, patients are prevented access to in-house information on harmful quality failures associated with their care.[67] Likewise, disclosure of error to patients is discouraged by in-house counsel. Many believe that the most comprehensive way to overcome such concerns about confidentiality and immunity – and to do so in a way that does *not* compromise the interests of the individual patient – is through a no-fault (or strict liability) compensation scheme for medical injuries. Although this idea has received considerable attention in the last ten years,[68] it dates back at least to the mid-1970s when the 'malpractice crisis' produced questions about the cost and effectiveness of the tort system.[69] It has been suggested that a no-fault scheme could be implemented through the mechanism of a patient compensation fund.[70] Such a fund could be financed by all members of society through some form of taxation or by a health insurance surcharge. A no-fault scheme would have a number of desirable benefits. Because it ignores fault, it provides the necessary background conditions for the reporting of quality failures. In addition, because it does not restrict compensation to injuries resulting from negligence, it can, in principle, compensate patients for a broader range of the harms they suffer as a result of their care. Moreover, in a no-fault system, individual patients would not have to pursue remedy through the costly, slow, and overburdened tort litigation system. The fact that the adjudication of medical liability claims can now take up to seven years may help to explain the Harvard Medical Practice study findings that only one in fifty patients with an identifiable negligent injury filed a claim for that injury.[71] Finally, in a no-fault system, neither individual patients nor individual providers would be burdened with the full impact of medicine's inevitable downsides. As we saw in Chapter 3, the justification for iatrogenic illness during the post World War II period relied on the utilitarian argument that these complications were 'the price of medical progress.' It is one of the moral advantages of a collectively funded, no-fault compensation scheme that it allows that if there *is* a price to be paid, it will be paid collectively, not selectively. If it is true that most harmful errors result from system failures, a no-fault scheme provides that neither individual patients (because of the onerous litigation process, lack of remedy for non-negligent harms, or lack of access to confidential information about their care) nor individual providers (through targeted fault-based negligence actions) will bear the full burden for harmful errors.

Although a no-fault scheme has these potential advantages, it also raises important questions regarding accountability and deterrence. How in a no-fault scheme for medical injury compensation would it be possible to sustain an ethos of individual accountability? And what, in such a system, would be the motivation for individuals to avoid poor performance? To respond to these questions, we need to examine the notion of collective accountability in the theory of CQI.

As we have said, CQI is premised on a model of collective agency – quality failures result from the inevitable complexity of overlapping domains and processes involving multiple individuals. The hospitalized patient's receipt of the correct drug at the correct time and in the correct dose depends upon reliable systems of drug information dissemination, ordering and transcribing, and drug delivery. Similarly, the prevention of nosocomial infection involves reliable systems for sterilization and hand-washing, wound dressing, catheter replacement, prevention of antibiotic resistance, and reduction of the susceptibility to infection through, for example, the maintenance of a patient's body temperature during surgery.[72]

The premise of collective agency in CQI is accompanied by an ethos of collective accountability. Attributions of moral responsibility are not

abandoned in the theory of CQI, they simply bear the stigma of accountability rather than blame. In essence, quality improvement is seen to depend
on cooperation and collaboration both in the achievement of primary
outcomes and in the ongoing improvement of outcomes and processes.
This is accomplished through supportive team work, competition for
quality, and statistical feedback on such complications as surgical wound
infection and nosocomial pneumonias.[73] Individuals (and organizations)
are expected to improve performance constantly, not simply in response to
complaints or crises.[74] In a system where everyone involved in the processes of care is accountable to everyone else in the services of the ultimate
end of patient well-being, the potential for 'free riding' – that is, the
potential for institutions or individuals to perform poorly without consequence – is limited. Collective accountability does not entail a dissipation
or diminution of individual responsibility, rather, every participant in a
process is fully morally responsible.[75] In CQI, 'free-riding' is inconsistent
with the moral demands of collective effort.[76] As those working in the field
of medical quality improvement have noted, the success and staying-power
of an ethos of CQI depends in large part on the willingness of leadership in
health care institutions and organizations to abandon the practice of
finger-pointing in favor of supportive and cooperative goal-setting. In such
a context, the incentive system will be oriented to rewards for cooperation
rather than penalties for non-compliance.

As far as institutional accountability is concerned, the incentive to
reduce compensable events might come from institutional benchmarking.
For example, if a particular hospital is found to be disproportionately
drawing down the compensation fund, its quality profile will make it less
appealing in a competitive market. One health services researcher has
suggested that an institution's demonstrated adherence to the principles of
continuous improvement – public reporting of error, patient follow-up
after discharge, and active mechanisms for improvement – should all be
conditions for participation in a no-fault system.[77]

As we saw in Chapter 1, the tradition of personal accountability in the
eighteenth and nineteenth centuries held that for the physician confronting
harmful error, there was 'no tribunal, other than his own conscience.'[78] In
medicine today, the potential for error extends far beyond individual
conduct to the design of systems and standards of practice. In the face of
the complex processes and collective efforts that comprise health care
today, individual practitioners can no longer plausibly argue that they are
accountable only to themselves. Likewise, it is no longer plausible to argue
that quality failures result from individuals alone. The theory of CQI is

promising because it emphasizes the broader system-related causes of patient harm and addresses them through an ethos of collective accountability. The success of CQI depends upon the creation of a non-threatening atmosphere in which practitioners can feel free to dissect and discuss the sources of harmful error. A no-fault compensation scheme for medical injuries, would foster such an atmosphere and would protect the interests of the injured patient by removing the incentive to conceal the circumstances surrounding his or her care.

Conclusion

In Part II we have emphasized ethical norms as fundamental mechanisms of accountability in health care. We have described a patient-centered ethos in which the norms of beneficence and nonmaleficence – themselves grounded in the nature of the healing relationship – are enriched by the democratic principle of respect for patient autonomy. The immediate implications of such an ethos for our understanding of medical harm is that the concept itself is informed not only by the values of the clinician as clinician but also by those of the patient. This observation supports efforts to make outcomes research more inclusive of patient-centered health-related quality of life measures, as well as efforts to understand and appreciate the effects of treatment from the point of view of the individual patient. We have also suggested that considerations of justice in the distribution of health care resources are inevitable in contemporary society and should be addressed through fair institutional procedures.

We have also discussed how the norms of beneficence, nonmaleficence, respect for patient autonomy, and justice are specified in the notion of due care, how they may be balanced to justify patient risk and harm and how they provide the necessary normative background conditions for the various circumstances that excuse patient harm. We have argued that in the face of new and specifically financial forms of accountability, appeal to these ethical norms should be decisive. Finally, as an alternative to the term 'iatrogenic,' we have introduced the term 'comiogenic' to capture the range of agents accountable for patient harm.

In Part III we look at three types of comiogenic harm: nosocomial infection, adverse drug reactions, and unnecessary surgery. In addition to presenting data on the incidence of these problems, we explore how formal mechanisms of accountability imposed by private and public regulatory bodies have influenced and shaped the practices of individual and institutional providers in these areas. We discuss how these formal mechanisms of accountability – including those that encourage more economically efficient and evidence-based practices – may effect the quality of patient care. We argue that those forms of accountability that coincide with ethical norms are the most promising and defensible guides to institutional and individual practice.

Endnotes

1 For example: Smith CR, Petty BG. Specific complications of medical management. In Harvey A, Johns RJ, eds. *The Principles and Practices of Medicine*, 21st edn. Norwalk, CT: Appleton-Century-Crofts, 1984.
   Preger L. *Iatrogenic Diseases*. Boca Raton: CRC Press, 1986.
   Horwitz NH, Rizzoli HV. *Postoperative Complications of Extracranial Surgery*. Baltimore: Williams and Wilkins, 1987.
2 Cluff LE, Thornton G, Seidl L, et al. Epidemiological study of adverse drug reactions. *Trans Assoc Am Physicians* 1965; 78:255–68.
3 Special thanks to Victoria Pedrick who provided the essential philological guidance needed to coin the term 'comiogenic.'
4 Levin LS. *Iatrogenics* 1991; 1(1):i.
5 In the case of the transplacental agents, thalidomide and diethylstilbestrol, harms accrued not to the patient herself but to her offspring, who were not technically speaking 'patients' in the context of these treatments. We do include the gestating fetusus/future offspring of patients as objects of iatrogenic harm because, like the patient, the fetus/future offspring is directly, rather than incidentally affected by the acts or omissions of providers. The balancing of medical risks and benefits to fetus and pregnant woman is a question that has generated considerable discussion.
   See for example McCullough LB, Chervenak FA. *Ethics in Obstetrics and Gynecology*. New York: Oxford University Press, 1994, ch. 6 (pp. 196–237).
6 For a discussion of the moral demands upon the clinician-researcher see Pellegrino ED. Beneficence, scientific autonomy and self-interest: Ethical dilemmas in clinical research. *Cambridge Quarterly Health Care Eth* 1992; 1:361–9.
7 Feinstein A. *Clinimetrics*. New Haven: Yale University Press, 1987.
8 For an appraisal of quality-of-life measures, see Gill TM, Feinstein AR. A critical appraisal of the quality of quality-of-life measurements. *JAMA* 1994; 272:619–26.
9 Wilson IB, Cleary PD. Linking clinical variables with health-related quality of life. *JAMA* 1995; 273:59–65.
   Guyatt GH, Cook DJ. Health status, quality of life, and the individual. *JAMA* 1994; 272:630–1.
10 Greenfield S, Nelson EC. Recent developments and future issues in the use of health status assessment measures in clinical settings. *Med Care* 1992; 30:MS23–MS41.
11 MacKeigan LD, Pathak DS. Overview of health-related quality-of-life measures. *Am J Hosp Pharm* 1992; 49:2236–45.
12 Reiser SJ. The era of the patient: using the experience of illness in shaping the missions of health care. *JAMA* 1993; 269:1012–17.

13 Caplan A, Engelhardt HT, McCartney J. *The Concepts of Health and Disease.* Reading, MA: Addison-Wesley, 1981.

14 Kleinman A. *The Illness Narratives: Suffering, Healing and the Human Condition.* New York: Basic Books, 1988, p. 5.

15 Faden RR, Beauchamp TL. *A History and Theory of Informed Consent.* New York: Oxford University Press, 1986, p. 31.

16 Gerteis M, Edgman-Levitan S, Daley J, Delbanco T (eds.). *Through the Patient's Eyes: Understanding and Promoting Patient-Centered Care.* San Fransisco: Jossey-Bass, 1993.

17 Feinberg J. *The Moral Limits of the Criminal Law.* vol 1. *Harm to Others.* New York: Oxford, 1984.

18 Feinberg J, p. 108 (see No. 17).

19 Many of the classic cases in medical ethics demonstrate that there is often conflict between respect for patient autonomy and a paternalistic interpretation of beneficence. It is not our purpose to discuss the resolution of such conflicts for this has been done with insight elsewhere. The history of medical harm does, however, offer a strong argument against physician paternalism. Even if we leave aside the fact that the physician's recommendation might not represent the patient's values or that the physician may be less risk-averse than the patient, there remains the equally compelling fact that the physician's judgments are subject to variability, uncertainty and error. Thus, medical fallibility and uncertainty mitigate against the justifiability of any unilateral decision on the physician's part to override the patient's autonomy for the patient's good.
See, for example: Beauchamp TL, Childress JF. *The Principles of Biomedical Ethics*, 4th edn. New York: Oxford, 1994.
McCullough LB, Chervenak FA. *Ethics in Obstetrics and Gynecology.* New York: Oxford University Press, 1994, pp. 42–8.

20 Morreim EH. *Balancing Act: The New Medical Ethics of Medicine's New Economics.* Washington, DC: Georgetown University Press, 1995, p. 2.

21 Beauchamp TL, Childress JF, p. 336 (see No. 19).

22 These conditions represent a modified version of those presented in: American College of Obstetricians and Gynecologists. Human immunodeficiency virus infection: Physician's responsibilities. ACOG Committee Opinion 85 (Washington, DC: ACOG, 1990).
Mathieu D. *Preventing Prenatal Harm: Should the State Intervene?* Dordrecht: Kluwer, 1991.
Beauchamp TL, Childress JF, pp. 337–41 (see No. 19).

23 American Medical Association. Principles of medical ethics. 1957. Reprinted in Reich WT, ed., *The Encyclopedia of Bioethics*, vol V. New York: Simon and Schuster/Macmillan, 1995, pp. 2648–9.

24 Wu AW, Folkman S, McPhee SJ, Lo B. Do house officers learn from their mistakes? *JAMA* 1991; 265(16): 2089–94.
Robins N. *The Girl Who Died Twice: Every Patient's Nightmare: The Libby Zion Case and the Hidden Hazards of Hospitals.* New York: Delacorte Press, 1995.

25 Beauchamp TL, McCullough LB. *Medical Ethics: The Moral Responsibilities of Physicians.* Englewood Cliffs, NJ: Prentice-Hall, 1984, p. 152.

26 Blumberg M. Provider price changes for improved health care use. In G Chacko, ed., *Health Handbook: An International Reference on Care and Cure.* Amsterdam: North Holland, 1979, p. 160.

27 Pellegrino ED. Words can hurt you: Some reflections on the metaphors of managed care. *J Am Bd Fam Prac* 1994; 7:508.

28 Gray BH. *The Profit Motive and Patient Care: The Changing Accountability of Doctors and Hospitals.* Cambridge, MA: Harvard University Press, 1991, p. 309.
    Wolf SM. Health care reform and the future of physician ethics, *Hastings Ctr Rep* 1994; 24:36.

29 Wolf SM, p. 36 (see No. 28).

30 Morreim EH (see No. 20).

31 Feinberg J, p. 108 (see No. 17).

32 Classen DC, Pestotnik SL, Evans RS, Burke JP. Computerized surveillance of adverse drug events in hospital patients. *JAMA* 1991; 266(20):2847–51.

33 Gorovitz S, MacIntyre A. Toward a theory of medical fallibility. *J Med Philos* 1976; 1:51–71.

34 Silverman WA. The lesson of retrolental fibroplasia. *Sci Am* 1977; 236(6):100–7.

35 Quoted in Smith R. The ethics of ignorance. *J Med Ethics* 1992; 18:117–8,134 (p. 117).

36 Kessler DA (for the Working Group). Introducing MEDWatch: A new approach to reporting medication and device adverse effects and product problems. *JAMA* 1993; 269:2765–68.

37 More often, however, they do so by claiming that cost-containment policies do not increase patient risk but may, in fact, reduce risk by reigning in unnecessary or inappropriate utilization. As we will see in Chapter 10, how one defines 'appropriateness' is pivitol in debates about utilization.

38 *Wickline* v. *State of California* 228 Cal. Reptr.661 (Cal. App.2Dist.1986).

39 Morreim EH, p. 117 (see No. 20).
    Despite absolving the state of liability in this case, the court did make it clear that the law would hold utilization review operators responsible: 'Third-party payers of health care can be held legally accountable when medically inappropriate decisions result from defects in the design or implementation of cost-containment mechanisms.' *Wickline* v. *State of California* 228 Cal. Reptr.661 (Cal. App.2Dist.1986), 670–1.
    See Hamborg CJ. Medical utilization review: The new frontier for medical malpractice claims? *Drake Law Rev.* 1992; 41:113–38.

40 Leape LL, Lawthers AG, Brennan TA, Johnson WG. Preventing medical injury. *Qual Review Bull* 1993; 19(5):144–9.

41 Bedell SE, Deitz DC, Leeman D, et al. Incidence and characteristics of preventable iatrogenic cardiac arrests. *JAMA* 1991; 265:2815–20.

42 Cooper JB, Newbower RS, Kitz RJ. An analysis of major errors and equipment failures in anesthesia management. Considerations for prevention and detection. *Anesthesiology* 1984; 60:34–42.

43 Websters College Dictionary. New York: Random House, 1991, pp. 867–8.

44 Leape LL. Error in medicine. *JAMA* 1994; 272:1851–7.

45 Ward GG. Audits measure our results. *Mod Hosp* 1947; 69:86–8.

46 Dans PE. Clinical peer review: Burnishing a tarnished icon. *Ann Intern Med* 1993; 118(7):566–8.

47 Leape LL, Bates DW, Cullen DJ, et al. for the ADE Prevention Study Group. Systems analysis of adverse drug events. *JAMA* 1995; 274:35–43.

48 Dearden CH, Rutherford WH. The resuscitation of the severely injured in the accident and emergency department – a medical audit. *Injury* 1985; 16:249–52.

49 Wu AW, Folkman S, McPhee SJ, Lo B (see No. 24).
50 Robins N, p. 101–3 (see No. 24).
51 Asken MJ, Raham DC. Resident performance and sleep deprivation: a review. *J Med Ed* 1983; 58:382–8.
Orton DI, Gruzelier JH. Adverse changes in mood and cognitive performance of house officers after night duty. *Br Med J* 1989; 298:21–3.
Asch DA, Parker RM. The Libby Zion case: One step forward or two steps backward? *N Engl J Med* 1988; 318:771–5.
52 Doctor who cut off wrong leg is defended by colleagues. *New York Times*, September 17, 1995, p. A28.
53 *Wickline* v. *State of California* 228 Cal. Reptr.661 (Cal. App.2Dist.1986).
54 Berwick DM. Continuous improvement as an ideal in health care. *N Engl J Med* 1989; 320(1):53–6.
55 Mizrahi T. Managing medical mistakes: ideology, insularity and accountability among internists in-training. *Soc Sci Med* 1984; 19:135–46.
56 Keeton P, Keeton R, Sargentich L, Steiner H. *Tort and Accident Law*. St. Paul:West Publishing Co., 1983, p. 1.
57 Leape LL, Bates DW, Cullen DJ, et al. for the ADE Prevention Study Group. Systems analysis of adverse drug events. *JAMA* 1995; 274:36.
58 Deming WF. *Out of the Crisis*. Cambridge, MA: MIT Center for Applied Engineering Studies, 1986.
59 Leape LL, Bates DW, Cullen DJ, et al. (see No. 57).
60 Codman EA. *The Shoulder*. Malabar, FL: RE Kreiger, 1984, p. xii. (first published 1934.)
61 Berwick DM. Continuous improvement as an ideal in health care. *N Engl J Med* 1989; 320(1):53–6.
62 Codman EA. A study in hospital efficiency as represented by product. *Trans Am Gynecol Soc* 1914; 39:60–100 (p. 62).
63 Joint Commission on Accreditation of Healthcare Organizations. The agenda for change. *Agenda Change Update* 1987; 1:1–3
64 Neuhauser D. Ernest Amory Codman, MD, and end results of medical care. *Int J Technol Assess Health Care* 1990; 6:307–25.
65 Codman EA. *A Study in Hospital Efficiency As Demonstrated by the Case Report of the First Five Years of a Private Hospital*. Oakbrook Terrace, IL: Joint Commission on Accreditation of Healthcare Organizations, 1996.
66 Leape LL, Bates DW, Cullen DJ, et al. (see No. 57).
67 Brennan T. Ethics of confidentiality: The special case of quality assurance research. *Clin Res* 1990; 35:551–7.
68 See, for example: Weiler PC, *Medical Malpractice on Trial*. Cambridge MA: Harvard University Press, 1991.
Weiler PC, Hiatt HH, Newhouse JP, et al. *A Measure of Malpractice: Medical Injury, Malpractice Litigation and Patient Compensation*. Cambridge, MA: Harvard University Press, 1993.
Abraham KS. Medical liability reform: a conceptual framework. *N Engl J Med* 1988; 260:68–72.
69 See, for example: Mills DH, Boyden JS, Rubsamen DS. *Medical Insurance Feasibility Study*. San Francisco, California Medical Association, 1977.
Keeton P. Compensation for medical accidents. 121 U. PA. Law Rev. 590 (1973).
Carlson R. A conceptualization of a no-fault compensation system for medical malpractice injuries. *Law and Society Review* 1973; 7:329–69.

70 Manuel BM. Professional liability: A no-fault solution. *N Engl J Med* 1990;
    322(9):627–31.
71 Weiler PC, Hiatt HH, Newhouse JP, et al. *A Measure of Malpractice: Medical
    Injury, Malpractice Litigation and Patient Compensation.* Cambridge, MA:
    Harvard University Press, 1993, p. 73.
72 Kurz A, Sessler DI, Lenhardt R et al. Perioperative normothermia to reduce
    the incidence of surgical-wound infection and shorten hospitalization. *N Engl
    J Med* 1996; 334:1209–15.
73 Haley RW, Gaynes RP, Aber RC, Bennett JV. Surveillance of nosocomial
    infections. In Bennett JV, Brachman PS. *Hospital Infections*, 3rd edn.
    Boston:Little, Brown, 1992, pp. 79–108.
74 McLaughlin CP, Kaluzny AD. Total quality management in health: Making
    it work. *Health Care Mgmt Rev* 1990; 15:7–14.
75 Zimmerman M. Sharing responsibility. In PA French, ed., *The Spectrum of
    Responsibility*. New York: St. Martin's Press, 1991, pp. 275–86.
76 See, Laffel G, Blumenthal D. The case for using industrial quality
    management science in health care organizations. *JAMA* 1989; 83:1031–7.
77 Neuhauser D (see No. 64).
78 AMA, Code of medical ethics, 1847, p. 3.

PART III

7

From hospitalism to nosocomial infection control

Historic debates: puerperal fever, antisepsis, and the germ theory of disease

What is now known as nosocomial[1] or hospital-based infection made its indelible mark on history during the childbed fever epidemics of the eighteenth and nineteenth centuries. During this period, puerperal deaths in hospitals and lying-in institutions were estimated to be as high as 150 per 1000 deliveries, whereas the same disease afflicted less than 20 in 1000 women delivering at home.[2] One of the first indications of the physician's role in the etiology of childbed fever was given by Alexander Gordon in 1795 in his account of 28 cases of the disease at the Aberdeen dispensary, Scotland. In this account, he expressed his conviction, based on empirical evidence from his own practice, that he and certain midwives had been the source of transmission.

The most significant epidemiological work on the physician's role in the transmission of puerperal fever was done in the mid-nineteenth century by Ignaz Semmelweis at the Allgemeines Krankenhaus in Vienna.[3] During this period, pathological anatomy was becoming an integral part of the medical curriculum, and medical students and physicians moved freely between the autopsy and delivery rooms. Based on astute clinical observation of the two obstetric wards at the hospital, Semmelweis identified physicians going from cadavers to parturient women as the main vector of the disease. In Ward 1, where deliveries were performed by physicians and students, 600 to 800 women or 20% died each year from childbed fever. In Ward 2, where deliveries were performed by midwives who did not participate in autopsies, the death rate was only 60 per year. After Semmelweis instituted a policy of hand disinfection with chlorinated lime, the death rate in Ward 1 dropped from 20% to 1.2%.[4] Despite the documented success of this antiseptic measure, Semmelweis's successor allowed hand

washing measures to decline. In the absence of continued surveillance and
control, the epidemic promptly resumed. With Pasteur's discovery in the
late 1850s of bacterial putrefaction, Semmelweis's theory that puerperal
fever deaths were the result of purulent, infectious matter carried on the
hands of medical practitioners received important substantiation. In the
face of this evidence, many conscientious obstetricians ceased their pathological experiments and began hand washing regimens.

Hand washing continues to be one of the cornerstones of nosocomial
infection control and prevention.[5] Ironically, though, in light of the dramatic history that led to hospital antiseptic and aseptic measures, recent
studies of hand washing precautions have found that on average, health
care professionals observe hand hygiene practices in less than half of
patient contacts.[6]

In the United States, the most famous debate on the physician's role in
the transmission of puerperal fever was between Oliver Wendell Holmes
and Charles Meigs. As we saw in Chapter 1, during the eighteenth and
nineteenth centuries, a gentleman effected moral improvement by bringing
his conduct 'to mental view' and privately committing himself to the
rectification of perceived failings. Meigs' response to the charge that he
might be the medium of transmission for puerperal fever reflected this ideal
of self-scrutiny:

I have practiced midwifery for many long years; I have attended some thousands of
women in labor, and passed through repeated epidemics of childbed fever, both in
town and in hospital. After all this experience, however, I do not, upon careful
reflection and self-examination, find the least reason to suppose I have ever
conveyed the disease from place to place in any single instance . . . In the course of
my professional life I have made many necroscopic researches of childbed fever,
but did never suspend my ministry as accoucheur on that account. Still, I certainly
was never the medium of its transmission.[7]

Underscoring the traditional view that the gentleman physician could not
be guilty of patient harms, Meigs offered an argument that he found to be
unassailably true, namely, that 'a gentleman's hands are clean.'[8] By contrast, Holmes advocated a more public form of accountability that challenged both the gentlemanly ideal of self-scrutiny and the growing call for
professional solidarity. In his 1843 essay on 'The Contagiousness of Puerperal Fever,' Holmes urged fellow physicians to accept that,

The time has come when the existence of a *private pestilence* in the sphere of a single
physician should be looked upon not as a misfortune but a crime; and in the
knowledge of such occurrences, the duties of the practitioner to his profession,
should give way to his paramount obligations to society.[9]

Resistance to the idea of contagion was also manifest in the response in the United States to antisepsis. The use of antiseptic techniques to prevent infection was pioneered by British surgeon Joseph Lister. Although the reigning explanation for putrefaction identified the presence of oxygen as the principle causal factor, Lister found this hypothesis unsatisfactory.[10] Based on his studies of coagulation and inflammation, he postulated that the cause must be some as yet unidentified foreign substance transmitted to a wound site. In 1865, Lister read Pasteur's papers on fermentation and immediately recognized Pasteur's microscopic organisms as this substance. 'When I read Pasteur's original paper, I said to myself, "Just as we may destroy lice on the head of a child who has pediculi, by poisonous applications which will not injure the scalp, so I believe we can use poisons on wounds to destroy bacteria without injuring the soft tissues of the patient."[11] To destroy the omnipresent microbes, which he believed were borne by air, Lister developed an elaborate system of disinfection with carbolic acid. The patient's wound was dressed with bandages dipped in carbolic acid solution; the solution was used to clean the hands and instruments of the surgical team and eventually was sprayed into the air of the operating suite. In his 1870 report in the *Lancet*, Lister summarized his results as follows: In 1864 before the use of antisepsis, 16 of 35 patients (46%) undergoing amputation died. In 1867–9, after the introduction of antiseptic techniques, there were only six deaths in 40 cases (15%)[12] Shortly before Lister came to the United States to address the International Medical Congress in Philadelphia, Samuel Gross, the city's and, indeed, the nation's most influential surgeon, had this to say about Lister's methods: 'Little if any faith is placed by any enlightened or experienced surgeon on this side of the Atlantic in the so-called carbolic acid treatment of Prof. Lister apart from the care which is taken in applying the dressing.'[13]

Several factors undergirded the resistance of practitioners in the United States to Lister's techniques. One was the enduring influence both here and abroad of the ancient Hippocratic doctrine that infection, or more specifically the suppuration of a wound, was essential to the healing process.[14] It was this view that prompted the description of certain types of wound drainage as 'laudable pus.'[15] Other factors generating skepticism to Lister's methods were unique to the United States.

In the mid-nineteenth century, the death rate for surgery was high in all of the hospitals in Europe. In Paris, postoperative mortality was 60%, in Glasgow, 34%, and in Zurich, 46%. As a result of these data, Sir James Simpson, the Scottish surgeon and inventor of chloroform anesthesia, coined the term 'hospitalism' to refer to the hygienic evils of institutional care.[16] Appalled by the mortality statistics associated with hospital surgery, Simpson declared that 'the man laid on the operating table in one of our surgical hospitals is exposed to more chances of death than the English soldier on the field of Waterloo.'[17] In the United States, by contrast, 'hospitalism' was not regarded as a serious problem.[18] A high percentage of surgeries was still performed in rural areas.[19] Hospitals in the United States were smaller and less crowded than the burgeoning charitable hospitals of Europe, and the largest hospitals had operative mortality rates around 25% – significantly lower than some of their European counterparts. After the Civil War, the former Virginia Army surgeon, Hunter McGuire, observed that although Lister's antiseptic techniques might be beneficially applied in the city hospitals, in rural Virginia, 'it is generally unnecessary, the pure country air . . . being in itself aseptic.'[20] For many in the United States, these conditions obviated any need for Lister's new and complicated antiseptic techniques.

Another reason in the United States for the resistance to surgical antisepsis was skepticism and even hostility to the germ theory – the 'animacular hypothesis'[21] – upon which antisepsis was based. In the mid- to late nineteenth century, the professional and moral identity of the American physician was linked essentially to practice and to an epistemology grounded in experience rather than theory. As one mid-nineteenth century doctor put it, 'in America, nothing theoretical is wanted, but only that which is practical.'[22] Thus, without definitive proof of germs as the causative agents in infection, American physicians were loathe to suggest that clinical experience could be traded for some theory imported from abroad. Opponents of the germ theory repeatedly reminded their colleagues that the words of Lister are 'those of a theorist.'[23] George Shrady, editor of the *Medical Record*, warned his colleagues not to abandon therapeutics for etiologic speculation: 'Judging the future by the past,' he said,

we are likely to be as much ridiculed in the next century for our blind belief in the power of unseen germs, as our forefathers were for their faith in the influence of spirits, of certain planets and the like, in inducing certain diseases.[24]

Henry Bigelow, Harvard's leading hospital surgeon expressed a similar skepticism regarding Lister's elaborate methods with carbolic acid spray: 'It flatters neither the vanity nor the scientific sense to exorcise an invisible enemy with something very like a censer.'[25]

In Europe, Florence Nightingale opposed the germ theory on similar grounds. Like her counterparts in the United States, she regarded antisepsis and disinfection as 'mystic rites.'[26] In her case, however, the notion that germs were responsible for disease threatened the prevailing assumption that disease was the result of moral turpitude and could best be treated through a regimen focusing on the moral as well as the physical health of the patient. Likewise, Nightingale believed that hospital-induced disease, although linked to bad air and overcrowding, was the direct result of institutional 'carelessness [and] ignorance.'[27] In her view, disease associated with hospitals could be prevented only by responsible, broad-based efforts at sanitation and hygiene. On the strength of this belief, Nightingale undertook her now famous reforms in nursing care and hospital design and construction. Appealing to the principle of nonmaleficence as the basis for her reforms, Nightingale introduced her *Notes on Hospitals*, with the following observation:

It may seem a strange principle to enunciate as the very first requirement in a Hospital that it should do the sick no harm. It is quite necessary, nevertheless, to lay down such a principle, because the actual mortality *in* hospitals, especially in those of large crowded cities, is very much higher than any calculation founded on the mortality of the same class of diseases among patients treated *out of* hospital would lead us to expect.[28]

By the end of the nineteenth century, bacteriology had found legitimacy in the canons of medical science. Not only had Koch's experiments in bacteria culture and induced infection provided experimental verification for the germ theory, but bacteriology had also provided objective criteria by which the efficacy of infection control measures could be assessed. With the development of the autoclave, sterile surgical gowns, and rubber gloves in the 1890s, onerous and seemingly indiscriminate antiseptic techniques were made obsolete by surgical asepsis. Therapeutic disinfection of the patient's wound was replaced by preventive sterilization of everything that came in contact with the site of an operation. During this period, hand washing and sterilizing instruments became standard surgical practice.

Over the next few decades, the practice of surgery reshaped the American hospital. The promise of surgical cures brought greater numbers of paying patients into the hospital setting and greater power and prestige to the surgeons whose expertise they sought. By the 1920s surgical admissions outnumbered medical admissions to the hospital and concerns were already being expressed that procedures such as appendectomy were performed excessively and unnecessarily.[29]

The infection control movement and hospital epidemiology
It was during this period that the incidence of hospital induced infection became the focus of study in the United States. In the 1920s and 1930s,

studies of clean surgical wound infection revealed an incidence of roughly 12% in hospital populations.[30] In the 1940s, the development and widespread use of antimicrobial agents such as penicillin induced many to believe that the problem of hospital infection would soon be solved. By the late 1940s and early 1950s, however, when a pandemic of staphylococcal infection swept through the hospitals in the United States, it was clear that these expectations could not be sustained. Hospital personnel became carriers of the epidemic strains and transmitted them to patients who then became carriers to the community.[31]

This staphylococcal pandemic catalyzed the first systematic efforts to understand and control hospital infection in the United States. Voluntary hospital infection control programs represented the earliest of these efforts. To respond to the growing interest and activity in these programs, the Communicable Diseases Center (CDC) in Atlanta[32] opened a Hospital Infections Branch. In 1965, the Joint Commission on the Accreditation of Hospitals (JCAH) included a standard requiring the establishment of hospital infection surveillance programs and by 1969 had added standards for isolation facilities, microbiology services, restricted duties for obstetrical nurses, and the prevention of food contamination.[33] In the intervening years, the American Hospital Association (AHA) issued the first edition of its manual *Infection Control in Hospitals*.[34] The original definition of nosocomial infection was published in 1970 by the CDC. Under that definition, which remains the standard, a nosocomial infection is 'one that develops in a patient after admission to a hospital; an infection that was neither present nor in the incubating stage at the time of the patient's admission unless related to a previous hospitalization.'[35] In the 1960s and 1970s the reported incidence of nosocomial infections ranged from 3.5% to 6% in general hospital patients.[36] By 1980, the Hospital Infections Branch of the CDC was responding to more than 10,000 inquiries per year from hospitals seeking to reduce their numbers of infection. Based on extensive, multi-site investigation by the CDC and others, it is now estimated that nosocomial infections affect approximately three million patients a year in the United States, cause 60,000 fatalities,[37] and result in an excess of $4 billion in direct health care costs.[38] The most comprehensive study to date estimates that almost one-third of these infections are preventable by effective infection control programs.[39]

Since the pioneering and often solitary work by Semmelweis, Lister, and Nightingale more than a century ago, infection control has become an integral part of hospital quality management. At the heart of this enterprise is the application of epidemiologic methods to the hospital population. Epidemiology is the study of the incidence, prevalence, source, and causes of disease in populations and is the scientific basis of public health practice. The distinct field of *hospital* epidemiology originated with nosocomial infection surveillance in the 1970s and is a promising approach to identifying and controlling comiogenic harm in general. In order to understand how lessons from the epidemiology of nosocomial infection may be applied to comiogenic harm generally, we need to examine the use of these methods in the study of infection control itself.

Leaders in the field of infection control identify epidemiologic surveillance of disease as a continuous process consisting of the following elements:[40]

(1) defining as concisely and precisely as possible the events to be surveyed;
(2) collecting the relevant data in a systematic way;
(3) consolidating or tabulating the data into meaningful arrangements;
(4) analyzing and interpreting the data;
(5) using the information to bring about change.

Infection surveillance has a number of important uses. These include the establishment of baseline rates of endemic infection; the identification of epidemics, the creation of a statistical basis for arguments supporting and reinforcing the institution of new preventive practices and the abandonment of those that are ineffective; the satisfaction of accreditation standards; and the achievement of hospital cost savings. The ultimate aim of infection surveillance, however, is the reduction of infection risk.[41]

Although surveillance methods are, as risk reduction strategies, applied to all types of hospital infection, it is important to emphasize the distinction between infection to patients and infection to providers. As we said above, a nosocomial infection is standardly defined as 'one that develops *in a patient* after admission to a hospital . . .'[42] (our emphasis added). Thus, although patient to provider transmission of infections such as tuberculosis, hepatitis B (HBV) or HIV is one of the legitimate foci of infection control efforts, these infections are not, technically speaking, 'nosocomial.' Notwithstanding this official definition, the term 'nosocomial infection' has come to be used indiscriminately to refer to *any* infection that is hospital-acquired or -associated. The reasons for this are clear. Methodologically, hospital epidemiology focuses on the entire hospital population, including providers. Historically, the AIDS epidemic and the risk of HBV have together raised considerable concern about provider safety. Nevertheless, this broader use of the term 'nosocomial infection' obscures an important ethical reality. As we argued in Chapter 5, the health care professional's obligation to do no harm is grounded in the vulnerability of the patient and the healer's promise to help. As a fiduciary, the caregiver is required to place his or her own interests secondary to those of the patient. At times, fulfillment of this obligation may require the health professional to assume some personal risk.[43] When the term 'nosocomial infection' encompasses infection to both providers and patients, however, it may have the practical effect of increasing patient risk. As evidence of this, experts in the field of infection control point out that caregivers have been confused about the aim of precautionary measures and have gone from patient to patient wearing the same pair of gloves.[44] Even in this era of standard precautions,[45] a health care professional may decide to forgo isolation precautions based solely on an assessment of risk to him or herself, forgetting that the precautions are intended to protect both parties from infection. As a matter of both practical and ethical significance, therefore, we would recommend that the term 'nosocomial infection' be used to refer strictly to infectious complications in patients. Hospital-related infections contracted by health care professionals should be termed 'occupational infections'. Preserving the conceptual distinction between nosocomial infection and infection to caregivers reflects the unique demands of the fiduciary relationship.

Until the mid-1970s, it was common practice for hospital infection control committees to perform routine microbiological samplings of the environment as part of their infection control programs. Early work by the CDC, however, indicated that this practice was inefficient and ineffective in reducing infection. During this period, CDC training programs discouraged routine environmental culturing in favor of active and site-specific surveillance.[46] Since the mid-1970s, surveillance of nosocomial infection has provided valuable insight into the nature and scope of the problem.

A 1976 study by Wenzel et al.[47] was based on one of the first state-wide nosocomial infection programs using active surveillance techniques. Overall, the study found a crude infection rate of 3% in 24,757 patients. A breakdown of infections revealed that the greatest proportion occurred in patients in critical care units. Thirty-three to 45% of all nosocomial bloodstream infections occurred in patients occupying only 8% of hospital beds. Intensive care unit (ICU) patients had bloodstream infections up to 24 times more frequently than patients on wards. Findings also indicated that the use of intravascular devices (such as arterial and central venous pressure catheters) in surgical intensive care (SICU) patients substantially increased infection risk. A 1978 study by Stamm[48] supported the correlation between devices and increased risk of infection. In his study, Stamm analyzed CDC reports from 1956 to 1975 to determine how frequently medical devices were involved in hospital epidemics. He found that device-related epidemics, while rare before 1965, increased in frequency from 1965 to 1975 during which period they were responsible for 42% of all hospital epidemics.

On the basis of these and similar findings, the concept of preventable nosocomial infection was developed. Preventable infections were defined as those related to a device or specific procedure[49] – in other words, infections whose risk profile could be rigidly controlled. In the late 1970s and early 1980s, studies of nosocomial infection as well as infection control measures reflected the lessons learned from the previous decades of research regarding high risk patients. During this period, studies emphasized ICUs as the single largest source of infections with rates three to four times higher than non-ICU patients.[50] Because they tend to be the sickest – the most immunocompromised – and undergo many invasive forms of therapy and monitoring, patients in critical care units continue to be the group at the greatest risk for infection.

In 1985, the results of the CDC's 11-year, nationwide Study on the Efficacy of Nosocomial Infection Control (SENIC) were published thus providing the most comprehensive information to date on rates of different types of infection as well as their preventability and relative costs.[51] In the study, data were collected from a representative sample of hospitals across two time periods: 1970 and mid-1975 to mid-1976. For each period almost 170,000 records of adult medical and surgical patients were reviewed. Results from the 1975–6 period revealed that surgical wound infection accounted for 24% of total infections. As an indicator of their severity, these complications, however, accounted for almost 60% of extra hospital days. Similarly, nosocomial pneumonia, although only 10% of the total number of infections, accounted for almost one-quarter of extra hospital days. SENIC investigators estimated that overall, 32% of nosocomial infections were preventable. (See Table 7.1.) Although the SENIC study provided valuable incidence data on hospital acquired infections, its principal objectives were to determine the extent to which surveyed hospitals had, between 1970 and 1975–6, adopted new infection surveillance and control programs and the extent to which these programs had reduced nosocomial infection rates in the country. The study revealed that between the two time periods, hospitals with infection control programs had achieved a 6% reduction in nosocomial infections. Hospitals without such programs, however, showed an increased rate of 18% over the five

Table 7.1. *Comparison of the relative frequency of the major types of nosocomial infections and alternative measures of their relative importance*[52]

Type of infection	Percent of all nosocomial infections	Total extra days (%)[a]	Total extra charges in US dollars (%)[a]	Percent preventable[b]
Surgical wound infection	24	889 (57)	102,286 (42)	35
Pneumonia	10	370 (24)	95,229 (39)	22
Urinary tract infection	42	175 (11)	32,081 (13)	33
Bacteremia	5	59 (4)	7,478 (3)	35
Other	19	69 (4)	8,680 (3)	32
Total (all sites)	100	1,562 (100)	245,754 (100)	32

[a]Data are drawn from SENIC pilot studies: R.W. Haley, Schaberg DR, Crossley KB, et al., Extra charges and prolongation of stay attributable to nosocomial infections: A prospective interhospital comparison. *Am J Med* 1981; 70:51. Note that all charges are in 1975 US dollars.
[b]Data are drawn from SENIC analysis of efficacy: R.W. Haley, Culver DH, White JW, et al., The efficacy of infection surveillance and control programs in preventing nosocomial infections in US hospitals. *Am J Epidemiol* 1985; 121:198–9.

years.[53] The data from SENIC have since been used to analyze the cost-effectiveness of infection control programs. In this way, nosocomial infection control has been one of the first patient care improvement strategies to confront the issue of economic accountability.

Cost-effectiveness and nosocomial infection control

Even in the earliest studies of nosocomial infection, cost and resource utilization arguments were marshaled to support infection control efforts. A 1977 study in the United States of post-operative wound infection pointed out that following surgery for appendectomy, hysterectomy, cesarean section, and coronary artery bypass graft, patients with infection had average lengths of stay from 6 to 11 days longer and costs from $500 to $2600 higher than those of controls.[54] A 1978 study based on the CDC's National Nosocomial Infection Study (NNIS) involving 83 hospitals estimated that overall, nosocomial infections accounted for more than six million extra hospital days and 10.5 billion extra dollars in 1977.[55]

Robert Haley, director of the SENIC project has observed that the reason for the consistent attention to the costs associated with hospital-acquired infection is that it has often otherwise been difficult to motivate hospital administrators to invest resources in infection control programs.[56] Under the dominant fee-for-service or retrospective payment system, hospitals were not liable or accountable for the cost of nosocomial infections. Rather, these costs were passed onto, and fully reimbursed by, insurance companies.[57] In addition, nosocomial infection control initiatives, like so many other preventive health programs, were perceived by administrators as cost rather then revenue centers for a hospital. Thus, without data on the cost-savings associated with infection control programs, it was difficult to inspire administrators to embrace such programs beyond the minimal requirements imposed by the JCAH. In the early 1980s, as health care expenditures exceeded 11% of the gross national product, hospital administrators had additional incentives to curtail or eliminate programs that could not justify their costs. At a cost of approximately $60,000 per year in a 250-bed hospital, infection control programs were an obvious target for cut-backs. One strategy during this period was to consolidate all infection control, utilization review, and risk management activities under the hospital's quality assurance program.

It was not until the advent of prospective payment in the 1980s that hospitals themselves became economically liable for nosocomial infections and thus recognized a financial incentive for their control. In the early 1980s, the United States federal government initiated hospital reimbursement for Medicare beneficiaries under the system of diagnostic-related groups (DRGs)[58] whereby hospitals are reimbursed on a fixed-fee basis tied to the patient's primary diagnosis. Although, in principle, DRG assignment provided for additional reimbursement for complications occurring during hospitalization,[59] a 1987 extrapolation of SENIC data[60] concluded that hospitals were actually reimbursed only 1% to 5% of the cost of treating a nosocomial infection. Based on an approximate cost of $1800 for treatment, hospitals under prospective payment would be liable for roughly $1710 to $1782 in extra costs for each infection. On the basis of SENIC's estimation that 32% of nosocomial infections are preventable, it was calculated that an effective infection control program could produce an annual net savings of $1000 per bed in the prospective-payment era. With these data on the financial benefits of infection control, hospital administrators have by and large come to support systematic infection control programs in their institutions. As Wenzel and Pfaller have observed, 'the DRGs represented a very important force in institutionalizing hospital epidemiology.'[61]

In the mid-1990s prospective payment through Medicare and managed care has become the dominant form of reimbursement for both individual and institutional providers. The financial incentives to reduce costly infections are thus greater than ever. For this reason, it is important to reemphasize the distinction made in Chapter 5 between cost-benefit and cost-effectiveness analysis.

In cost-benefit analysis (CBA), both costs and benefits are understood and measured in monetary terms. From the point of view of a CBA, the nosocomial infection control program costs roughly $60,000 per year but results in a gross savings of approximately $305,000. In strictly financial terms, an infection control program not only pays for itself but results in a net annual gain of roughly $250,000 for a 250-bed hospital. In this way, nosocomial infection control makes good economic sense; the economic benefits justify the costs.

In cost-effectiveness analysis (CEA), by contrast, benefits are measured in non-monetary terms such as health, life, quality of life, or harm prevention. With CEA, non-economic goals are valued for their own sake as policy objectives. In CEA, unlike CBA, economic efficiency is valued only as a means to the achievement of goals valued for their own sake. Thus, from the point of view of CEA the principal value of infection control is not its potential for cost-savings (or net gain) but in its ability to prevent patient harms. Indeed, the history of nosocomial infection control suggests that the goal of patient welfare provided the sustaining motivation for infection control efforts long before they were perceived to be financially advantageous by hospital administrators in the United States.[62] After decades of work to determine the success and the cost-effectiveness of infection control programs, nosocomial infection control holds a unique position among strategies for preventing medical harm generally. As Haley has observed, 'reducing nosocomial infections appears to be one of the only proven methods for reducing unreimbursed resource utilization while improving patient care.'[63]

Thus, in nosocomial infection control today, the financial incentive to contain costs coincides with the moral imperative to protect patient welfare. As concerns about cost increasingly drive and reshape the delivery of health care in the United States, it is clear that these imperatives will not always so elegantly coincide. Of greatest concern in this regard are the cost-based restrictions that health care plans place on needed services. From a moral point of view, therefore, CBA is appropriate only after important values have been respected. CEA, by contrast depends in the first instance upon an articulation of those values that will be pursued in the most efficient manner. The most appropriate way of identifying the values that we want to sustain in our institutional and public policies regarding health care resources is through a public and democratic discussion of our ethical and cultural priorities. This is also the most appropriate way to modify our goals given the economic and technical constraints that may prevent us from achieving them.[64] Our choice of the particular values that will guide us in shaping our health care priorities will determine the extent to which we can sustain the foundational demands of healing. This difficult moral task will be greatly aided by the kind of empirical analyses performed in nosocomial infection control, analyses that clarify the relationship between economic efficiency, and the prevention and control of comiogenic harm.

Nosocomial infection control and quality improvement

In our brief discussion of the history of nosocomial infection control in the United States, we observed that cost containment efforts by hospitals in the early to mid-1980s resulted in the decision to consolidate infection control and risk management activities under the direction of the hospital's quality assurance (QA) program. According to Robert Haley, this initiative threatened the survival of the epidemiologic approach to infection control.[65] To understand why, recall that, as we noted in Chapter 5, QA operates on a number of fundamental assumptions, among them that harmful quality failures are unusual events, fundamentally linked to individual error, and best prevented by a system of standards and oversight. The epidemiologic orientation of infection control (epitomized by the SENIC study), however, is systematic in its emphasis. Its population-based approach assumes the inevitable occurrence of infectious complications. Its comprehensive strategy of data collection and analysis goes beyond a model of individual agency to systems analysis in order to understand and control the occurrence of these complications.

Since the release of the SENIC results in the mid-1980s, the value of the epidemiologic orientation for determining the efficacy of infection control has been increasingly acknowledged. In addition, the promise of a more outcomes-based quality assessment demonstrated in the infection control literature is now a central feature of the Joint Commission for the Accreditation of Healthcare Organisations' (JCAHO) new orientation to continuous quality improvement (CQI). With the introduction of indicators in anesthesiology, obstetrics, cardiology, oncology, trauma, and medication use as well as infection control,[66] the JCAHO is, for the first time in its history, evaluating health care quality on the basis of data regarding actual patient outcomes. This information can enhance the risk profile of hospital services by enabling hospitals to establish baseline rates on infection and related complications. These data can, in turn, become an essential component of the patient's decision-making process. For example, if a patient is informed either through the informed consent process or through publicly available sources that a hospital's risk-adjusted infection rate is elevated, he or she can choose to postpone a hospital stay or obtain care at another facility.

Nosocomial infection control: a model for prevention of comiogenic harms?

Although infection control is distinctive, particularly insofar as infection represents its only dependent variable, there are, nevertheless, insights from the field that can be effectively applied to the control of comiogenic harms generally. First, is the superiority of active, continuous surveillance over passive voluntary reporting. Passive voluntary reporting relies solely on the initiative of individual health care professionals to record in the chart, and/or in a database, infection data, adverse drug reaction data, or any other information about hospital-related complications. This data collection method is inevitably weakened by the unsystematic and incomplete nature of the reporting. In the field of infection control, the limitations of passive voluntary reporting provided the impetus for the implementation of active, intensive surveillance by nurse and physician epidemiologists.[67] Unlike passive, voluntary reporting, which tends to be retrospective, intensive surveillance is proactive, and as such, aims to anticipate nosocomial infection and ameliorate its effects on particular patients. A similar approach is now used to identify and prevent adverse drug reactions.[68]

From the method of active, intensive surveillance itself, additional insights have been gained. One is that the most effective surveillance is oriented to the investigation of the *specific* types of infection and their *specific* manifestations rather than to the identification of a hospital's *overall* infection rate. In infection control, this insight led to the development of separate surveillance systems with specific preventive strategies for surgical wound infection, pneumonia, urinary tract, and bloodstream infections. Insights gained from this approach could be applied to the design of surveillance techniques and preventive measures for other comiogenic hazards such as falls and decubitus ulcers as well as for certain drug-related and procedure-related adverse effects. In the arena of health care quality assessment, this approach is currently reflected in the JCAHO outcomes indicators.[69]

Another insight gained from the implementation of intensive surveillance in infection control is that data from such surveillance can be analyzed in combination with data from other infection control programs to determine the best achievable rates for specific types of nosocomial infection. In addition, this type of surveillance can also make use of multivariate analysis for a more accurate determination of important risk factors for nosocomial complications. The experience of infection control suggests that the determination of baseline data, risk factors, and optimal rates may be essential components in the empirical framework required for the effective prevention and control of other types of comiogenic complication.[70]

Ethical issues in hospital epidemiology and quality improvement research

As we consider the contributions of nosocomial infection control to health care quality, we must also recognize the unique ethical issues raised by the epidemiologic method. The epidemiologic method is essentially population-based and, as such, is oriented to public safety, or, in other words, to the goal of *overall* risk reduction. In some cases, the achievement of this goal may require measures that compromise the interests of the individual patient. These measures may include quarantine of a patient colonized with a resistant and highly communicable infection, or the posting of notices on a patient's door, or labels in the chart to alert providers to a patient's infection status.[71] These are classic examples of the dilemma of public health – where the public good may be safeguarded only at the expense of the individual patient's interests. In Chapter 6, we discussed the conditions that might together justify compromise to the patient's interests in confidentiality and autonomy. Given that such tensions are inherent to the institutional treatment of infection, patients should, upon admission to the hospital or as soon as their infection status is known be made aware of the possibility that public safety concerns may require limits on their autonomy and privacy.

The practice of infection control highlights another way in which a hospital's commitment to overall risk reduction may come into conflict with the interests of the individual patient. At issue is whether there is a duty to disclose to the patient information about his or her care that may be damaging to the hospital and that may, in turn, threaten the viability of the infection control program. The nurse or physician who functions in the dual role of clinician and hospital epidemiologist is at the center of this conflict. As a clinician, the nurse- or physician-epidemiologist has a traditional fiduciary obligation to act on behalf of individual patients, As an epidemiologist, however, the practitioner has a primary duty to the hospital population in aggregate. Inevitably, this second duty is intertwined with the epidemiologist's obligation to the hospital which supports the infection control program. In their paper on ethical issues in infection control, Chavigny and Helm[72] use a series of cases to illustrate the dilemma. In one representative case, the authors report on the care of a 20-year-old man who twisted a knee while skiing. Effusion to the knee joint required that the man be hospitalized and the knee joint be surgically drained. On the day of discharge the patient had some purulent discharge from the knee and was readmitted to the hospital within 24 hours with systemic *Staphylococcus aureus* infection. The organism was resistant to penicillin and osteomyletitis developed in the knee joint and tibia. Subsequent tissue destruction required plastic surgery and extensive rehabilitation. Assuming that the infection control practitioner discovers the source of transmission of this infection to have been improper hand washing, should he or she provide this information to the patient? Although such moral dilemmas are heightened for the hospital epidemiologist who may have direct contact with the patient in question, the issue of disclosure is also pertinent to health services researchers and researchers in the field of quality improvement.

As in public health, the goal of health services or quality improvement research is benefit to an aggregate population through the development of medical knowledge. Troyen Brennan, a principle investigator in the Harvard Medical Practice Study writes of the dilemma regarding disclosure in this research on hospital-related adverse events.[73] In order to gain access to hospital records, the researchers had to promise to destroy all identifying codes thereby making them unavailable to potential plaintiffs in malpractice litigation. Highlighting the dilemma, Brennan asks whether 'the quality of care researcher [has] any duty to inform an individual patient about substandard care that has caused injury . . . or [whether it is permissable] to remain silent about substandard care that leads to injury, even if this silence leaves the costs of the accident for the patient to bear?'[74]

In 1978, the broader question of patients' access to information was raised in nosocomial infection control research when the CDC requested a limited exemption from the Freedom of Information Act (FOIA) for hospitals participating in data collection for the SENIC project. The CDC requested that the Public Health Services Act be amended to protect the identity of participating hospitals on the theory that the assurance of anonymity would encourage greater involvement by hospitals in infection surveillance and control. The Ethics Advisory Board took up the question and concluded that the public's right to know outweighed the hospital's interest in keeping nosocomial infection data confidential.[75]

There are a number of approaches to resolving these conflicts regarding disclosure and patient access to information. For infection control, or quality improvement officers, or researchers torn between obligations to a patient and to the public health, it may be appropriate to disaggregate their roles as clinician and epidemiologist thereby alleviating direct conflicts of obligation. This solution will not however, resolve the conflict that may remain for the epidemiologist or researcher whose sense of obligation to the patient is not based on a fiduciary role but, rather, on a more general sense of fairness and truthtelling.

Another approach, therefore, might be to assume that hospitalized or other patients whose treatment information is used to conduct infection control or quality surveillance are in fact participating in research. In this case, protections now extended to subjects in standard research protocols would be extended to patients as well. Patients would be informed about the anticipated use of information regarding their care and their consent would be required as a condition of the research.[76] As Brennan points out, such an approach to the problem of quality improvement research would emphasize that the research 'is intended to benefit all patients, not just individual patients.'[77] If patients were so informed at the outset and waived their right of access to research records, then destruction of identifiers would be legitimate. There are a number of obvious problems with this approach. First, patients seeking care would be in a potentially coercive situation if they are asked to waive their right to information regarding their care prior to receiving that care. Secondly, the information provided to the patient in the consent process could be so innocuous (e.g. 'we will be conducting research regarding the processes and outcomes of health care delivery') as to preclude the possibility of genuine consent. Thirdly, if a substantial number of patients or former patients refused to waive their right to information regarding their care then such research could not go forward and data essential for quality improvement would be lost.

The idea that patients may legitimately be denied access to potentially damaging information so long as that information is used to improve subsequent performance is not new. Indeed, this was precisely the view espoused in Percival's 1803, *Medical Ethics.* where he counseled physicians that 'good intentions and the imperfections of human skill . . . will sufficiently justify what is past provided the failure be made conscientiously subservient to future wisdom and rectitude in professional conduct.'[78] Although today, the mandate for infection control and quality improvement is no longer strictly a matter of *personal* honor and accountability but, rather, is imposed by accreditors and regulators, the ethical issue remains the same: do the demands of health care quality improvement justify the concealment of potentially damning information from the patient?

In Chapter 5 we offered an alternative solution to this conflict and one that we reiterate here: the success of quality improvement and infection control programs cannot be guaranteed only at the expense of injured patients. One way in which the interests of the injured patient (in access to information) and future patients (in high quality care) can be simultaneously respected is through a compensation scheme that transcends the malpractice framework. If nosocomial infections and other hospital-related harms can be compensated from a fund outside of the framework of malpractice then in principle, the most compelling incentive that hospitals have to seek anonymity and confidentiality regarding the quality of health care delivery would be removed.

Endnotes

1 In the Byzantine world, the name *Nosocomeion*, literally, a place where diseases are cared for, was used to refer to institutions treating the sick. The phrase 'nosocomial infection' was first used in its current sense in the mid-nineteenth century.
   See Schadewaldt H. Hospitalinfektionen im Wandel. *Zentralbl Bakteriol Mikrobiol Hyg* 1986; 183:91–102.
2 Nightingale F. *Introductory Notes on Lying-In Institutions.* London: Longman, Green, 1871.
3 Semmelweis I. *The Etiology, Concept, and Prophylaxis of Childbed Fever.* (Ed. and trans. K. C. Carter.) Madison: University of Wisconsin Press, 1983.
4 Carter KC, Tate GS. The earliest-known account of Semmelweis's initiation of disinfection at Vienna's Allgemeines Krankenhaus. *Bull Hist Med* 1991; 65:252–7.
5 Larson E. A causal link between handwashing and risk of infection? Examination of the evidence. *Infect Control* 1988; 9:28–36.
6 Larson E, Kretzer EK. Compliance with handwashing and barrier precautions. *J Hosp Infect* 1995; 30(supp.):88–106.
   Albert RK, Condie F. Hand-washing patterns in medical intensive-care units. *N Engl J Med* 1981; 304:1465–6.
   Doebbeling BN, Stanley GL, Sheetz CT, et al. Comparative efficacy of alternative hand-washing agents in reducing nosocomial infections in intensive care units. *N Engl J Med* 1992; 327(2):88–93.
7 Meigs C. *On the Nature, Signs, and Treatment of Childbed Fever.* Philadelphia, 1859, p. 102.
8 Meigs C, p. 104 (see No. 7).
9 Holmes OW. The contagiousness of puerperal fever. *N Engl Q J Med.* 1843:1–23. (Reprinted in *Medical Classics*, vol. 1. Baltimore: Williams and

Wilkins, 1937, p. 243.)
10 Lister J. On the antiseptic principle in the practice of surgery. *Lancet* 1867; 1:741–5.
11 Nuland, SB. *Doctors: The Biography of Medicine.* New York: Vintage, 1988, p. 364.
12 Lister J. Effects of the antiseptic system of treatment upon the salubrity of a surgical hospital. *Lancet* 1870; 1:4–6; 40–2.
13 Garipey TP. The introduction and acceptance of Listerian Antisepsis in the United States. *J Hist Med Allied Sci* 1994; 49:167–206 (p. 181).
14 Lawrence G. Surgery (traditional). In BynumWF, Porter R, eds. *Companion Encyclopedia of the History of Medicine.* New York: Routledge, 1993, ch. 41, p. 963.
15 Nuland, SB, p. 344 (see No. 11).
16 Simpson JY. *Anaesthesia, Hospitalism, Hermaphrodism and a Proposal to Stamp Out Small-pox and other Contagious Diseases.* Edinburgh: Adam & Charles Black, 1871.
17 Nuland, SB, p. 346 (see No. 11).
18 Earle AS. The germ theory in America: Antisepsis and asepsis (1867–1900). *Surgery* 1969; 65:508–22.
19 Rosenberg CE. *The Care of Strangers:The Rise of America's Hospital System.* New York: Basic Books, 1987.
20 Cited in Earle AS, p. 510 (see No. 18).
21 Richmond PA. American attitudes toward the germ theory of disease (1860–1880). *J Hist Med and Allied Sci* 1954; 9:428–54.
22 Cited in Richmond PA, p. 83n (see No. 21).
23 Cited in Brieger GH. American surgery and the germ theory of disease *Bull Hist Med* 1966; 40:135–45 (p. 139).
24 Cited in Brieger GH, p. 139 (see No. 23).
25 Cited in Earle AS, p. 513 (see No. 18).
26 Cited in Larson E. Innovations in health care: Antisepsis as a case study. *Am J Pub Health* 1989; 79:92–9 (p. 96).
27 Nightingale F. *Notes on Hospitals,* 3rd edn. London: Longman, Green, 1863, p. 22.
28 Nightingale F, p.1 (see No. 27).
29 Rosenberg CE, p. 149–50 (see No. 19).
30 Goff BH. An analysis of wound union *Surg. Gyn. Obstet* 1925; 41:728–39. Meleney FL. Infection in clean operative wounds. A nine year study. *Surg Gyn Obstet* 1935; 60:264–75. Eliason EL, McLaughlin C. Post-operative wound complications. *Ann Surg* 1934; 100:1159–76.
31 Wise RI, Ossman EA, Littlefield DR. Personal reflections on nosocomial staphylococcal infections and the development of hospital surveillance. *Rev Infect Dis* 1989; 11:1005–19.
32 Now the Centers for Disease Control and Prevention.
33 Eickhoff TC. The third dicennial international conference on nosocomial infections: Historical perspective: The landmark conference in 1970. *AM J Med* 1991; 91:3B–5S.
34 American Hospital Association. *Infection Control in Hospitals.* Chicago, AHA, 1968.
35 CDC Proceedings of the International Conference on Nosocomial Infections. August 3–6, Atlanta: CDC, 1970, p. 42.

36 Eickhoff TC, Brachman PW, Bennett JV, et al. Surveillance of nosocomial
   infections in community hospitals. I. Surveillance methods, effectiveness and
   initial results. *J Infect Dis* 1969; 120(3):305–17.
   Wenzel RP, Osterman CA, Hunting KJ. Hospital acquired infections II.
   Infection rates by site, service and common procedures in a university
   hospital. *Am J Epidemiol* 1976; 104:645–51.
   Haley RW, Shactman RH. The emergence of infection surveillance and
   control programs in US hospitals: An assessment. *Am J Epidemiol* 1980;
   111:574–91.
37 Public health: Surveillance, prevention and control of nosocomial infections.
   Morb Mort Week Rep 1992; 41:783–7.
38 Haley RW, Culver DH, White JW, et al. The efficacy of infection surveillance
   and control programs in preventing nosocomial infections In US hospitals.
   Am J Epidemiol 1985; 121:182–205.
39 Haley RW, Culver DH, White JW (see No. 38).
40 Haley RW, Gaynes RP, Aber RC, Bennett JV. Surveillance of nosocomial
   infections. In Bennett JV, Brachman PS, eds. *Hospital Infections*, 3rd edn.
   Boston:Little, Brown, 1992, pp. 79–108.
41 Haley RW, Gaynes RP, Aber RC, Bennett JV, p. 85 (see No. 40).
42 CDC Proceedings of the International Conference on Nosocomial Infections.
   August 3–6, Atlanta: CDC 1970, p. 42.
43 The degree of risk demanded by this obligation has been the subject of
   considerable argument at least since the Middle Ages when physicians were
   confronted with the choice of fleeing plague ridden cities or staying to treat
   patients. Since the advent of the AIDS epidemic these questions have again
   come to the fore. Because our project focuses exclusively on harm to patients,
   we will not address the important and complex ethical issues surrounding
   patient to provider transmission of infectious disease.
   See, Amundsen DW. Medical deontology and pestilential disease in the late
   middle ages. *J Hist Med* 1977; 32:403–21.
   Childress J. Hospital acquired infections: Some ethical issues. In Wenzel RP,
   ed. *Prevention and Control of Nosocomial Infections.* Baltimore: Williams and
   Wilkins, 1987, pp. 49–55.
44 Patterson JE, Vecchio J, Pantelick EL et al. Association of contaminated
   gloves with transmission of *Acinetobacter calcoaceticus* var. *anitratus* in an
   intensive care unit. Am J Med 1991 Nov; 91(5):479–83.
   Goldman D, Larson E. Hand-washing and nosocomial infections. *N Engl J
   Med* 1992; 327:120–2.
45 Garner JS and the Hospital Infection Control Practices Advisory Committee.
   Guideline for isolation precautions in hospitals. *Am J Infect Control* 1996;
   24:24–52.
46 Eickhoff TC. Microbiological sampling. *Hospitals* 1970; 44:86–7.
   Committee on Infections within Hospitals, American Hospital Association.
   Statement on microbiological sampling in the hospital. *Hospitals* 1974;
   48:125–6.
47 Wenzel RP, Osterman CA, Hunting KJ. Hospital acquired infections II.
   Infection rates by site, service and common procedures in a university
   hospital. *Am J Epidemiol* 1976; 104:645–51.
48 Stamm WE: Infections related to medical devices. *Ann Intern Med* 1978;
   89:764–8.
49 Wenzel RP, Thompson RL, Landry SM, et al. Hospital-acquired infections in

intensive care unit patients: An overview with emphasis on epidemics. *Infect Control* 1983; 4:371–5.
50 Chandrasekar PH, Kruse JA, Matthews MF. Nosocomial infection among patients in different types of intensive care units at a city hospital. *Crit Care Med* 1986; 14:508–10.
51 Haley RW, Culver DH, White JW, et al. (see No. 38).
52 Chart and notes reproduced from Haley RW, Gaynes RP, Aber RC, Bennett JV. Surveillance of nosocomial infections. In Bennett JV, Brachman PS, eds., p. 101 (see No. 40).
53 Haley RW, Culver DH, White JW, et al. (see No. 38).
54 Green JW, Wenzel RP. Postoperative wound infection: A controlled study of the increased duration of hospital stay and direct costs of hospitalization. *Ann Surg* 1977; 185:264–8.
55 Dixon RE: Effect of infections on hospital care. *Ann Intern Med* 1978; 89:749–73.
56 Haley RW. Measuring the costs of nosocomial infections: methods for estimating economic burden on the hospital. *Am J Med* 1991; 91(Supp. 3B):32S–38S.
57 Wenzel RP, Pfaller MA. Infection control: The premier quality assessment program in United States hospitals. *Am J Med* 1991; 91(Supp. 3B):27S–31S.
58 Inglehart JK. Medicare begins prospective payment of hospitals. *N Engl J Med* 1982; 368:1482–3.
59 Dixon RE. Costs of nosocomial infections and benefits of infection control programs. In Wenzel RP, ed. *Prevention and Control of Nosocomial Infections.* Baltimore: Williams and Wilkins, 1987, pp. 19–25.
60 Haley RW, White JW, Culver DH, et al. The financial incentive for hospitals to prevent nosocomial infections under the prospective payment system. An empirical determination from a nationally representative sample. *JAMA* 1987; 257(12):1611–14.
61 Wenzel RP, Pfaller MA. Infection control: The premier quality assessment program, p. 28S (see No. 57).
62 Wenzel RP, Pfaller MA (see No. 57).
63 Haley RW, p. 32S (see No. 56).
64 Sagoff M. *The Economy of the Earth.* New York: Cambridge University Press, 1988, p. 14.
65 Haley RW. The development of infection surveillance and control programs. In Bennett JV, Brachman PS, eds., pp. 63–78 (see No. 40).
66 Joint Commission on Accreditation of Health Care Organizations. *Accreditation Manual for Hospitals.* Chicago: JCAHO, 1993, Appendix D.
67 Haley RW (see No. 65).
68 Classen DC, Pestotnik SL, Evans RS, Burke JP. Computerized surveillance of adverse drug events in hospital patients. *JAMA* 1991; 266(20):2847–51.
69 Joint Commission on Accreditation of Health Care Organizations (see No. 66).
70 Haley RW (see No. 65).
71 Herwaldt LA. Ethical aspects of infection control. *Infect Control Hosp Epidemiol* 1996; 17:108–13.
72 Chavigny KH, Helm A. Ethical dilemmas and the practice of infection control. *Law Med Health Care* 1982; 10:168–71,174.
73 Brennan TA. Ethics of confidentiality: The special case of quality assurance research. *Clin Research* 1990; 38(3):551–7.

74 Brennan TA, p. 552 (see No. 73).
75 See Dept. of Health and Human Services, Ethics Advisory Board. The request of the Center for Disease Control for a limited exemption from the freedom of information act. Washington, DC: US Government Printing Office, 1980.
76 In *administrative* continuous improvement, there is a consensus that a 'prior notification' statement adequately affords patients the opportunity to decline participation in a hospital's ongoing self-evaluation. Here, the absence of patient refusal to have records open to review, is taken to imply consent. The specific question of the patient's access to research findings does not, however, seem to be included in prior notification statements. See Goldberg HI. Ethical issues in administrative continuous improvement. *Med Care* 1990; 28:822–33.
77 Brennan TA, p. 557 (see No. 73).
78 Percival T. *Medical Ethics or A Code of Institutes and Precepts adapted to the Professional Conduct of Physicians and Surgeons.* Manchester: S. Russell, 1803) p. 107.

8

Adverse effects of drug treatment

Sir William Osler said that, 'a desire to take medicine is, perhaps, the great feature which distinguishes man from other animals.'[1] Unfortunately, no medicinal agent is without potential side-effects. The noxious actions of drugs were well-recognized in early nineteenth-century medicine in the United States and even before; indeed, drugs were often chosen precisely for such effects during the era of counter-irritant/depletion therapy promulgated by Rush and his disciples.[2] Medicinal remedies often included toxic minerals, such as mercury, arsenic, and antimony.[3] Use of patent medicines, popular in the eighteenth century, expanded considerably after the revolutionary war, in part due to extensive advertising.[4] Even as promoters of patent medicine criticized regular practitioners for using mercury-containing purgatives, they also not uncommonly included mercury in their nostrums, as well as substantial amounts of opium and alcohol.[5,6]

Since the mid-nineteenth century, government legislation and regulation relating to drugs have served to reduce consumer and physician control of drug choices. Until the Drug Import Law of 1848, the majority of medications were imported into the United States. The Federal Food and Drug Act of 1906, and the Federal Food, Drug, and Cosmetic Act of 1938 to standardize medicinal preparation and availability, with the intent of protecting the consumer. However, prescription drug use since the late-1920s has increased dramatically. From 1929 to 1949, prescription drug expenditures increased five-fold, and prescription drugs as a percentage of expenditures for all drugs climbed from 32% to 57%; Between 1949 and 1969, expenditures for prescription drugs again increased more than five-fold, comprising more than 80% of total drug expenditures.[7] This increase in prescription drug sales reflected, to a substantial degree, the accelerated introduction of new drugs into the marketplace: five-year averages were 14 new drugs per year for the period 1941–45; 29 for the period 1946–50; 43 for the period 1951–55; and 53 in the period 1956–60.[8]

The marked increase in drug development and utilization after World War II, particularly the use of antibiotics such as penicillin, underscored the potential dangers of pharmacotherapy. Increased interest in iatrogenic illness generally during this period, combined with the observation that adverse drug effects comprise the single largest category of iatrogenic complications, focused attention on the scope and magnitude of this problem. Complications of drug treatment are remarkably frequent, accounting for 5–10% of all hospitalizations and contributing to in-hospital morbidity in 20–25% of patients. As one observer has noted, 'No one has a better chance to live dangerously than the ill who must take their medicine.'[9]

The objective of public policy initiatives relating to drug regulation has been to improve the safety of those who take medications. Unfortunately, even the strongest regulations cannot eliminate adverse drug reactions, which are inherent in drug use. Adverse drug effects may follow appropriate or inappropriate use; even in recommended doses, all drugs carry potential side-effects. These are often divided into two types.[10] Type A reactions reflect the usual pharmacological effects of a drug, but which are exaggerated; they tend to be predictable, relatively common, often dose-related, and typically less serious. The usual treatment is to reduce the drug dose. Type B reactions tend to be idiosyncratic and less common; they are usually not dose-related but are often serious. Of course, misuse of drugs – inappropriate dosing, administration frequency or timing – by the patient or by the provider, may also contribute to adverse drug effects. Adverse drug reactions (ADRs) may be precipitated or compounded by multiple drug use (polypharmacy) and/or by the extensive use of unprescribed over-the-counter medications.[11]

Beginning in the mid-1960s, a large number of studies have addressed the incidence of ADRs in the inpatient and outpatient settings, as well as the incidence of drug-related hospital admissions. However, there has been little consistency across studies with regard to definition, study design, or even objectives. In their critical review of the early literature on this subject, Karch and Lasagna observed that published studies were 'incomplete, unrepresentative, uncontrolled, lacking in operational criteria ...'[12] Because of these failings, the incidence range for ADRs in those studies has varied by as much as several orders of magnitude. The restrictiveness of the definition used, the data collection process (retrospective versus prospective, degree of surveillance), or the type of research setting (intensive care unit, general medical ward, general surgical ward, etc.) markedly affect the incidence rates that have been described. Each of these methodological issues deserves discussion in an attempt to address the scope of the problem of ADRs.

Definitions: adverse drug reaction and adverse drug event

The most inclusive definition of an ADR is 'any undesirable effect produced by a drug.'[13] This would include intentional overdose and drug abuse, which are qualitatively different from consequences related to medicinal use. However, a number of reported studies do include intentional overdoses or poisonings, as well as the effects of drug and alcohol abuse. Such a broad definition, which includes use of drugs for diagnostic as well as therapeutic purposes, has been employed in a number of early papers addressing the incidence of adverse drug effects, particularly in the hospital setting. Schimmel (1964) defines an adverse drug effect as a 'noxious response accompanying the use of therapeutic drugs.'[14] For Ogilvie and Ruedy, the definition is 'any undesired consequence of drug therapy.'[15] Borda et al. describe an adverse drug reaction 'as any unintended or undesired effect of a drug in a patient.'[16]

In contrast, other authors have used more restrictive definitions, in which physician intent or the severity of side-effects are specified. For Seidl et al., the definition is 'any noxious change in a patient's condition which a physician suspects may be due to a drug, which occurs at dosages normally used in man, and which (i) requires treatment, or (ii) indicates decrease or cessation of therapy with the drug, or (iii) suggests that future therapy with the drug carries an unusual risk.'[17] Even more limited was Reidenberg's definition of ADR as 'those responses unintended and undesired by the physician which were severe enough to be commented on in the progress notes.'[18] Relatively restrictive definitions have also been proposed by the World Health Organization (WHO) and the Food and Drug Administration (FDA), which are widely cited. For the WHO, an ADR is a response to a drug 'which is noxious and unintended and which occurs in doses used in man for prophylaxis, diagnosis, or therapy.'[19] Only slightly modified is the FDA definition of an adverse drug reaction as one 'that is noxious, unintended, and occurs in doses normally used in man for the prophylaxis, diagnosis, or therapy of disease.'[20]

In general, the very restrictive definitions do not include intentional overdose or accidental poisonings; nor do they include drug abuse, ethanol abuse, or therapeutic failures. Karch and Lasagna in their critical analysis suggest a slight modification of the WHO or the FDA definitions to clarify the exclusion of therapeutic failures: 'An adverse drug reaction is any response to a drug that is noxious and unintended, and occurs in dosages used in man for prophylaxis, diagnosis or therapy, excluding failure to accomplish the intended purpose.'[21] Not surprisingly, studies that have used the more restrictive definitions tend to report incidence rates for ADRs in the outpatient or inpatient setting that are substantially below those employing more inclusive definitions.

One of the problems with restrictive definitions like that proposed by the WHO or the FDA is that they refer only to the appropriate use of drugs, whereas most drug-related harms result from errors in medication use.[22] For this reason, Bates and colleagues have broadened the definition referring to an adverse drug *event* (ADE) as 'an injury resulting from medical intervention related to a drug.' Not only is such a definition more comprehensive, but it appears to be more clinically relevant.

Methodological issues

A number of studies have used retrospective methods to assess ADRs in a variety of settings. These have included chart reviews, evaluation of discharge summaries, or assessment of patient recollections. In general, such retrospective methods tend to substantially underestimate the incidence of ADRs. In contrast, prospective studies typically use active surveillance methods, either by study investigators, research nurses, or pharmacists. Use of multiple, parallel systems of surveillance appears to decrease the false-negative rates. Schumock et al. compared pharmacy-based concurrent surveillance methods to traditional retrospective medical record reporting of ADRs.[23] The active surveillance method identified 14 of 15 adverse drug reactions as compared to only four by the retrospective technique. Prosser and Kamysz report on the consequences of establishing a multidisciplinary adverse drug reaction surveillance program in a community hospital setting – the number of ADR reports increased from zero to 134 in the first 11 months of the program.[24] Borda et al. suggest that the relatively high incidence of adverse drug reactions identified by them may have reflected their active drug surveillance program.[25] Classen and colleagues compared a newly-established computerized surveillance method for ADEs in hospitalized patients to traditional detection methods – 731 ADEs were observed using computerized techniques as compared to only nine with traditional methods.[26]

Several algorithms have been created to enhance the active surveillance process. Naranjo and colleagues developed a ten-question ADR probability scale to enhance inter-observer reliability in estimating its probable occurrence.[27] In a study to evaluate the consistency of assessment among a group of physicians and pharmacists, they demonstrated the validity and reliability of their instrument. A more sophisticated algorithm was developed by Kramer, Hutchinson, Leventhal and colleagues, which provided well-defined operational criteria for assessing the probability of suspected ADR.[28] Their scoring system used six 'axes of decision strategy' including previous experience with the drug, etiologic alternatives, timing, drug levels/evidence of overdose, dechallenge, and rechallenge. In their carefully constructed study, these authors demonstrated both the validity and effectiveness of their instrument – pairwise agreement between experts in clinical pharmacology increased from 47% to 63% when the algorithm was used.[29]

Ultimately, any probabilistic scaling or scoring method will divide ADRs into three main categories – definite, probable or possible. Evaluations of ADRs based upon only the former category generally report a lower incidence, whereas inclusion of possible events tends to report a higher incidence.[30]

As we will see later in reviewing specific studies, the patient population studied substantially affects reported incidence rates. Thus, intensive care unit settings and general medical environment appear to show the highest incidence, whereas obstetrical units, surgical units, and pediatric units appear to show lower rates. Therefore, one should be cautious in extrapolating rates from one clinical setting to another. Moreover, epidemiological data have suggested that the incidence of ADRs are higher in the elderly and in women. Thus, studies that have excluded women may show a lower incidence rate, whereas those studying geriatric populations may demonstrate relatively higher rates.

Adverse drug reactions in the outpatient setting

A number of studies have addressed the incidence of ADRs or ADEs in the outpatient environment. Clearly, in assessing these data one must be mindful of the methodological issues that have been previously raised, in particular the definitions used and whether active surveillance or retrospective methods were employed.

Kellaway and McCrae studied 200 subjects in New Zealand discharged from acute medical wards.[31] They used follow-up interrogation of patients during their outpatient visits, or if the latter were infrequent, supplemented this by telephone questioning or questionnaire. The authors adopted the WHO definition of ADR. They do not describe how they assessed the probability value for an ADR, nor do they report which categories (i.e., 'definite', 'probable', 'possible') they included. An ADR rate of 31.5% was reported as compared to 17% from their previous unpublished inpatient study. They found a higher incidence in women, in the young and elderly, and in those exposed to multiple drugs. One of the earliest outpatient studies was by Stewart and Cluff[32] as part of a series of reports on the epidemiology of ADRs. This was a retrospective survey of 75 patients from a general medical clinic of the University of Florida teaching hospital. Patient interviews were complemented by pharmacy data. Medication histories involved a 30-day period prior to the interview. Possible drug interactions were noted in 51.7% of patients who took an average of 9.5 chemicals (prescription plus non-prescription) in the preceding 30 days. Forty-three percent of prescription drug users obtained the drug from multiple prescribers; 12% 'borrowed' prescription medications. More than 50% of patients reported ADRs at some time in the past. Although the small patient sample and retrospective method used do not permit meaningful conclusions about the incidence of outpatient ADRs, the study does underscore the important issues of polypharmacy and non-prescription drug use.

Campbell and colleagues reported a study population that consisted of a 5% random sample of Kaiser Foundation Health Plan members in Portland, Oregon, USA.[33] The investigators employed a retrospective review of patient treatment codes using the International Classification of Disease and subsequently identified approximately 100 codes as reflecting an undesirable effect of the drug used in the treatment/cure, prevention, or diagnosis of disease. The operational definition they used was similar to that proposed by Karch and Lasagna, and excluded intentional and accidental overdose, as well as drug abuse and treatment failures. The paper did not reveal what probability scaling or scoring method was used to assess the likelihood of an ADR. The mean ADR prevalence rate for the six-month study period as 2.97, with a mean incidence rate of 3.19. These relatively low percentages undoubtedly reflect the restrictive nature of the definition they used and the retrospective scoring method. Another significant problem with the study design was that the investigators used individual physician's clinical judgment to establish a likely causal relationship between morbidity and a drug, rather than using an objective instrument or algorithm.

Martys reported the results of a two-year prospective study using a general practice outpatient population of approximately 3300 patients in Great Britain.[34] Patients administered a drug for the first time completed a questionnaire in which they were asked whether, in their own opinion, they developed any symptoms that may have reflected a side-effect of the drug that was prescribed. The patients were subsequently questioned directly about any specific symptoms, and whether they were using self-medications. This survey was restricted to patients administered single drug treatment for the first time and thus reflects only a small percentage of patients in a general medical practice. Using the questionnaire and follow-up data, the investigator determined which events appeared to be 'definitely' or 'probably' due to the drug prescribed. Of the 817 patients evaluated, 41% were thought to have a reaction to the prescribed drug. It should be noted that despite the high percentage figures reported, the author used the relatively restrictive WHO definition of an ADR.

In the United States, Klein and colleagues identified 299 randomly selected medical outpatients from Johns Hopkins general medical clinics and used a structured multiple choice survey to identify drug treatment compliance, as well as the percentage of patients who associated adverse symptoms with their drug use.[35] They report that 30% of their subject pool noted at least one medication causing an 'undesirable symptom.' Surprisingly, they observed that subjects 65 years of age or older reported a lower mean incidence rate of adverse symptoms, as compared to younger subjects. While the authors appear to have used a well-constructed survey process and reasonable data analysis, they fail to provide information about how they assigned probabilities of an adverse drug effect. Moreover, treatment failures were not included, nor was information provided regarding self-medications.

Hutchinson and colleagues reported the frequency of ADRs, using intensive telephone-based surveillance methodology, in 1026 patients followed by an internal medicine group practice during a one-year period.[36] They used the carefully constructed algorithm developed by their group to assess the probability that an adverse reaction was due to a drug effect. They reported a rate of probable or definite ADRs in 5% of patients and in 2% of each drug course. The percentage of possible ADRs was more than three times higher than the rate of probable/definite reactions. The authors noted that although the number of ADRs was related to the number of drugs being used, use of multiple drugs *per se* did not appear to increase the reaction rate for an individual patient. More drug reactions were found in elderly patients as compared to younger ones, this difference could be explained nearly entirely by the larger number of drugs used. This study is exceptionally well conducted and includes both active surveillance and an objective algorithm for determining the probability for an ADR. As stated by the authors, the true ADR rate probably lies somewhere between the rate of probable/definite reactions and possible reactions.

More recently, a study by Schneider and colleagues assessed the incidence of ADRs in elderly outpatients attending either an inter disciplinary geriatric clinic or a general medical clinic during 1988.[37] A retrospective approach was employed and subjects were identified as having an ADR if this was documented by the physician, or if a relevant symptom was observed in the record. An ADR Probability Scale was used to assess the likelihood that an ADR was due to a drug effect. The authors used the ADR definition of Naranjo et al.,[38] which is restrictive and excludes therapeutic failure, intentional and accidental poisoning, and drug abuse. Subjects were noted as having an ADR only if the physician documented this or if the relevant complaint was documented in the record with a score of '1' or greater on the ADR Probability Scale. The authors report 107 events in 97 patients (21%); 12 of the 97 patients were hospitalized as a direct result of the ADR. Of the patients with ADR, 50 were listed as 'possible', 44 'probable' and 3 'definite'. Thus, 10% of the patients exhibited a definite or probable ADR. The authors admit that their relatively low rate of ADRs reported likely reflected the conservativeness of their method for determining an ADR. Moreover, the retrospective chart review method of identifying ADRs also may have accounted in part for this lower incidence rate. In this study, age *per se* did not appear to influence ADR risk, although the use of drugs with potential interactions and drugs requiring monitoring appeared to increase the relative incidence.

In summary, the findings from these various outpatient studies suggest a highly variable rate of ADRs ranging from under 3% to over 40%. These differences appear to be explained in large part by differing definitions of ADRs, various methods used to collect data, such as active surveillance versus retrospective reporting, or the use of algorithms to determine the probability of ADR occurrence. In general, the findings support an increased incidence of ADRs in women and in those administered multiple drugs. The higher incidence of ADRs reported in the elderly appears to be largely a function of the increased number of drugs used in this population.

Drug related hospital admissions

Drug-related hospital admissions have been studied by a large number of investigators. Most of these studies are prospective and use active surveillance techniques. However, the definitions employed vary considerably – some report only ADRs whereas others include ADRs, therapeutic failures, and/or intentional overdose (including alcohol abuse). Several studies incorporate restrictive definitions that refer to 'normal doses' of drugs and 'appropriate use,' whereas others interpret the definition broadly to reflect any adverse reaction to a drug. With more restrictive definitions and including only definite/probable ADRs, the percentage of drug-related hospital admissions as a function of total admissions is approximately 3–4%.[39] Using a broader definition of ADR but still excluding intentional overdose and therapeutic failures more than doubles the incidence to 6–11%.[40–48] A far higher incidence rate yet is found in studies that examine drug-related 'adverse events' or 'drug-related problems' associated with hospital admission.[49] The latter include self-poisoning or intentional overdose, as well as therapeutic failures. Incidence rates in these groups ranged from 16% to more than 30%.

In general, there is little consistency across studies with regard to definitions or methodology. However, if one examines the various studies using same definitional criteria and probability scaling methods, the data are remarkably consistent. For example, studies by Cluff et al., Hurwitz et al., Caranosos et al., Lakshmanan et al., and Miller et al. in the Boston Collaborative Drug Surveillance Program used similar restrictive definitions for admission rates related to ADRs, as well as similar probability scaling methods.[50] A consistent incidence rate of 2.9–3.9% was found across diverse patient populations from different geographical areas. Moreover, if one takes the high rates reported by Levy et al. but includes only definite/probable reactions, the ADR rate leading to hospitalization is less than 5%.[51] Similarly, McKenny and Harrison report a rate of 7.9% ADRs resulting in hospitalization, but if only definite/probable ADRs are included, effective rate drops to slightly over 5%.[52] The 5.6% ADRs leading to hospitalization reported by Bergman and Wiholm includes patient noncompliance in nearly 50% of cases; thus their modified rate would only be approximately 3%.[53] The 7% incidence rate reported by Bero et al. is reduced to approximately 4% using more restrictive ADR definitions.[54] Finally, the study by Hallas et al. indicating a 10.6% incidence rate includes both therapeutic failures and 'possible' events; with more restrictive definitions, these rates also approach those indicated above.[55]

A number of other consistent findings can be drawn from these studies. As with many of the outpatient ADR studies, the majority found an increased incidence in women and in the elderly.[56–58] It is also important to recognize that although much of the literature excludes therapeutic failures, noncompliance appears to account for between one-quarter and one-half of all drug-related hospital admissions.[59,60] Unlike idiosyncratic reactions to drugs, noncompliance may be a suitable target for aggressive patient and physician education strategies. Patients who are admitted to the hospital because of ADRs have a much higher probability of sustaining another ADR in the hospital as compared to other patients; for example, Ogilvie and Ruedy noted a 31% incidence of second reactions in patients admitted with an ADR.[61] Like the outpatient ADR studies described previously, certain specialties and/or wards are more likely to have patients hospitalized because of an ADR. For example, Hallas et al. found that patients on the general medicine or geriatrics services had substantially higher incidences than other services.[62]

Adverse drug effects in the hospital setting

A substantial number of studies have examined the incidence of drug-induced illness in hospitalized patients. As in outpatient studies and drug-related hospitalizations, the definitions used, patient populations studied, probability instruments/algorithms employed, and survey methodology are all critical determinants of the incidence rates reported. Retrospective studies, restrictive definitions, or less active surveillance methods were all associated with lower reported incidence rates. The lowest rates reported (0.5%, 0.6%) were in two retrospective studies.[63,64] One used a particularly restrictive definition that included side-effects only if they were significant enough to prolong hospital stay or cause disability at discharge. A rate of 1.5% from a Veteran's Administration study reflected the absence of women patients and the relatively young average patient age (~59 years), as well as the restrictive definition used.[65]

The similar rate of 1.76% reported by Classen et al. was based upon the restrictive WHO definition and excluded therapeutic failures, poisoning, and intentional overdose.[66] In this latter study, virtually all the reported adverse events were in the moderate and severe range, suggesting that many mild reactions may have been omitted; moreover, all services of a community hospital were sampled, which would tend to yield lower rates than found on general medical wards.

Smidt and McQueen noted a relatively low rate of 2.7% across all services of a general hospital with the highest rate of 6% found on the general medical service.[67] However, the surveillance method used required medical and nursing personnel to fill out ADR notification sheets, which may have caused under-reporting. They also used a restrictive definition that excluded side-effects of drugs occurring during the process of maximizing the therapeutic dose, unless these side-effects were especially severe.

Higher rates (in the range of 6–9%) have been reported by other investigators. Shumock et al. noted a rate of 7.5% although an ADR was only listed if it required a major change in patient management.[68] For Burnum, the rate of 8.6% was observed in a population that included all services in a community hospital.[69] Although the more recent study by Bates et al. defined an ADE more broadly, they observed a rate of only 6.5% across 11 medical and surgical units in two university hospitals.[70] However, the rates were considerably higher in the acute medical and intensive care units.

A larger number of studies found incidence rates in the range of 10–18%; most of these involved general medical services.[71–75] Among this group, the highest reported rate was in a study that used a relatively broad definition, that included both diagnostic and therapeutic effects, and that had an especially high degree of surveillance.[76]

The highest incidence rates were found by Dorda (35%)[77] and Levy et al. (27% and 28%).[78] Borda's was a prospective study that utilized a broad definition that included 'possible' cases and had a high degree of surveillance. If one includes only those patients with definite or probable ADRs, the calculated rate is substantially less, approximately 22%. Studies by Levy and colleagues used a broad definition and included 'possible' ADRs. Limiting the findings to only 'probable' or 'definite' cases reduces the incidence to 21%.

As with the outpatient related studies, an increased incidence was found in women and the elderly.[79,80] Once again, higher rates were found in patients on general medical services.[81] Patients who suffered an ADR in the hospital appeared to have longer stays.[82–83] In addition to patients suffering ADRs in the hospital, a considerable number of patients are subjected to medication errors. This issue has been best studied by Bates et al., who observed nearly as many potential (5.5%) as probable/definite (6.5%) ADEs.[84] Potential events were defined as incidents with the potential for producing injury related to a drug, with a major category being medication errors.

The severity of ADRs occurring in the hospital is difficult to compare across studies because of differing definitions. However, the most serious reactions, which are categorized as either 'major' or 'serious' in many of the studies, shows a remarkably wide range of incidences ranging from approximately 0.3% of all patients up to 9%. Median values across studies are approximately 1% for severe reactions. The percentage of fatal reactions due to ADEs likewise varies considerably. Studies by Seidl et al. and

Ogilvie and Ruedy in the 1960s showed the highest rates of drug-related deaths at 1.1% and 2.3% respectively, of all patients.[85,86] In contrast, studies in the 1970s have been lower, ranging from approximately 0.07% to 0.44%.[87,88] Clearly, as for the other categories of ADRs or ADEs, the inclusiveness of the definitions and the rigor of the methodology explains much of the apparent discrepancy in the incidence of serious or reported episodes. Inclusion of overdoses, poisonings and drug abuse or 'possible' reactions markedly affect the reported figures. In addition, the type of active surveillance methods used would be expected to have a considerable impact on the adverse reactions observed. For example, the studies by Bates et al. observed that only 8% of the ADEs noted by them would meet the more restrictive criteria used in their earlier medical practice study by the *same* group.[89]

Costs of adverse drug events

The cost of ADRs or ADE appears to be considerable. Evans et al. have suggested that each ADE in the United States adds approximately $2,000 per patient hospital cost.[90] Not included in this figure are the costs to the patient *per se* in terms of lost work days or the degree of suffering or disability. Malpractice costs relating to iatrogenic illness in general, and to ADRs in particular, are also considerable; drug-induced injuries result in the largest costs for all procedure-related injuries.[91]

How many deaths each year may be attributed to ADRs clearly depends upon the incidence figures utilized. For example, using the median value across studies (which are those reported by Levy and colleagues), more than 150,000 deaths each year may occur in hospitalized patients alone. Insufficient data are available from outpatient studies to determine the number of such individuals who die from ADRs. However, given the number of patients using drugs, both prescription and over-the-counter, thus number must be substantial. No current figures are available with regard to costs relating to hospitalizations caused by ADEs, but if one accepts that 5–10% of hospitalizations are caused by ADRs, approximately two to four million hospitalizations per year are likely to occur on this basis.

Preventability of adverse drug events

Few studies have directly addressed the issue of preventability of ADRs or ADEs. The most rigorous analysis is that by Bates and colleagues, who reported that 28% of ADEs were thought to be preventable, with a notably higher percentage (42%) considered preventable in the class of life-threatening and serious ADEs.[92] Nine out of ten preventable ADEs result from errors in the stages of medication ordering and drug administration. Inadequate knowledge of drug use and dosage, particularly by physicians, accounted for nearly a third of observed errors. Moreover, the majority of errors resulted from systems failures that could potentially be corrected through improved information systems.[93]

Why so many adverse drug events?

The causes of comiogenic drug harm are multifactorial, including the increased use of pharmaceuticals and the frequent administration of multiple drugs to patients with consequent additive or superadditive (synergistic) consequences.

During the past 20 years there has been a diminished role for primary care physicians, who can provide a coordinating role for drug treatment prescribed by multiple health professionals. Many patients are treated by multiple physicians, of whom not one may be aware of the full portfolio of drugs used by a given patient. Moreover, patients may fill prescriptions at different pharmacies, and even in the same pharmacy, the still largely inefficient use of computerized drug screening may fail to alert the patient or the pharmacist to the potential adverse drug–drug, drug–food, or drug–disease reactions. This was shown in a recent study by Cavuto et al., in which nearly a third of pharmacies filled prescriptions with two drugs, the combination of which is known to lead to potentially fatal drug–drug interactions.[94] Of the 48 pharmacies with computerized drug interaction programs, 14 (29%) were ineffective in identifying this well-recognized drug–drug interaction.

Drug compliance by patients remains a major problem; both under-utilization and over-utilization of drugs, particularly in the setting of polypharmacy may be a significant cause of treatment failures and complications of treatment.[95] Use of unprescribed over-the-counter medications in combination with prescription drug-use may also prove hazardous.[96] In addition, a significant number of individuals 'borrow' prescriptions from friends or family members.[97]

Unfortunately, inadequate training of medical students and physicians in clinical pharmacology appears to be a significant contributing factor. Not only are most physicians poorly trained in clinical pharmacology, they also have relatively little knowledge about the pharmacokinetics and pharmacodynamics, or even potential side-effects, of the drugs they are prescribing. Moreover, the source of much information used by physicians in choosing drug treatment is suspect. Indeed, although physicians often report that most of the information about the drugs they use comes from critically reviewed literature and peer-reviewed journals, careful studies do not support this view.[98] Rather, physicians appear to derive most of the information about the drugs they prescribe from pharmaceutical company advertisements or from pharmaceutical company representatives. Thus, selection of drugs used to treat patients often does not reflect careful consideration of treatment options.

Reducing adverse drug events

The systems analysis approach probably provides the best means for reducing the incidence of ADEs, particularly serious ones. Addressing systems errors, rather than individual errors, has become an increasingly accepted strategy used in quality improvement programs in many non-health-related industries. Leape et al. suggest that the same approach should be used to address iatrogenic adverse events, particularly relating to drug use.[99] Employing such methods, they observed that most drug treatment errors resulted from problems with access to and dissemination of information. Computerized ordering systems could be used to alert physicians, nurses, and pharmacists to errors in dosing or to a history of allergic reactions, as well as possible drug–drug, drug–food or drug–disease interactions. Such ordering systems could also be used to limit the options of prescribing physicians, such as requiring unit dosing or limit the doses that can be accepted. Because people make fewer errors when given only appropriate alternatives, standardization of drug treatment to limit choices of doses, frequencies of administration, or routes of administration, would likely reduce treatment mistakes.[100,101]

A relatively high percentage of errors occurs at the time of drug administration by nurses. These errors are less likely to be intercepted and thus prevented than those related to drug ordering, transcription, or dispensing. Such errors would probably best be handled by improved training.[102] Physician education, particularly in the area of clinical pharmacology is also important.[103] During training, medical students often receive most of their education regarding the pharmacokinetics and mechanisms of drug use during their preclinical years. Enhanced and integrated clinical pharmacology during the clinical training years would be useful. It has also been suggested that centers for education and research in therapeutics be established in experimental therapeutics, to provide information as well as pharmacology education to physicians on an ongoing basis; such information mechanisms would serve as a counterbalance to the present system in which information regarding new drugs is being provided predominantly through representatives of pharmaceutical companies.[104]

Summary

In summary, ADEs are the leading cause of iatrogenic illness in the hospitalized patient, and may account for nearly 10% of hospitalizations. Use of systems approaches, which utilize continuous quality improvement strategies adapted from successful non-health-related industries, may help to reduce this problem. Improved access to and dissemination of information, greater standardization of treatments, and improved education/training should also serve to address this frequent type of iatrogenic harm.

Endnotes

1 Strom BL, Tugwell P. Pharmacoepidemiology: Current status, prospects, and problems. *Ann Intern Med* 1990; 113:179–81.
2 Warner JH. *The Therapeutic Perspective: Medical Practice, Knowledge and Identity in America 1820–1885*. Cambridge, MA: Harvard University Press, 1986.
3 Young JH. *Pure Food*. Princeton University Press, 1989, p. 29.
4 Young JH. The marketing of patent medicines in Lincoln's Springfield. *Pharmacy in History* 1985; 27:98–102.
5 Young JH (see No. 3).
6 Estes SW. Public pharmacology: modes of action of nineteenth century "patent" medicines. *Medical Heritage* 1986; 2:218–28.
7 Temin P. *Taking Your Medicine: Drug Regulation in the United States*. Harvard University Press, 1980, p. 1–10.
8 Temin P (see No. 7).
9 Temin P (see No. 7).
10 Rawlins MD. Clinical pharmacology: Adverse Reactions to drugs. *Br Med J* 1981; 282:974–6.
11 Melmon KL. Preventable drug reactions: Causes and cures. *N Engl J Med* 1971; 284:1361–8.
12 Karch FE, Lasagna L. Adverse drug reactions: A critical review *JAMA* 1975; 234:1236–41.
13 Karch FE, Lasagna L (see No. 12).
14 Schimmel EM. The hazards of hospitalization. *Ann Intern Med* 1964; 60:100–10.
15 Ogilvie RI, Ruedy J. Adverse drug reactions during hospitalization. *Can Med Assn J* 1967; 97:1450–7.
16 Borda IT, Slone D, Jick H. Assessment of adverse reactions within a drug surveillance program. *JAMA* 1968; 205:645–7.

17 Seidl LG, Thornton GF, Smith JW, Cluff LE. Studies on the epidemiology of adverse drug reactions. III: Reactions in patients on a general medical service. *Bull Johns Hopkins Hosp* 1966; 119:299–315.
18 Reidenberg MM. Registry of adverse drug reactions. *JAMA* 1968; 203(1):31–4.
19 World Health Organization. International drug monitoring – the role of the hospital. World Health Organization Drug Intelligence. *Clin Pharm* 1970; 4:101.
20 Pearson KC, Kennedy DC. Adverse drug reactions and the Food and Drug Administration. *J Pharm Pract* 1989; 2:209–10.
21 Karch FE, Lasagna L (see No. 12).
22 Bates DW, Cullen DJ, Laird N, et al. Incidence of adverse drug events and potential adverse drug events. *JAMA* 1995; 274:29–34.
23 Schumock GT, Thornton JP, Witte KW, et al. Comparison of pharmacy-based concurrent surveillance and medical record retrospective reporting of adverse drug reactions. *AJHP* 1991; 48:1974–6.
24 Prosser TR, Kamysz PL. Multidisciplinary adverse drug reaction surveillance program. *Am J Hosp Pharm* 1990; 47:1334–9.
25 Borda IT, Slone D, Jick H (see No. 16).
26 Classen DC, Pestotnik SL, Evans RS, Burke JP. Computerized surveillance of adverse drug events in hospital patients. *JAMA* 1991; 266(20):2847–51.
27 Naranjo CA, Busto U, Sellers EM, et al. A method for estimating the probability of adverse drug reactions. *Clin Pharmacol Ther* 1981; 30:239–45.
28 Kramer MS, Leventhal JM, Hutchinson TA, et al. An algorithm for the operational assessment of adverse drug reactions. *JAMA* 1979; 242:623–32.
29 Kramer MS, Leventhal JM, Hutchinson TA, et al. (see No. 28).
30 Karch FE, Lasagna L (see No. 12).
31 Kellaway GSM, McCrae E. Intensive monitoring for adverse drug effects in patients discharged from acute medical wards. *NZ Med J* 1973; 78:525–8.
32 Stewart RB, Cluff LE. Studies on the epidemiology of adverse drug reactions: VI: Utilization and interactions of prescription and non-prescription drugs in outpatients. *Johns Hopkins Med J* 1971; 129:319–31.
33 Campbell WH, Johnson RE, Senft RA, Azevedo DJ. Treated adverse effects of drugs in an ambulatory population. *Med Carer* 1977; 15:599–608.
34 Martys CR. Adverse reactions to drugs in general practice. *Br Med J* 1979; 2:1194–7.
35 Klein LE, German PS, Levine DM, et al. Medication problems among patients: a study with emphasis on the elderly. *Arch Int Med* 1984; 144:1185–8.
36 Hutchinson TA, Flegel KM, Kramer MS, et al. Frequency, severity and risk factors for adverse drug reactions in adult out-patients: A prospective study. *J Chron Dis* 1986; 39(7):533–42.
37 Schneider JK, Mion, LC, Frengley JD, et al. Adverse drug reactions in an elderly outpatient population. *Am J Hosp Pharm* 1992; 49:90–6.
38 Naranjo CA, Busto U, Sellers EM, et al. (see No. 27).
39 Miller RR. Hospital admissions due to adverse drug reactions. *Arch Intern Med* 1974; 134:219–23.
40 Levy M, Nir I, Birnbaum D, et al. Adverse reactions to drugs in hospitalized medical patients. *Isr J Med Sci* 1973; 9:617–26.
41 Black AJ, Somers K. Drug related illness resulting in hospital admissions. *J R Coll Physicians London* 1984; 18:40–1.

42 Ghose K. Hospital bed occupancy due to drug related problems. *J Roy Soc Med* 1980, 73:853–6.
43 Davidsen F, Hughfelt T, Gram LF, Brøsen K. Adverse drug reactions and non-compliance as primary causes of admission to a cardiology department. *Eur J Clin Pharmacol* 1988; 34:83–86.
44 Ives TJ, Bentz EJ, Gwyther RE. Drug related admissions to a family medicine inpatient service. *Arch Intern Med* 1987; 147:1117–20.
45 Colt HG, Shapiro AP. Drug-induced illness as a cause for admission to a community hospital. *J Am Geriatr Soc* 1989; 37:323–6.
46 Hurwitz N. Admissions to hospital due to drugs. *Br Med J* 1969; 1:539–40.
47 Caranasos GJ, Stewart RB, Cluff LE. Drug-induced illness leading to hospitalization. *JAMA* 1974; 228:713–17.
48 Grymonpre RE, Mitenko PA, Sitar DS, et al. Drug associated hospital admissions in older medical patients. *J Am Geriatr Soc* 1988; 36:1092–8.
49 Black AJ, Somers K. Drug related illness resulting in hospital admissions. *J R Coll Physicians London* 1984; 18:40–1.
50 Miller RR. (see No. 39).
51 Levy M, Nir I, Birnbaum D, et al. (see No. 40).
52 McKenny JM, Harrison WL. Drug-related hospital admissions. *Am J Hosp Pharm* 1976; 33(8):792–5.
53 Bergman U, Wiholm B-E. Drug related problems causing admission to a medical clinic. *Eur J Clin Pharmac* 1981; 20:193–200.
54 Bero LA, Lipton HL, Bird JA. Characterization of geriatric drug-related hospital readmissions. *Med Care* 1991; 29(10):989–1003.
55 Hallas J, Gram LF, Grodum E, Damsbo N, et al. Drug related admissions to medical wards: a population based survey *Br J Clin Pharmacol* 1992; 33(1):61–8.
56 Miller RR (see No. 39).
57 Hallas J, Gram LF, Grodum E, Damsbo N, et al. (see No. 55).
58 Colt HG, Shapiro AP. Drug-induced illness as a cause for admission to a community hospital. *J Am Geriatr Soc* 1989; 37:323–6.
59 Miller RR (see No. 39).
60 Davidsen F, Hughfelt T, Gram LF, Brçsen K (see No. 43).
61 Ogilvie RI, Ruedy J (see No. 15).
62 Hallas J, Gram LF, Grodum E, Damsbo N, et al. (see No. 55).
63 Reidenberg MM (see No. 18)
64 Leape LL, Brennan TA, Laird N, et al. The nature of adverse events in hospitalized patients. Results of the Harvard Medical Practice Study II. *N Engl J Med* 1991, 324(6): 377–84.
65 Wang RIH, Terry LC. Adverse drug reactions in a Veterans Administration Hospital. *J Clin Pharmacol* 1971; 11:14–18.
66 Classen DC, Pestotnik SL, Evans RS, Burke JP. Computerized surveillance of adverse drug events in hospital patients. *JAMA* 1991; 266(20):2847–51.
67 Smidt NA, McQueen EG. Adverse reactions to drugs: A comprehensive hospital inpatient survey. *NZ Med J* 1972; 76:397–401.
68 Schumock GT, Thornton JP, Witte KW, et al. (see No. 23).
69 Burnum JF. Letter: Preventability of adverse drug reactions. *Ann Intern Med* 1976; 85(1):80–1.
70 Bates DW, et al. (see No. 22).
71 Schimmel EM. The hazards of hospitalization. *Ann Intern Med* 1964; 60:100–10.

72 Borda IT, Slone D, Jick H (see No. 16).
73 Ogilvie RI, Ruedy J (see No. 15).
74 Miller RR (see No. 39).
75 Simmons M, Parker JM, Gowdy CW, et al. Adverse drug reactions during hospitalization (letter). *Can Med Assoc J* 1968; 98175.
76 Ogilvie RI, Ruedy J (see No. 15).
77 Borda IT, Slone D, Jick H (see No. 16).
78 Levy M, Nir I, Birnbaum D, et al. (see No. 40).
79 Hurwitz N. Predisposing factors in adverse reactions to drugs. *Brit Med J* 1969; 1:536–9.
80 Seidl LG, Thornton GF, Smith JW, Cluff LE. Studies on the epidemiology of adverse drug reactions. III: Reactions in patients on a general medical service. *Bull Johns Hopkins Hosp* 1966; 119:299–315.
81 Smidt NA, McQueen EG. Adverse reactions to drugs: A comprehensive hospital inpatient survey. *NZ Med J* 1972; 76:397–401.
82 Ogilvie RI, Ruedy J (see No. 15).
83 Evans RS, Classen DC, Stevens LE, et al. Using a hospital information system to access the effects of adverse drug reactions. *Bull Johns Hopkins Hosp* 1966; 1191:299–315.
84 Bates DW, Cullen DJ, Laird N, et al. (see No. 22).
85 Ogilvie RI, Ruedy J (see No. 15).
86 Seidl LG, Thronton GF, Smith JW, Cluff LE. Studies on the epidemiology of adverse drug reactions. III: Reactions in patients on a general medical service. *Bull Johns Hopkins Hosp* 1966; 119:299–315.
87 Smidt NA, McQueen EG. Adverse reactions to drugs: A comprehensive hospital inpatient survey. *NZ Med J* 1972; 76:397–401.
88 Porter J, Jick H. Drug related deaths among medical in-patients. *JAMA* 1977; 237:879.
89 Bates DW, Cullen DJ, Laird N, et al. (see No. 22).
90 Evans RS, Classen DC, Stevens LE, et al. Using a hospital information system to access the effects of adverse drug reactions. *Bull Johns Hopkins Hosp* 1966; 1191:299–315.
91 National Association of Insurance Commissioners. Medical Malpractice Closed Claims, 1975–1978. Brookfield, WI: National Association of Insurance Commissioners; 1980.
92 Bates DW, Cullen DJ, Laird N, et al. (see No. 22).
93 Leape LL, Bates DW, Cullen DJ, et al. Systems analysis of adverse drug events. *JAMA* 1995; 274:35–43.
94 Cavuto NJ, Woosley RL, Sale M. Pharmacies and the prevention of fatal drug interactions. *JAMA* 1996; 275:1086–8.
95 Melmon KL. Preventable drug reactions: Causes and cures. *N Engl J Med* 1971; 284:1361–8.
96 Melmon KL (see No. 95).
97 Melmon KL (see No. 95).
98 Avorn J, Chren M, Hartley R. Scientific versus commercial sources of influence on the previous behavior of physicians. *Am J Med* 1982; 73:4–8. McGettigan P, Chan R, McManus J, et al. Sources of drug information in prescribing in general practice. *Br J Clin Pharmacol* 1994; 7:512–3.
99 Leape LL, Bates DW, Cullen DJ, et al. Systems analysis of adverse drug events. *JAMA* 1995; 274:35–43.
100 Melmon KL (see No. 95).

101 Leape LL, Bates DW, Cullen DJ, et al. (see No. 93).
102 Leape LL, Bates DW, Cullen DJ, et al. (see No. 93).
103 Melmon KL (see No. 95).
104 Woosley RL. Centers for education and research in therapeutics. *Clin Pharm Therap* 1992; 55:249–55.

9

Unnecessary surgery

In the context of surgery, the term 'iatrogenic illness' or 'iatrogenic complication' has been reserved for surgical mishaps and adverse surgical outcomes. Although these outcomes may secondarily give rise to an assessment that a procedure was itself unnecessary or inappropriate,[1] unnecessary surgery *per se* has not traditionally been recognized as an iatrogenic harm. One explanation for this may be that attention to unnecessary surgery has primarily come from private or governmental insurers who have tended to focus on the direct aggregate economic costs of the phenomenon rather than on its indirect or intangible human costs in morbidity, mortality, pain, suffering, or loss of livelihood to individuals. In other words, from the point of view of health policy, unnecessary surgery has been understood principally as a problem of 'surgical overuse' rather than iatrogenic harm. Another reason why unnecessary surgery has not itself been regarded as a patient harm may be a general skepticism about even the occurrence of unnecessary surgery. If we understand an unnecessary surgery to be one that offers no anticipated preponderance of benefit to the patient, then many would argue that no doctor would perform such a surgery. This view is of course countered by another common impression that such surgeries do occur and that the only identifiable benefits that accrue from them are remunerative ones to the physician.

In this chapter, we explore both what is meant by the term unnecessary surgery and the evidence that has been offered to explain the scope and nature of the problem. Our identification of unnecessary surgery as a form of iatrogenic harm presupposes that surgery, as an invasive intervention, is *de facto* harmful. One of the essential justifying conditions for this harm (as well as the associated risks of nosocomial infection and adverse anesthesia events) is a greater anticipated benefit to the patient. When a surgery is unnecessary, this justifying condition is absent.

Historical antecedents

In 1910, Abraham Flexner's survey of medical education in the United States revealed that members of the overcrowded surgical profession were poorly educated and poorly trained. Flexner also described how fierce competition for surgical patients resulted in fee splitting and unnecessary surgery.[2] In response to these findings, the American College of Surgeon's (ACS) proposed to institute reforms in surgical practice and the quality of hospital care. The core of the ACS program was Codman's End-Result System. Although Codman's proposal had focused on the processes and outcomes of hospital and surgical care, the Minimum Standard instituted by the ACS in 1918 shifted the emphasis to an institution's organizational structure. The implicit assumption of this emphasis was that a hospital in compliance with key structural standards, such as staff credentialing, systematic medical record keeping, the establishment of internal committees, and diagnostic and therapeutic facilities, would, accordingly, furnish good quality surgical and medical care.

This indirect assessment of quality was consonant with the established tradition of strictly personal accountability. By stressing the hospital and staff's capacity to do good work – reflected in criteria of organizational structure and educational qualifications – rather than *the work itself* – reflected in criteria for evaluating technical competence, patient outcomes, and surgical necessity – the Minimum Standard left undisturbed the ethos of professional autonomy. This intensive focus on structural guidelines also supplanted Codman's original and more contentious question of a hospital's rates of unnecessary operations and surgical failures.

By the late 1940s, medical and surgical advances used on the battlefield began to be applied in great numbers to the civilian patient population. This development, coupled with the achievement of desired uniformity in hospital structure, led to a renewed attention to the problem of unnecessary surgery. In the 1940s and 1950s this attention was manifested in the United States in medical audits and the establishment of hospital tissue committees.[3] Arguing in favor of the medical audit to determine the rates of surgical mortality and morbidity associated with individual surgeons, one New York physician made oblique reference to prevailing indirect standards of quality saying, that because a hospital has 'socially prominent trustees, and large elaborate buildings with beautiful surroundings, it does not follow that the patients of that hospital have received the skillful treatment they have a right to expect.'[4]

Early methods to curb unnecessary surgery

In the 1950s, audits of gynecological surgery revealed that normal ovaries were routinely removed[5] and that as many as 36% of hysterectomies failed to meet explicit criteria indicating the need for the surgery.[6] During this same period, studies of tonsillectomy and adenoidectomy revealed that over 50% of children in a general patient population had had one or both of these procedures before their teenage years, with the majority of these surgeries conferring no benefit to the patient.[7]

During this period in the United States, the hospital tissue committee was initiated to provide a method of evaluating the quality of presurgical diagnosis and the appropriateness of surgical intervention. The removal of tissue determined to be normal was believed to provide direct evidence that a surgery was unjustified. The prevalence of inappropriate surgery was then gleaned from the reduction in targeted procedures that followed feedback on normal pathology. In 1952, Weinert and Brill reported a 15% reduction in appendectomies following two years of surveillance by a tissue committee.[8] In 1958, Verda and Platt reported that appendectomies decreased by 60% following the establishment of tissue review.[9]

The evidence provided by tissue committees proved of limited use in determining the extent of unnecessary surgery. According to one 1947 account, pathology reports tended to contain euphemistic terms apparently in an effort to avoid the outright declaration that a surgeon had removed essentially normal tissue.[10] Tissue committee data were also called into question by the practice of postponing the recording of postoperative observations until after the operation and pathology report had been done. Evidence from pathologic review was also ultimately acknowledged to be a logically insufficient basis for conclusions regarding the prevalence of unnecessary surgery. One cannot validly argue from a correlation between pathologic review and reduction in surgeries, that the surgeries foregone were inappropriate. In addition, by targeting only those surgeries that involved the removal of tissue, pathologic evidence provided, at best, only a narrow picture of surgeries that might be called into question.

Tissue review and medical audits were also seriously hindered by the definition of unnecessary surgery under which they operated. In the 1950s, the ACS defined an unnecessary or unjustified surgery as one 'not supported by clinical reasoning and judgment and which is not confirmed in diagnosis by disease actually found.'[11] One weakness of this definition was its exclusion of procedures such as cesarean section that did not result in tissue subjected to pathologic confirmation. In addition, for those surgeries that did result in tissue removal, the definition failed to allow an error rate for the removal of normal tissue where preoperative symptoms indicated the presence of abnormality. Finally, the definition turned on the imprecise expression 'clinical reason and judgment.' and, in this way, the definition sidestepped the question of *conflicting* professional judgment and how such conflicts should be resolved.

In the United States during the 1940s and 1950s, the establishment of industrial and other employer-sponsored medical programs and commercial insurance and indemnity plans such as Blue Cross and Blue Shield solidified the role of the third party payer in health care. As the cost and utilization of surgical services increased over the following two decades, third party payers, including the federal government under Medicare, sought to address the problem of unnecessary surgery through surgical second opinion programs and other indirect controls on surgical utilization. Payers were galvanized in their attention to unnecessary surgery by two provocative studies in the early 1970s. One study by Bunker[12] showed a much higher per capita utilization of surgical services in the United States than in Britain. A 1974 study by McCarthy and Widmer[13] showed a high rate of surgeries to be unconfirmed by surgical second opinion.

The study by Bunker reported that in 1967 there were twice as many surgeons in proportion to population in the United States as in England and Wales and that American surgeons performed twice as many operations as their British counterparts. Although these data did not definitively support an interpretation of overuse on the part of American physicians, non-clinical factors such as fee-for-service reimbursement, solo practice, and a more aggressive therapeutic approach by American surgeons was correlated with the greater number of operations in the United States.

The McCarthy and Widmer study was the first report of a surgical second opinion program. Based on their study of elective operations in members of the Storeworker's union, these authors reported that the proportion of cases unconfirmed by second opinion was 16.4% for general surgery, 31.4% for gynecology, 40.3% for orthopedics, 16.3% for ear, nose, and throat, 28.2% for ophthalmology, and 35.8% for urology. Based on an overall non-confirmation rate of 24%, McCarthy and Widmer estimated that the total savings represented by unconfirmed (and, therefore, unperformed) surgeries was approximately $580,000. Although the authors stated that the purpose of the program was 'to help patients make a more informed decision,'[14] and cautioned that their findings could not be extrapolated to the general population, the data were used in a House

Subcommittee on Oversight and Investigation to estimate the national rate of unnecessary surgery. Based on the McCarthy and Widmer data, the Moss subcommittee conjectured that in 1974, 17% or nearly two and a half million of the surgeries in the United States were unnecessary. These surgeries, the committee concluded, resulted in 12,000 preventable deaths and cost roughly $3.9 billion.[15]

As Leape[16] points out, the prospect of fewer unnecessary surgeries and enormous anticipated savings motivated the prompt institution of second opinion programs by the US Department of Health, Education and Welfare and many private insurers and employers. By 1988, in the United States 148 large firms had instituted coverage limits if a patient failed to obtain a second opinion.[17] These programs were intended to curb surgical overuse and, in the process, to provide indirect evidence of the extent of the problem. Surgical second opinion programs (SSOPs) have failed in both of these respects. First, many studies since McCarthy and Widmer, have repeatedly shown a confirmation rate of 90% or better. Second, a 1985 study of the Massachusetts Medicaid SSOP found that although targeted operations were reduced by 24%, only 2% of the reduction was the direct result of nonconfirmation. The other 22% was, Leape says, due to the 'sentinel effect' – physicians recommended fewer surgeries when they learned that second opinions would be obtained. In addition, few if any controlled studies have been done to assess the health status of patients whose decisions have been influenced by second opinion programs.

The usefulness of SSOP in measuring unnecessary surgery is limited also by the inherent shortcomings of unstructured implicit review – the type of review most common in SSOPs. In implicit review, the second surgeon, like the first, bases the recommendation on his or her own experience and clinical judgment. Without the use of explicit criteria, however, there is no a priori reason to assume that the second opinion was any better than the first. In other words, difference of opinion is not a sufficient basis on which to evaluate a surgery as unnecessary.[18] Ironically, the use of implicit criteria by independent reviewers may in fact increase one's chance of a surgical recommendation.[19] In a 1934 study of tonsillectomy – a surgery whose indications were at that time a subject of controversy – 60% of a sample of 1000 New York school children had already had their tonsils removed. Of the remaining 40% examined by a school physician, close to half were recommended for the surgery. Those not recommended were then re-examined by a second set of physicians and again close to half were recommended for the procedure. In their commentary on the study, Wennberg et al. report that 'after three successive "second opinions," only 67 out of the original 1000 were spared a recommendation for tonsillectomy.'[20]

During the mid-1970s, the ACS and the American Surgical Association jointly offered a revised definition of unnecessary surgery in their *Study on Surgical Services for the United States*. The study defined six categories of operation that might be termed unnecessary:[21]

(1) Completely discretionary operations for asymptomatic, non-pathologic, non-threatening disorders.
(2) Operations where no pathological tissue is removed.
(3) Operations where indications are a matter of difference in judgment and opinion among experts.
(4) Operations to alleviate endurable and tolerable symptoms
(5) Operations formerly performed [but] . . . now considered outdated, obsolete, or discredited.
(6) operations for which there is little justification by clinical, X-ray or laboratory study, that are done primarily for the personal gain of the surgeon, wherein the weight of informed opinion would deny any indication to be present.

This classification identified some useful parameters: an unnecessary intervention was one that was unsupported by clinical and laboratory evidence; one whose main objective was the surgeon's personal gain; or one that has been discredited. Not so helpful, however, was the identification of discretionary or 'comfort' surgeries as 'unnecessary' without some preliminary determination of the *legitimate* purposes or aims of surgical intervention. Perceptions of medical need are not motivated solely by biological values but may be closely linked to aesthetic or social norms or personal preferences. The third category of unnecessary operations as those in which indications are a 'matter of difference in judgment among experts' anticipates the consensus review approach that emerged in the 1980s as the authoritative basis for surgical indications. The evidentiary value of expert consensus continues, however, to be the subject of considerable debate – its greatest challenge coming from those who hold randomized controlled trials to offer evidentiary superiority.

Geographic variations

Since the 1970 study by Bunker, a large literature has emerged documenting geographically-based variations in the utilization of medical and surgical services. Variations similar to those reported by Bunker have been demonstrated in studies by Wennberg,[22] Leape[23] and others.[24] Wennberg and Gittleson's 1973 study of surgical rates in 13 Vermont hospital service areas, for example, found that the number of procedures performed per 10,000 persons ranged from 13 to 151 for tonsillectomy, 10 to 32 for appendectomy, and from 30 to 141 for dilation and curettage.[25] In a study of Medicare enrollees, Leape at al.[26] found that use rates per 10,000 enrollees varied from 13 to 150 for coronary angiography, 5 to 41 for carotid endarterectomy and 42 to 164 for upper gastrointestinal tract endoscopy. In a recent study of coronary artery bypass surgery (CABS) in the United States and Canada, Anderson et al.[27] found that in 1989, the age-adjusted rate of CABS in California was 27% higher than in New York and 80% higher than in three Canadian provinces combined.

These data support a number of different theories both on the factors contributing to an area's total rate of surgical utilization and on the factors contributing to rate variations between areas. Regarding total use within an area, studies have repeatedly shown that the supply of surgical resources (surgeons, surgeon's time, operating rooms, hospital beds) is a major determinant of utilization.[28] In a 1969 study, C. E. Lewis referred to this phenomenon as a 'medical variation of Parkinson's law: patient admissions for surgery expand to fill beds, operating suites and surgeons' time.'[29]

Although *utilization* within a region seems to be positively related to the supply matrix, there is conflicting evidence regarding the effect of supply on rate *variations* between regions. Wennberg and Gittelsohn found no correlation between regional rate variations and the number of physicians or the supply of hospital beds.[30] By contrast, Mitchell and Cromwell[31] and Vayda et al.[32] found as much as 62% of variation to be attributable to bed and specialist supply.

The most intuitively plausible explanation for regional variation in surgical use is epidemiological – surgical rate variations are attributable to the difference in disease incidence of regional populations. Greater medical need demands proportionally greater provision of services. In the studies that have been done to test this hypothesis, however, no such correlation has been found. In studies by Roos et al., there was no association between tonsillectomy rates and rates of respiratory infection, or between high hysterectomy rates and clinical need.[33] In a narrower study of practice variations and cesarean section, there was no correlation between patient obstetric risk and high cesarean rates.[34] As for demographic predictors of demand for surgical services, Leape points out that although surgical utilization is higher in older patients, in women, in doctors and their families, and in those with higher incomes, these predictors account for only a small fraction of rate variation.[35]

The most compelling explanation for differences in surgical utilization rates is not the matrix of supply or demand but, rather, professional uncertainty regarding the indications for surgical treatment. Based on decades of research, Wennberg and others have concluded that professional uncertainty regarding the value of a procedure and the indications for its use give rise to practice styles that favor high or low use. The best evidence for this hypothesis is that higher rates of variation are associated with procedures that lack professional consensus as to their efficacy and clinical indications (such as carotid endarterectomy). Where there is overall professional agreement about the efficacy and indications for a procedure (such as inguinal hernia repair or fractured hip) variation is least.[36]

Although the phenomenon of geographic variation raises a number of interesting questions, the one that is of direct concern here is to what extent rate variation is indicative of unnecessary surgery. As many investigators have pointed out, sheer variation itself does not reflect the *extent* of surgical overuse. Indeed, surgical rate variation may be an indicator *either* of overuse or underuse.[37] The more specific question of whether high use rates are indicative of overuse was investigated by the RAND Corporation in the 1987 Health Services Utilization Study (HSUS).[30] In this study, over 75 million Medicare payment claims provided the data base for measuring the rates of use for six common procedures. These were carotid endarterectomy, coronary angiography, upper gastrointestinal endoscopy, coronary bypass surgery, colonoscopy, and cholecystectomy.

The RAND study represents a watershed in the conceptualization of the problem of surgical utilization. By shifting the focus of research from unnecessary surgery to 'appropriateness' the RAND study makes it explicit that judgments about surgical overuse and the provision of unnecessary services depend on *prior* judgments about the criteria for *appropriate* use. In short, the RAND study operates on the logical assumption that we cannot determine whether something is being done incorrectly until we know the parameters for doing it correctly. The implications of this shift are profound. In the problematic of 'unnecessary surgery,' the implicit assumption is that an intervention is effective (necessary) until proven otherwise (unnecessary). The problematic of 'appropriateness,' however, shifts the burden of proof and in so doing mandates a more rigorous attention to the evidentiary basis of surgical practice.

From the 1940s to the 1960s, control of surgical utilization occurred largely through the *indirect* means of tissue committee review, surgical audits, and SSOPs. During this time, the authority of the medical profession was largely preserved by the fee-for-service reimbursement structure.[39] Since the mid-1970s, however, fee-for-service has declined and third party payers have become more involved in utilization decisions. In the process, surgeons have increasingly been subject to *direct* controls through utilization review and approval. The shift in the evidentiary justification for practice has become a fundamental element of cost containment efforts in the changing structure of health care financing and delivery. As Relman has observed, medicine has entered an era of 'assessment and accountabiliy.'[40] As institutional payers increasingly seek to guarantee that they are getting value for their health care dollars, they demand evidence that benefits actually accrue from the services for which they pay. But, as Relman says, the phenomenon of geographic variation unaccompanied by discernible differences in outcome 'has led to the suspicion that in many cases [medicine] still has much to learn about the indications for a given course of action or the reasons for choosing one procedure over another.'[41] The findings of the RAND appropriateness research added to this suspicion.

Findings from the RAND Health Services Utilization Study

In the HSUS, RAND researchers defined an appropriate procedure as,

one in which the expected health benefits of doing a procedure (i.e. increased life expectancy, relief of pain, reduction of anxiety, improved functional capacity) exceed the expected negative consequences (i.e. mortality, morbidity, anxiety of anticipating the procedure, pain produced by the procedure, time lost from work) by a sufficiently wide margin that the procedure [is] worth doing.[42]

This definition has two important components. First, unlike earlier definitions of unnecessary surgery, it assesses the appropriateness of surgery in terms of patient benefit as the explicitly stated endpoint of care. In this way, it hearkens back to Codman's original criterion of therapeutic efficiency. Secondly, by introducing the notion of a surgery's 'worth' it signals the fundamentally evaluative nature of the concept of appropriateness. The appropriateness of a surgical procedure is not *simply* a function of its expectation of net clinical benefit to the patient but also of the way in which benefit is understood and valued by patients and others in the decision-making process.

The RAND HSUS was a consensus review of care in 13 large geographic areas. This study identified substantial levels of inappropriate use for three procedures: 17% for coronary angiography and upper gastrointestinal endoscopy, and 32% for carotid endarterectomy. For two of these procedures, rates of inappropriate use were consistent over high- and low-use areas, for the third (coronary angiography) 28% of rate variation was attributable to inappropriate use although this variance was identified with a single outlier county. Although the RAND findings failed to support the hypothesis that rate variations are caused by inappropriate overuse of services in high-use areas,[43] they provide little consolation regarding the overall incidence of inappropriate surgery, at least for certain controversial procedures. At rates of inappropriateness between 15% and 40%, consistent over *both* high- and low-use areas, the extent of overuse identified by RAND was considerable. The RAND studies provide some of the best evidence to date on the incidence of inappropriate or unnecessary surgery. The strength of these studies lies in their use of explicit, rather than implicit, criteria for the assessment of each procedure. Table 1 summarizes data gathered from RAND and other explicit criteria studies from 1977 to 1993. Although particular procedures were studied often precisely because they had been identified as controversial rather than representative, the findings can reasonably support the conclusion that at least 10% of invasive interventions are unnecessary.

Why does unnecessary surgery occur?

Financial incentives

There are numerous theories that have been offered to explain the occurrence of unnecessary surgery. Perhaps the one dominant in popular culture is that physician greed leads to unscrupulous practices. Although greed may certainly motivate some individuals, the financial incentives built into reimbursement systems may constitute a broader, systemic impetus for the provision of unnecessary care. In the 1911 preface to his play *The Doctor's Dilemma*, G. B. Shaw deplores how the pecuniary incentives created by fee-for-service arrangements encourage bad practice: 'It is not the fault of our doctors,' he says,

that the medical service of the community, as at present provided for, is a murderous absurdity. That any sane nation, having observed that you could provide for the supply of bread by giving bakers a pecuniary interest in baking for you, should go on to give a surgeon a pecuniary interest in cutting off your leg, is enough to make one despair of political humanity. But that is precisely what we have done. And the more appalling the mutilation, the more the mutilators is paid. He who

Table 9.1. *Explicit criteria studies addressing unnecessary or inappropriate procedures*[44]

Year	Procedure	Number	Unnecessary/ inappropriate (%)	Reference number
1977	Tonsillectomy	3072	86	45
1986	Carotid Endarterectomy	107	13	46
1987	Coronary angiography	1677	17	47
1987	Gastrointestinal endoscopy	1585	17[††]	48
1988	Carotid endarterectomy	1302	32[††]	49
1988	CABG*	386	14[††]	50
1988	Pacemaker	382	20	51
1990	Hysterectomy	257	8	52
1990	Coronary angiography	320	21[††]	53
1990	CABG*	319	16[††]	54
1991	Carotid endarterectomy	2200	17	55
1993	CABG*	1388	2[††]	56
1993	PTCA[†]	1306	4[††]	57
1993	Coronary angiography	1355	4[††]	58
1993	Hysterectomy	642	16[††]	59

*Coronary artery bypass graft
[†]Percutaneous transluminal coronary angioplasty
[††]Indicates RAND studies

corrects the ingrown toe-nail receives a few shillings: he who cuts your inside out receives hundreds of guineas.[60]

Although the data are scant, there is some evidence to support Shaw's concern. In a review of organizational and financial influences on patterns of surgical care, LoGerfo found that economic incentives contribute to a higher rate of unnecessary surgery in fee-for-service arrangements than in pre-paid systems of care.[61] In a related study, a decrease in Colorado Medicare reimbursement rates resulted in an increase of the provision of more intensive and complex services.[62] Unnecessary surgery may also be encouraged in fee-for-service arrangements which tend to disproportionately reward procedures rather than cognitive services.[63] In comparisons of fee-for-service and prepayment structures it is important to keep in mind that these different financial incentives may encourage either overuse or underuse respectively.[64] A complementary finding in LoGerfo's comparative analysis of fee-for-service and prepayment arrangements is that although they are appropriate candidates for surgery, some HMO (Health Maintenance Organization) patients may not be offered the surgical option because of its high cost.[65] As prepayment and capitation strategies increase under managed care, the incentives for unnecessary surgery may well be eclipsed by those that encourage surgical underuse. From the point of view of comiogenic illness, in other words, harms associated with the inappropriate performance of surgery may well be overtaken in this area by the harms associated with the omission of indicated surgeries.

Structures of the medical marketplace – supply and demand

As noted in our discussion above, the supply side of health care delivery has also been suspected of contributing to surgical overuse. The data, however, are mixed on the extent to which physician or hospital supply encourages unneeded operations. On the demand side, 'ritualistic surgeries' and fad operations have been held partially accountable for surgical overuse. Writing in 1969, Bolande[66] observed that tonsillectomy, widely practiced despite its meager scientific justification, was performed much more often in the children of wealth. This, he speculated, might have reflected parent's equation of tonsillectomy with social status. Indeed, sociologists have observed that as a culture rises above the poverty level, it tends to value goods more for their social or cultural meaning than for their use.[67] Although ritualistic and 'fad' operations may be responsible for some percentage of unnecessary surgery, these motivations raise the central conceptual question of how to define 'necessity' in this context. To claim that surgeries inspired by ritual beliefs, or by consumer demand are 'unnecessary' is to beg the question of appropriateness or the legitimate aims of surgical care. As Eisenberg has pointed out, medical need is manifested not only as a biological phenomenon but also as a matter of tastes and preferences, the price that patients and providers pay and the resources available to them.[68] Accordingly, any attempt to define medical necessity or appropriateness must attend to these diverse sources of value that inform medical decision-making. As we will see in our next chapter, how and by whom appropriateness is defined has important practical and ethical implications that bear on the subject of patient harm and the assumption of risk. Before we turn to this conceptual question, however, we look at two more theories on why unnecessary surgery occurs.

Defensive medicine

The term 'defensive medicine' is typically understood to refer to instances where a health care provider's practice decisions are motivated primarily by the desire to protect him- or herself from the risk of legal liability. Defensive practice strategies may take at least two forms – risk avoidance and risk reduction.[69] *Risk avoidance* involves refraining from practices that are accompanied by a high degree of perceived malpractice risk. Thus, providers may cut back on the care of 'high-risk' patients or on the use of specific 'high-risk' procedures such as we saw in the case of nineteenth-century bone-setting. Both of these risk avoidance strategies have been recently identified in the practice of obstetrics. Fewer physicians now provide obstetric services at all and concerns about bad outcomes to infants delivered vaginally have played a part in the four-fold increase in cesarean sections from 5.5% of all deliveries in the United States in 1970 to 24% in 1989.[70]

Risk reduction involves the implementation of practice strategies that are intended as safeguards against litigation. These include the use of more diagnostic tests, enhanced record-keeping, increased follow-up visits, and increased communication with patients regarding the risks and benefits of procedures. Although some of these defensive practices, such as increased communication with patients, might lead to improved quality of care, others may be nonproductive and harmful. For example, the defensive use of electronic fetal monitoring – a diagnostic procedure which, although widely used has repeatedly failed to improve outcomes for high-risk deliveries – may be associated with higher rates of cesarean section.[71]

Although studies have shown that physician practice patterns are indeed influenced by concerns about legal liability,[72] there is no data available to answer the question whether the documented increases in defensive tests and services are beneficial for patients or unnecessary and harmful. As Tancredi and Barondess[73] have pointed out, the answer to this question depends upon the establishment of standards of care based on the efficacy and effectiveness of different procedures. Only when we know what works under particular clinical conditions, will we be able to determine its appropriateness in particular clinical contexts. This brings us to the final and perhaps most compelling explanation for the occurrence of unnecessary surgery, namely, inadequacies in the knowledge base of clinical practice and inadequacies in the dissemination and use of medical information.

Inadequacies in the knowledge base of surgical practice

As a corollary to the uncertainty hypothesis in surgical rate variation, it has been conjectured that unnecessary or inappropriate surgeries may be largely attributable to deficiencies in the knowledge base of surgical practice and in the dissemination and use of medical information.[74] Because there is no agency like the Food and Drug Administration that regulates and authorizes the introduction of new invasive procedures, many surgical innovations are disseminated into practice without the benefit of large or controlled clinical trials. As a result, the benefits and harms of a procedure may be gleaned slowly and unsystematically as a procedure is used in clinical practice. From the point of view of patient harm, this practice has two obvious drawbacks. Firstly, patients exposed to unproven interventions face unknown risks. Secondly, unless the patient is informed of the speculative nature of the procedure, she or he is denied the right to informed consent regarding the risks and benefits associated with the care.

Absent a strong evidentiary basis for the efficacy and effectiveness of a procedure, surgeons must and do rely on an array of other sources of information for decision-making. These include information gained through medical training, journal reports, and regional or local standards of care – each of which has its particular weaknesses. Information gained in medical training may quickly became outdated. Journal reports may be biased toward favorable outcomes and so tend not to report negative findings or inefficacious applications of a procedure. In addition, information in journal articles is often fragmented and difficult to evaluate – so much so that community physicians may dismiss the scientific literature in favor of local norms and word of mouth endorsements by colleagues. As surgical rate variation studies have shown however, regional or local standards are equally handicapped by the absence of strong outcomes data and may, therefore, be unreliably idosyncratic.

Increasingly, medical and surgical practices have become the subject of guidelines which delineate the indications and contraindications for particular forms of treatment. These standards are promulgated by licensing boards, specialty societies, agencies such as Agency for Health Care Policy and Research (AHCPR) and increasingly by third-party payers. While many of these standards are backed by outcomes data, others may be less rigorous. Even if consensus does develop on indications for a procedure, however, it may take years before this new knowledge is absorbed into practice. Researchers have found that without repeated feedback and review, or endorsement of a practice by local opinion leaders, physicians can be unaware of the new information or simply reluctant to embrace it if it means abandoning more familiar practice strategies.[75] Recent follow-up studies on the utilization of AHCPR guidelines reveal that clinician resistance was one of the major obstacles to their implementation. In particular, these guidelines were regarded variously as 'cookbook medicine' and as a form of government interference in clinical work.[76]

Summary

As we have discussed, there are a number of complex reasons why patients may be subjected to procedures that are clinically useless or non-beneficial. These include characteristics of supply, of demand, and of defensive medicine. Although public perception and regulatory strategies such as sanctions by medical licensing boards, tissue committee review and SSOPs have tended to concentrate on the deviant practitioner, there is compelling evidence that another and more far reaching explanation of the problem lies in deficiencies in the production, dissemination, and application of medical knowledge.[77] The shift in the burden of proof from unnecessary surgery to assessments of a procedure's appropriateness represents an attempt to address this problem. This shift also reveals, however, the fundamentally evaluative nature of the concept of appropriateness; appropriateness is not only or chiefly an evidentiary issue – to be scientifically discovered – but rather, one that is also informed by the values of the patient and inevitably by those of third-party payers. Having said this, we nevertheless find it useful in a discussion of comiogenic harm to highlight the importance of sound clinical determinations for it is safe to assume that in seeking medical care, the patient accepts actual and potential harm only in anticipation of some greater identified clinical benefit to be gained.

The profession of medicine is guided by its moral commitment to avoid harm to patients and to aid them in maintaining or improving their health. On this basis, physicians have an obligation not to provide treatments whose clinical harms and benefits are unknown or whose harms are anticipated to outweigh their benefits. A correlative obligation falls on the profession as a whole to determine the efficacy and effectiveness of procedures before they are offered as clinical therapies. The inclusion of patient-centered health status measures, such as the impact of a procedure on role and social function, recuperation time, days lost from work, into assessment of efficacy and effectiveness will provide a more comprehensive range of relevant information as a basis for individual decision-making. Provision of this information in the informed consent process may aid the patient in assessing the desirability of an intervention and may also serve to minimize surgical risk. In the next chapter we discuss the evidentiary basis of clinical practice and the meaning of appropriateness in patient care.

Endnotes

1 Caplan RA, Posner KL, Cheney FW. Effect of outcome on physician judgments of appropriateness of care. *JAMA* 1991; 265:1957–60.
2 Lembcke PA. Evolution of the medical audit. *JAMA* 1967; 199:534–50.
3 Lembcke PA. Measuring the quality of medical care through vital statistics based on hospital service areas. I. Comparative study of appendectomy rates. *Am J Pub Health* 1952; 42:276–86.
 Klicka KS. Control of Surgery. *Mod Hosp* 1948; 71:84–6.
4 Ward GG. Audits measure our results. *Mod Hosp* 1947; 69:86.
5 Doyle JC. Unnecessary ovariectomies. *JAMA* 1952; 148:1105–11.
6 Doyle JC. Unnecessary hysterectomies: Study of 6,248 operations in thirty-five hospital during 1948. *JAMA* 1952; 151(5):360–6.
 Miller F. Hysterectomy: Therapeutic necessity or surgical racket. *Am J Obstet Gyn* 1946; 51:804–10.
7 Bawkin H. The tonsil-adenoidectomy enigma. *J Pediatrics* 1958; 52:339–61.
8 Weinert HV, Brill R. Effectiveness of a hospital tissue committee in raising surgical standards. *JAMA* 1952; 150:992–6.
9 Rutkow IM, Zuidema GD. Unnecessary surgery: An update. *Surgery* 1978; 84:671–8 (p. 673).
10 Lembcke PA, p. 547 (see No. 2).
11 Rutkow IM, Zuidema GD (see No. 9).
12 Bunker JP. Surgical manpower: A comparison of operation and surgeons in the United States and in England and Wales. *N Engl J Med* 1970; 282:135–44.
13 McCarthy EG, Widmer GW. Effects of screening by consultants on recommended elective surgical procedures. *N Engl J Med* 1974; 291:1331–5.
14 McCarthy EG, Finkel ML. Second opinion elective surgery programs: Outcome status over time. *Med Care* 16:984–94.
15 US Congress, House Subcommittee on Oversight and Investigation. *Cost and Quality of Health Care: Unnecessary Surgery.* Washington DC: USGPO, 1976.
16 Leape LL. Unnecessary Surgery. *Annu Rev Publ Health* 1992; 13:363–83 (see p. 370).
17 Peebles RJ. Second opinions and cost-effectiveness: The questions continue. *Am Coll Surg Bull* 1991; 76:18–25.
18 Emerson R, Creedon JJ. Unjustified surgery dilemma: second opinion versus preset criteria. *NY State J Med* 1977; 77:779–85.
19 Leape LL, p. 372 (see No. 16).
20 Wennberg JE, Barnes BA, Zubkoff M. Professional uncertainty and the problem of supplier induced demand. *Soc Sci Med* 1982; 16:811–24.
21 Stroman DF. *The Quick Knife: Unnecessary Surgery.* New York: Kennikat, 1979.
22 Wennberg J, Gittelsohn A. Variations in medical care among small areas. *Sci Am* 1982; 246:120–34.
 Wennberg JE, Freeman JL, Culp WJ. Are hospital services rationed in New York or over-utilized in Boston? *Lancet* 1987; 1:1185–9.
23 Leape LL, Park RE, Solomon DH, et al. Relation between surgeons' practice volumes and geographic variation in the rate of carotid endarterectomy. *N Engl J Med* 1989; 314:653–7.
24 Chassin MR, Kosecoff J, Park RE, et al. Does inappropriate use explain geographic variations in the use of health care services? *JAMA* 1987; 258(18):2533–7.

Lu-Yao GL, Mclerran D, Wasson J, et al. An assessment of radical prostatectomy: Time trends, geographic variation, and outcomes. *JAMA* 1993; 269:2633–6.

Paul-Shaheen P, Clark JD, Williams D. Small area analysis: a review and analysis of the North American literature. *J Health Polit Policy Law* 1987; 12:741–809.

25 Wennberg J, Gittelsohn A. Small-area variations in health care delivery. *Science* 1973; 182:1102–8.

26 Leape LL, Park RE, Solomon DH, et al. Does inappropriate use explain small area variations in the use of health care services? *JAMA* 1990; 263:669–72.

27 Anderson GM, Grumbach K, Luft HS, Roos LL, Mustard C, Brook R. Use of coronary artery bypass surgery in the United States and Canada. Influence of age and income. *JAMA* 1993; 269:1661–6.

28 Lembcke PA. Measuring the quality of medical care through vital statistics based on hospital service areas I. Comparative study of appendectomy rates. *Am J Pub Health* 1952; 42:276–86.

Bunker JP (see No. 12).

Wennberg J, Gittelsohn A (See No. 22).

29 Lewis CE. Variations in the incidence of surgery. *N Engl J Med* 1969; 281:880–4.

30 Wennberg J, Gittelsohn A (see No. 22).

31 Mitchell JB, Cromwell J. Variations in surgical rates and the supply of surgeons. In Rothberg DL, ed., *Regional Variations in Hospital Use.* Lexington, MA: Lexington books, 1982.

32 Vayda E, Anderson GD. Comparison of provincial surgical rates in 1968. *Can J Surg* 1975; 18:18–26

Vayda E, Barnsley JM, Mindell WR, Cardillo B. Five year study of surgical rates in Ontario's counties. *Can Med Assn J* 1984; 131:111–15.

33 Roos NP, Roos LL, Jr, Henteleff PD. Elective surgical rates – do high rates mean lower standards?: Tonsillectomy and adenoidectomy in Manitoba. *N Engl J Med* 1977; 297:360–5.

Roos NP, Roos LL, Jr. Surgical rate variations: Do they reflect the health or socioeconomic characteristics of the population? *Med Care* 1982; 20:945–58.

Roos NP. Hysterectomy. Variations in rates across small areas and across physicians' practices. *Am J Public Health* 1984; 7:327–35.

34 DeMott RK, Sandmire HF. The Green Bay cesarean section study. I. The physician factor as a determinant of cesarean birth rates. *Am J Obstet Gynecol* 1990; 162(6):1593–9.

35 Leape LL, p. 368 (see No. 16).

36 Eddy DM. Variations in physician practice: The role of uncertainty. *Health Affairs* 1984; 3(4):74–89.

37 LoGerfo JP, Efird RA, Diehr PK, Richardson WC. Rates of surgical care in prepaid group practices and the independent setting. *Med Care* 1979; 17:1–10.

Chassin M, Brook R, Park R, et al. Variations in the use of medical and surgical services by the Medicare population. *N Engl J Med* 1986; 314:285.

38 Chassin MR, Kosecoff J, Park RE, et al. Does inappropriate use explain geographic variations in the use of health care services? *JAMA* 1987; 258(18):2533–7.

39 Starr P. *The Social Transformation of American Medicine.* New York: Basic Books, 1982.

40 Relman A. Assessment and accountability: The third revolution in medical care. *N Engl J Med* 1988; 319:1220–2.
41 Relman A, p. 1221 (see No. 40).
42 Park RE, Fink A, Brook RH, Chassin MR, et al. Physician ratings of appropriate indications for six medical and surgical procedures. *Am J Public Health* 1986; 76:766–72.
43 Leape LL, Park RE, Solomon DH, et al. (see No. 26).
44 This table is a modified and expanded version of the one presented in Leape LL, p. 374 (see No. 26).
45 Roos NP, Roos LL, Jr, Henteleff PD (see No. 33).
46 Peebles RJ. Second opinions and cost-effectiveness: The questions continue. *Am Coll Surg Bull* 1991; 76:18–25.
47 Chassin MR, Kosecoff J, Solomon DH, Brook RH. How coronary angiography is used. Clinical determinants of appropriateness. *JAMA* 1987; 258:2543–7.
48 Chassin MR, Kosecoff J, Park RE, et al. (see No. 38).
49 Chassin MR, Kosecoff J, Park RE, et al. (see No. 38).
50 Winslow CM, Kosecoff JB, Chassin M, et al. The appropriateness of performing coronary artery bypass surgery. *JAMA* 1988; 260(4):505–9.
51 Greenspan AM, Kay HR, Berger DC, et al. Incidence of unwarranted implantations of permanent cardiac pacemakers in a large medical population. *N Engl J Med* 1988; 318:158–63.
52 Gambone JC, Reiter RC, Lench JB. Quality assurance indicators and short-term outcome of hysterectomy. *Obstet Gynecol* 1990; 76:8412–45.
53 Gray D, Hampton JR, Bernstein S, et al. Audit of coronary angiography and bypass surgery. *Lancet* 1990; 335:1317–20.
54 Gray D, Hampton JR, Bernstein S, et al. (see No. 53).
55 European Carotid Surgery Trialists' Collaborative Group. MCR European Carotid Surgery Trial: interim results for symptomatic patients with severe (70–99%) or with mild (0–19%) carotid stenosis. *Lancet* 1991; 227:1235–43.
56 Leape LL, Hilborne LH, Park RH, et al. The appropriateness of use of coronary artery bypass graft surgery in New York State. *JAMA* 1993; 269:753–60.
57 Hilborne LH, Leape LL, Bernstein SJ, et al. The appropriateness of use of percutaneous transluminal coronary angioplasty in New York State. *JAMA* 1993; 269(6):761–5.
58 Bernstein SJ, Hilborne LH, Leape LL, et al. The appropriateness of use of coronary angiography in New York State. *JAMA* 1993; 269(6):766–9.
59 Bernstein SJ, McGlynn EA, Siu AL, et al. The appropriateness of hysterectomy. *JAMA* 1993; 269:2398–402.
60 Shaw GB. *The Doctor's Dilemma: A Tragedy.* New York: Brentano's, 1923, p. v.
61 LoGerfo JP. Organizational and financial influences on patterns of surgical care. *Surg Clin N Am* 1982; 62:677–84.
62 Rice TH. The impact of changing Medicare reimbursement rates on physician-induced demand. *Med Care* 1983; 21:803–15.
63 Franks, P, Clancy CM, Nutting PA. Gatekeeping revisited: protecting patients from overtreatment. *N Engl J Med* 1992; 217(6):424–9.
64 Relman AS. Salaried physicians and economic incentives. *N Engl J Med* 1988; 319:784.
65 LoGerfo JP (see No. 61).

212   *Medical Harm*

66 Bolande RP. Ritualistic surgery – circumcision and tonsillectomy. *N Engl J Med* 1969; 280:591–6.
67 Sagoff M. *The Economy of the Earth*. New York: Cambridge University Press, 1988, p. 106.
68 Eisenberg J. *Doctor's Decisions and the Cost of Medical Care*. Ann Arbor, MI: Health Administration Press, 1986, p. 67.
69 Weisman CS, Morlock LL, Teitelbaum MA, Klassen AC, Celantano DD. Practice changes in response to the malpractice litigation climate: results of a Maryland physician study. *Med Care* 1989; 27:16–24.
70 Keeler EB, Brodie M. Economic incentives in the choice between vaginal delivery and cesarean section. *Milbank Q* 1993; 71:365–404.
   Heilbrunn JZ, Rolph J. *Cesarean Sections as Defensive Medicine*. Santa Monica, CA: RAND, 1993.
71 Freeman R. Intrapartum fetal monitoring. A disappointing story. *N Engl J Med* 1990; 322(9):624–6.
72 Reynolds RA, Rizzo JA, Gonzales ML. The cost of medical professional liability. *JAMA* 1987; 257:2776–81.
73 Tancredi LR, Barondess JA. the problem of defensive medicine. *Science* 1978; 200:879–82.
74 Leape LL, p. 378 (see No. 16).
75 Wennberg JE, Blowers L, Parker R, et al. Changes in tonsillectomy rates associated with feedback and review. *Pediatrics* 1977; 59:821–6.
   Lomas J, Enkin M, et al. Opinion leaders vs. audit and feedback to implement practice guidelines: Delivery after previous cesarean section. *JAMA* 1991; 265:2202–7.
76 HHS Office of Inspector General Report cited in *Health News Daily* October 23, 1995, p. 5.
77 Leape LL (see No. 16).

10

The concept of appropriateness in patient care

Appropriateness, values and risk

The shift to appropriateness in health services research underscores that judgments about surgical overuse and the provision of unnecessary services depend on *prior* judgments about the criteria for *appropriate* use. This shift is, in other words, an acknowledgment that clinically sound utilization decisions depend on a sound evidentiary basis regarding what works in clinical practice. Because only a small minority (15 to 20%) of treatments have been evaluated in rigorous scientific trials,[1] however, this is a daunting task. It is also one that raises important and controversial questions about what counts as an authoritative form of evidence in determinations regarding efficacy, effectiveness, and safety – or in other words, regarding clinical benefit and harm. The shift to appropriateness also raises important questions regarding the values that do and should guide medical decision making. To say that something is 'appropriate' is to say that it is 'suitable or fitting for a particular purpose, occasion, or person.'[2] The term 'appropriate' is, thus, fundamentally evaluative; it implies the endorsement of some goal. 'Appropriate for what and whom?' and 'appropriate to what and whose ends?' are questions that must be answered, therefore, if the term is to be made meaningful.[3]

Traditionally, the authority for clinical decision-making has rested with the physician; the physician was believed to know what was best or appropriate for a patient and due deference was paid to medical judgment. The shift to appropriateness research, however, comes at a time when other values, in particular, those of the patient and those of third-party payers, play a central role in the process of health care decision-making. In addition to questions of evidentiary justification, determinations of appropriateness now inevitably touch on questions of the desirability and cost-worthiness of treatment. In this chapter, we identify four sources of value that give meaning to appropriateness in patient care: the clinical point of view; the point of view of the individual patient; the point of view of the third-party payer; and the social point of view.[4] Based on this analysis, we discuss some of the practical and ethical issues surrounding patient risk.[5]

Clinical appropriateness – what evidence is authoritative?

The RAND Health Services Utilization Study, used a modified Delphi form of consensus methodology to determine appropriateness. A procedure was deemed appropriate (i.e., its anticipated benefits for a particular patient scenario exceed its anticipated harms) if it was judged by a nine-member panel of physician-experts to be within a specified median range with no more than two physicians rating the procedure as inappropriate. Although panelists' evaluations were based in part on a synthesis of the relevant literature, only 10% of the available studies on coronary angiography, gastrointestinal endoscopy, carotid endarterectomy, and coronary artery bypass graft (CABG) were based on randomized controlled clinical trials. Moreover, RAND researchers made 'no attempt . . . to score the quality of journals, articles, or [article] contents' that formed the empirical basis for their recommendations.[6] The RAND method, therefore, was not based on an explicit linkage between recommendations and the quality of supporting evidence. For those who advocate for randomized controlled trials (RCT) as the best method for determinations of appropriateness, this represents a weakness of the RAND approach.[7]

The RCT also has its shortcomings, however, as a method for determining appropriateness. RCTs do not provide evidence for a procedure's effectiveness (the level of benefit achievable under ordinary clinical conditions), but, rather, for its possible efficacy (the level of benefit achievable under ideal clinical conditions). RCTs are often extremely expensive and their results may not be available for years. Moreover, many RCTs use a narrow range of outcome measures and ignore quality of life and other health status variables that are relevant in health care decision-making.[8] There are also ethical challenges to randomization itself – it exposes research subjects to unknown risk and may call for subjects in therapeutic research to forgo treatments which, in current practice, are believed to be beneficial.[9]

The RAND modified Delphi approach and randomized trials are only two in a growing number of sophisticated methods proposed to assess clinical appropriateness. The Agency for Health Care Policy and Research

(AHCPR) Patient Outcomes Research Team (PORT) studies, for example, provide a hybrid evidence-based approach that also relies on expert assessments. Another approach, meta-analysis, is an analytic method for synthesizing a range of sometimes disparate evidence from multiple studies.[10] The types and quality of evidence required to establish appropriateness are the subjects of on-going debate. As Eddy has pointed out, the resolution of these methodological questions will establish new standards for determining what works in medical practice, and this, in turn, will have an enormous influence on the utilization and reimbursement decisions of third-party payers.[11] In what follows, we look at a number of proposals that have been offered on the evaluation and ranking of evidence. We offer suggestions on how the evidentiary basis of treatment – and correlatively on the probability that clinical benefit and harm – might be conveyed to patients in the informed consent process.

Clinical assessment – correlating evidence and efficacy

In the context of patient care, the recommendation of a procedure is based on at least four interrelated clinical factors: (1) the patient's clinical profile; (2) the physician's (and team's) skill; (3) the quality of the evidence supporting a procedure; and (4) the procedure's clinical benefit/harm ratio,[12] understood in terms of the empirical evidence that is available on the intervention's clinical efficacy and effectiveness. From the physician's point of view, the *clinical* benefit/harm ratio represents one way of assessing the potential effects of a procedure in terms of such empirical and population-based variables as morbidity, mortality, and quality of life indicators. If an intervention is inconsistent with the patient's clinical presentation or if the physician or team is insufficiently skilled to carry out the intervention (e.g., has a high complication rate), then the intervention is *de facto* inappropriate and should not be recommended.

Evidentiary judgments are understood in terms of degree and thus are able to be roughly classified as a basis for clinical recommendations. Proposed rules of evidence for such classifications have recently come from a number of quarters. As reported by Sackett,[13] participants in a conference on the use of antithrombotic therapy have distinguished five levels of evidence. They are:

(1) Large RCTs with clear-cut results (and low risk of error) [low false positive errors and high power].
(2) Small RCTs with uncertain results (and moderate to high risk of error)

[high false positive errors and/or low power].
(3) Non-randomized, concurrent cohort comparisons.
(4) Non-randomized, historical cohort comparisons.
(5) Case series without controls.

Participants subsequently classified clinical recommendation into three grades, depending on their supporting levels of evidence. Grade A recommendations are those supported by Level 1 evidence. Those in grade B are supported by evidence level 2. Grade C recommendations are based on evidence from levels 3, 4 or 5.

This classificatory framework parallels that put forward by the US Preventive Services Task Force in its evaluation of the effectiveness of clinical preventive services.[14] The Task Force proposed a hierarchical ranking of evidentiary quality which gave greater weight to study designs whose methodology made them less subject to bias and inferential error. In descending order they are: well-designed RCTs followed by non-randomized controlled trials, cohort studies, case control studies, comparisons between time and place, uncontrolled experiments, and, finally, descriptive studies and expert opinion. Using this hierarchy, recommendations were graded on a five-point scale.

In what follows we provide a framework for correlating evidence and efficacy as a basis for clinical recommendations and informed consent. Our hierarchical ranking of evidence is similar to those discussed above. In addition, we use this framework to suggest terminological distinctions that can be used in place of the ambiguous terms 'appropriate' and 'necessary.'

The *possibly beneficial* intervention is one thought to be preponderantly beneficial but only on the basis of evidence that is provided largely by case reports or based on uncontrolled clinical impressions or uncontrolled studies. In other words, such inferences about the benefit of an intervention are rationally plausible but have only been subjected to the weakest empirical scrutiny. An example would be radical prostatectomy for well differentiated, localized prostate cancer in patients less than 75 years old.[15] Cases where uncontrolled studies provide the evidence for an intervention's efficacy include photorefractive keratectomy as a surgical treatment for myopia[16] and CABG in asymptomatic patients or patients with ischemia or mild angina/ischemia with three vessel disease, no severe left anterior descending (LAD) stenosis and normal left ventricular (LV) function.[17] It should be made clear to the patient that procedures in this category are based on the weakest empirical support.

Indicated and *highly indicated* interventions are supported by proportionally superior empirical evidence as to their benefit. The evidence supporting an indicated intervention should be derived from at least one randomized, controlled clinical trial, from a broad meta-analysis of sound studies[18] or from a systematic consensus methodology or outcomes review such as the AHCPR PORT projects.[19] An example would be conventional lumbar laminectomy/discectomy for patients with uncomplicated herniated discs.[20]

The *highly indicated* procedure is one whose benefit has been unequivocally established through either definitive or replicated randomized, controlled trials. Additionally, the highly indicated intervention is one whose expected benefits have been clearly shown to exceed the anticipated benefits of alternative therapies. Examples include carotid endarterectomy for patients with transient ischemic attacks (TIAs) and greater than 70% stenosis[21] or CABG for patients with left main artery disease and chronic stable class III angina.[22]

Just as the evidence regarding efficacy and effectiveness reveals the relative clinical benefits of an intervention, so too does it reveal the relative clinical harms. Accordingly, we recommend that the overly broad terms 'inappropriate' and 'unnecessary,' be replaced by the more specific designations described below. As with the previous distinctions regarding benefit, these terms have as their primary reference point the degree of empirical evidence substantiating a procedure's benefit/harm ratio. Again, these distinctions become relevant only when a procedure is consistent with a patient's clinical presentation and when the physician (and team) are adequately skilled. If *these* conditions are not met, then a procedure is contraindicated regardless of the strength of evidence for its general efficacy.[23]

When a procedure is thought to be preponderantly harmful based only on anecdotal evidence, case reports or uncontrolled studies, the procedure should be termed *possibly harmful*. Examples would include lumbar fusion for back pain[24] and decalcification for degenerative aortic stenosis.[25] These lower levels of evidence also support the *equivocal* intervention, one whose ratio of benefit to harm is roughly equal. An equivocal designation indicates above all, the need for more study on the particular intervention and its clinical uses. Examples include carotid endarterectomy for TIAs and 30–70% stenosis[26] or for asymptomatic bruit.[27]

Important ethical limits on human subjects research prevent the performance of rigorous trials to prove that a drug or procedure's burdens are indeed disproportionate to its benefits. Thus the evidentiary requirements to establish a procedure as *contraindicated* will not be as demanding as those placed on determinations of care that is indicated or highly indicated. Accordingly, when good evidence from controlled trials, from a broad meta-analysis of studies or from a systematic consensus methodology or outcomes review reveals that the harms outweigh the benefits of a procedure, that procedure should be termed 'contraindicated.' Examples of contraindicated procedures are extracranial–intracranial bypass for stroke prevention,[28] CABG in patients with mild stable angina and single-vessel disease,[29] radical prostatectomy for well-differentiated localized cancer in patients older than 75 years,[30] and carotid endarterectomy in patients with TIAs and less than 30% stenosis.[31] When superior evidence has established that the possibility of benefit and harm from an intervention is roughly equivalent, that is, when there is clearly no favorable benefit/harm ratio, that intervention should be classed as *non-indicated*.

Figure 10.1 represents the distinctions just described as they appear along the spectrum of evidence and the spectrum of benefit and harm that can be associated with a procedure. As represented by the vertical axis, evidence may be weak or strong depending on study methodology and scope. As represented by the horizontal axis, the efficacy (and/or effectiveness) of an intervention may extend from clearly preponderant benefit to clearly preponderant harm. Although this axis represents only magnitudes of benefit and harm, probability assessments are also relevant to the judgment process. The probabilities of benefit and harm are data that should be elicited from the available evidence and transmitted to the patient in the informed consent process.[32]

The shaded area in Figure 10.1 encompasses interventions that, because of insufficient evidence, should be identified as unproven. When any such intervention is contemplated, the fact that it is unproven should be made clear to the patient in the informed consent process. Ideally, interventions of unproved benefit should be undertaken, when ethically permissible, only within the context of a research protocol. Figure 10.2 is a sample plotting of the interventions described above.

The classifications represented in Figure 10.1 provide a degree of specificity not captured by the broad terms 'medically necessary,' or 'clinically appropriate.' As such, they can provide a coherent and meaningful vocabulary for medical practitioners and patients as they deliberate on the right course of treatment. These classifications can also serve as a useful analytic framework for practice guidelines. Specialty societies might, for example, use Figure 10.1 as a model to identify, in an on-going way, the correlation between evidence and the clinical benefit/harm ratio for the interventions particular to their specialties. This information would ideally

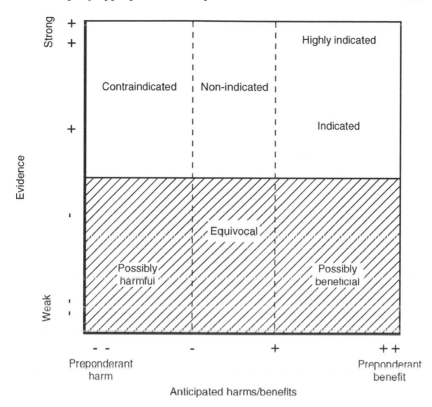

Figure 10.1   Clinical assessment: correlating evidence and efficacy

NOTE: shaded area denotes classes of interventions whose efficacy and effectiveness are as yet unproven

be supplemented by broader outcomes data on the comparative efficacy, effectiveness and safety of alternative treatments. Further, as evolving informed consent law recognizes their availability, these data may also increasingly be regarded as material information that *must* be disclosed to patients.[33]

In the following sections we discuss two different ways in which patient considerations should inform determinations about the appropriateness of an intervention. In the context of outcomes research, data about the *average* patient should be incorporated into patient-centered outcome measures. In the therapeutic context, considerations of the *individual* patient should determine the *desirability* of an intervention.

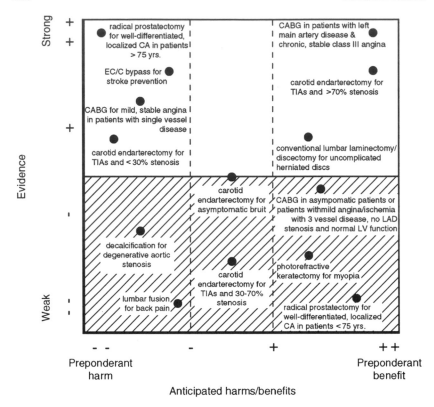

Figure 10.2 A sample plotting of interventions

NOTE: shaded area denotes classes of interventions whose efficacy and effectiveness are as yet unproven

Efficacy, effectiveness, and patient-centered outcome measures

Many of those in health services research believe that if clinical trials are to be the optimal source of evidence for clinical decision making, the measures used within these trials to determine a procedure's efficacy, effectiveness, and safety must be as broad as possible and should include well-standardized patient-centered quality of life and health status measures such as anxiety, impact on role and social function, recuperation time, and days lost from work.[34] To date, as Geigle, Brook and others point out, the narrow focus on mortality and morbidity or change in a physiologic variable and the attendant omission of quality of life measures has left the patient largely on the periphery of most outcomes assessment and outcome-oriented quality measurement.[35] By incorporating patient-centered health status measures such as these in their overall assessment of efficacy, effectiveness, and safety, recent studies have been able to provide a more comprehensive range of relevant information as the basis for informed health care decision-making.[36] In the best-case scenario, all of this information on survival rate, states of physical, emotional, and social function and patient satisfaction would be available to individual patients and physicians in the clinical setting and would provide a comprehensive basis for informed consent or refusal. Eddy[37] has suggested that a distinction be made in health services research between such 'intermediate outcomes' as test results or biological or physiological indicators and the ultimate 'health outcomes' of a procedure. He argues that health outcomes – those effects that patients experience and care about such as pain, anxiety, death, disfigurement, and disability – should be the primary focus of informed medical decision-making.

The patient's perspective and the desirability of treatment

Historically, the medical profession has tended to view appropriateness in strictly clinical terms. As one spokesman for this view has stated, 'The patient's attitude should have no influence on what the physician advises as appropriate therapy for the patient's illness. The . . . risks to benefit ratio, as stated by the physician, should be the only consideration when making a therapeutic decision.'[38] The fact that there may be incongruities between patient and physician perceptions of the appropriateness of treatment, however, is one of the bases of informed consent. Empirical evidence of such incongruities has also been demonstrated in a number of studies. In a comparison of risk preferences regarding prostatectomy, for example, Barry et al. have shown that patients presented with an analysis of risks and benefits, tend to decide in favor of the procedure less often than their physicians.[39] Similar differences have been observed in physician and patient perceptions of the appropriateness of laryngectomy as a treatment for throat cancer.[40] These observations underscore the evaluative nature of the concept of appropriateness. Given this, determinations of the appropriateness of a procedure therefore should not be regarded simply or even primarily as an evidentiary problem but rather as a problem of value assessments.

We have argued that the appropriateness of an intervention is to be understood in terms of potential benefits and harms that it offers to the patient. Given this, the concept of appropriateness must take into account not only the 'clinical' benefits and harms – understood both narrowly in terms of morbidity and mortality and more broadly in terms of overall quality of life for the 'average' patient – but also the *relevance* of clinical and 'non-clinical' benefits and harms for the *individual patient* in the context of medical decision making. This includes individual quality of life decisions and individual assessments of acceptable risk and cost. Of course, as outcomes measures become more patient-centered, the notion of a 'clinical' benefit will be correspondingly enlarged. Nevertheless, in the context of care, an individual patient's values, risk-preferences and financial and social circumstances introduce considerations that are essential to the decision-making process, and that cannot be captured by aggregate data about health outcomes. In short, it is the *individual patient* who determines the ultimate desirability of an intervention for him or herself. For instance, although surgery might be regarded as highly indicated, from the point of view of relative medical risks and benefits, it might also be regarded as undesirable by a patient who is either risk-averse or who rejects anticipated medical benefit in favor of other more highly valued goals.[41] Albert Einstein, for example, refused surgery for an aortic aneurysm (which ultimately killed him) because he was committed to a life based on simplicity. He judged the recommended surgery as undesirable because increased longevity was, in his view, outweighed by the inconvenience of the intervention.[42] In order to honor the values that the individual patient brings to the decision making process, we recommend that an intervention be termed *desirable* if it is freely accepted by the informed patient or valid surrogate.

Interpreting appropriateness in the clinical context – some ethical considerations

Avoiding conflict through the process of informed consent

The distinctions that we have made between a procedure's clinical merit and its desirability to the patient are an attempt to explicate how both clinical and patient values inform the concept of appropriateness and may lead to different understandings of the goals of care and the means to achieve them. In the process of clinical decision-making, the informed consent process is the means by which these different values and goals become enunciated. The process of informed consent is also the means by which a recommended intervention becomes meaningful to the patient as 'desirable' or 'undesirable' and as one, therefore, that she/he will choose to accept or forgo. As such, a key ingredient of the process of informed consent is a discussion between physician and patient of the relative clinical benefits and harms of different treatment options and on the quality of evidence that supports these judgments. Insofar as it allows the rough location of a procedure within the related spectra of evidence and benefits and harms, Figure 10.1 can serve as a useful tool in the decision-making process. Finally, the process of informed consent is the means by which the patient should be informed of non-clinical factors that influence treatment recommendations.

With changes in health care financing and delivery, there is another set of values that is increasingly informing interpretations of appropriateness in health care decision-making. These include the values of cost-containment and economic efficiency. Within this framework, the utilization of services and resources stands out as a key value in treatment determinations by third-party payers. As we discussed in Part II, treatment decisions, traditionally made within the confines of the physician-patient relationship, are increasingly influenced by administrative limits on care through utilization review and treatment authorization. In light of these developments, we would suggest that when treatment decisions are based on considerations of social distribution, rationing, or cost-containment, the proper term would be the *cost-worthiness* of an outcome, an intervention, or a likelihood of success, rather than its 'appropriateness.' This terminology makes explicit the economic values upon which a decision rests. As Tomlinson and Brody[43] observe, in this era of cost-containment, providers must maintain a clear distinction between the clinically non-beneficial operation and one that is simply judged not cost-worthy. When financial considerations by doctors or third-party payers influence treatment recommendations they may substantively affect the patient's risk profile. For this reason, candor regarding financial influences is essential in the informed consent process.

Ethical guides for conflict resolution

Cases will at times arise when patient, physician and/or third-party payer will disagree about the appropriateness of specific treatments. In cases concerning the withdrawal and withholding of treatment, for instance, a patient may refuse undesired care that physicians or hospitals deem clinically indicated. Likewise, a third-party payer may refuse to cover potentially beneficial treatments because they are not considered cost-worthy. Some ethical guidelines are useful when reflecting on conflicts of this sort.

First, based on the fundamental liberty of patients as persons, physicians have no unilateral right to implement a decision about what they consider necessary or unnecessary in the context of individual patient care. Rather, their legitimate domain is the assessment of clinical efficacy, estimation of the probable effects of alternative modes of therapy versus no therapy, and the discussion of this information and recommendations with the patient or valid surrogate. In the context of non-emergency care, the physician's authority to perform an intervention derives from the patient's (or surrogate's) consent to a procedure which he or she deems desirable. Because financial restrictions or incentives may increase the risk of patient harm, or compromise the patient's ability to make an informed choice among beneficial treatments, they must be disclosed in the informed consent process.

Secondly, the profession of medicine is guided by its moral commitment to avoid harm to patients and to aid them in maintaining or improving their health. On this basis, clinicians have a presumptive obligation not to provide treatments that are unproven or contraindicated. In addition, physicians are moral agents and as such, cannot be compelled to violate his or her personal moral convictions. For these reasons, a patient's demand for unproven or contraindicated care that he or she deems desirable is not sufficient to impose upon providers an obligation to provide that care. In cases where administrative and/or financial limits on care threaten the patient's health interests, the physician has an obligation to advocate on behalf of the patient.

Thirdly, third-party payers must clearly state the broad coverage exclusions and the specific financial restrictions that influence decision-making and must justify to both physician and patient the denial of coverage for services that doctor and patient believe to be in the patient's health interests.

The societal dimension of appropriateness

As growing concern over access to health care and the escalation of health care costs has made clear, individual and professional aims are not pursued within a vacuum. They are pursued within the context of health care institutions – hospitals, health maintenance organizations, third-party insurance – and within the larger societal context where the diverse aims of health care, education, defense, environmental protection, etc. must compete for limited social resources. In the institutional context, the issues of appropriateness and futility are embedded within the practices of gatekeeping and utilization review and they have found there way into new hospital policies on futility.[44] In the larger context of health policy, the societal meanings of appropriateness and futility are manifested in debates about 'global budgets,' a 'decent' minimum level of health care,[45] 'essential' and 'non-essential' services,[46] and health care rationing.[47] For better or worse, health care decisions are tied to the marketplace and the wider context of social policy.

As the United States and the individual states deliberate about society's obligation to provide health services, it will be our task as citizens to determine what goals are and are not worth pursuing given the forces of human need and market economics.[48] This determination is fundamentally based on the values we hold rather than on any 'facts' that can be supplied to us by scientific investigation. We concur, therefore, with a British National Health Service working group on appropriateness that the management of conflict regarding the cost-worthiness of potential outcomes is not a professional responsibility but a political one.[49]

As Daniel Callahan has observed, 'life was easier when we thought medical "necessity" and "futility" were scientifically discoverable.'[50] Knowing now that necessity, futility, and appropriateness are not so much discovered as *decided upon* on the basis of certain value commitments (of physicians, patients, third-party payers, and citizens) we must turn our attention to the difficult task of establishing a public standard that determines the boundaries of what society may offer and require in the arena of health care. Callahan suggests that such a standard should incorporate at least six elements,[51]

(1) medical need defined in some general way;
(2) the efficacy of available treatments in meeting that need;
(3) the comparative costs and benefits of those treatments;
(4) the necessity of setting health care priorities;
(5) a political process capable of making the combined medical and moral judgments that will unavoidably be encountered along the way;
(6) the stimulation of public and professional debate on the substantive content of the moral judgments.

Until we have begun to gain some clarity on these issues we would be wise to refrain from the uncritical use of the ambiguous and often misleading terms 'necessary,' 'unnecessary,' 'appropriate,' 'inappropriate,' and 'futile.' The use of more specific terminology by providers, patients, and policy makers may prevent mistaken assumptions, enhance the informed consent process and advance the public discourse.

Endnotes

1 Office of Technology Assessment. *The Impact of Randomized Clinical Trials on Health Policy and Medical Practice.* Washington, DC: US Government Printing Office, 1983.
2 *The Random House College Dictionary.* New York: Random House, 1980, p. 66.
3 Truog RD, Brett AS, Frader J. The problem with medical futility. *N Engl J Med* 1992; 326:1560–4.
4 See also Hopkins A, Fitzpatrick R, Foster A, et al. What do we mean by appropriate health care? *Quality in Health Care* 1993; 2:117–23. This working group of the British National Health Service offers a compatible framework for specifying the concept of appropriateness. We are grateful to Dr. Hopkins for alerting us to this report.
5 This chapter is drawn from Sharpe VA, Faden AI. Appropriateness in patient care: A new conceptual framework. *Milbank Q* 1996; 74:115–38.
6 Fink A, Brook RH, Kosecoff J, Chassin M, Solomon DH. The sufficiency of the clinical literature for learning about the appropriate use of six medical and surgical procedures. *West J Med* 1987; 147:609–15.
7 Woolf SH. Practice guidelines, a new reality in medicine. *Arch Intern Med* 1992; 152:946–52.
8 Guadagnoli E, McNeil BJ. Outcome research: Hope for the future or the latest rage? *Inquiry* 1994; 31:14–24.
9 Because the question of clinical benefit is precisely at issue in this evidentiary debate, the ethical problem associated with randomized controlled trials (RCTs) is somewhat odd. To assume that someone in the experimental arm of a protocol is deprived of the benefits of standard treatment or that someone in the control group is deprived of potential benefits as an experimental subject is to take for granted precisely what is unknown and therefore the subject of study. If, however, one believes that only a RCT can definitively establish clinical benefit, then any provision of treatments that have *not* been proven preponderantly beneficial in a RCT would be ethically suspect.
10 Chalmers TC. Meta-analysis in clinical medicine. *Trans Am Clin Climatol Assn* 1987; 99:144–50.
11 Eddy DM. Three battles to watch in the 1990s. *JAMA* 1993; 270:520–6.
12 We use the terms 'benefit' and 'harm' advisedly here, cognizant of the fact that, like the term 'appropriate,' these, are evaluative terms whose meanings are legitimately shaped by the values of patient and clinician.
13 Sackett DL. Rules of evidence and clinical recommendations on the use of antithrombotic agents. *Chest* 1989; 95(2 suppl):2s–4s.
14 US Preventive Services Task Force. *Guide to Cinical Preventive Services: An Assessment of the Effectiveness of 169 Interventions.* Baltimore: Williams and Wilkins, 1989.
15 Fleming C, Wasson JH, Albertsen PC, Barry MJ, Wennberg JE. A decision analysis of alternative treatment strategies for clinically localized prostate cancer. *JAMA* 1993; 269:2650–8.
North American Symptomatic Carotid Endarterectomy Trial Collaborators. Beneficial effect of carotid endarterectomy in symptomatic patients with high-grade carotid stenosis. *N Engl J Med* 1991; 325:445–53.
European Carotid Surgery Trialists' Collaborative Group. MRC European carotid surgery trial: interim results for symptomatic patients with severe

(70–99%) or with mild (0–29%) carotid stenosis. *Lancet* 1991; 337:1235–43.

16 Gartry DS, Kerr MG, Marshall J. Excimer laser photorefractive keratectomy. *Ophthalmology* 1992; 99:1209–19.
Salz JJ, Maguen E, Nesburn AB, et al. A two-year experience with excimer laser photorefractive keratectomy for myopia. *Ophthalmology* 1993; 100:873–82.

17 American College of Cardiology/American Heart Association Task Force on Assessment of Diagnostic and Therapeutic Cardiovascular Procedures (Subcommittee on coronary artery bypass graft surgery). Guidelines and indications for coronary artery bypass graft surgery. *J Am Coll Cardiol* 1991; 17:543–89.

18 L'Abbé KA, Detsky AS, O'Rourke K. Meta-analysis in clinical research. *Ann Intern Med* 1987; 107:224–33.

19 Clinton JJ. From the Agency for Health Care Policy and Research. *JAMA* 1991; 266:2057.

20 DATTA Report. Laminectomy and microlaminectomy for treatment of lumbar disk herniation. *JAMA* 1990; 264:1469–72.
DATTA report. Reassessment of automated percutaneous lumbar diskectomy for herniated disks. *JAMA* 1991; 265:2122–5.

21 North American Symptomatic Carotid Endarterectomy Trial Collaborators (NASCET). Beneficial effect of carotid endarterectomy.
Mayberg MR, Wilson SE, Yatsu F, et al. Carotid endarterectomy and prevention of cerebral ischemia in symptomatic carotid stenosis. *JAMA* 1991; 266:3289–94.

22 American College of Cardiology (see No. 17).

23 An important exception is the performance of procedures by physicians and nurses in training. Society allows for supervised intervention by residents and medical and nursing students because the future availability of medical care is viewed as a significant social good. Whether patients are informed of the risks attendant upon care by students and whether or not these risks are equitably distributed remain important ethical and public policy questions.

24 Turner JA, Ersek M, Herron L, Haselkorn J, Kent D, et al. Patient outcomes after lumbar spinal fusion. *JAMA* 1992; 268:907–11.
Franklin GM, Haug J, Heyer N, McKeefrey SP, Picciano J. Outcome of lumbar fusion in Washington state worker's compensation. *Spine* 1994; 19:1897–903.

25 Freeman WK, Schaff HV, Orszulak TA, Tajik AJ. Ultrasonic aortic valve decalcification: serial Doppler echocardiographic follow-up. *J Am Coll Cardiol* 1990; 16:623–30.

26 North American Symptomatic Carotid Endarterectomy Trial Collaborators. Beneficial effect of carotid endarterectomy; European Carotid Surgery Trialists' Collaborative Group. MRC European carotid surgery trial (see No. 15).

27 Barnett HJM, Haines SJ. Carotid endarterectomy for asymptomatic carotid stenosis. *N Engl J Med* 1993; 328:276–9.
Bornstein NM, Norris JW. Evolution and management of asymptomatic carotid stenosis. *Cerebrovasc Brain Metab Rev* 1993; 5:301–13.

28 The EC/IC Bypass Study Group. Failure of extracranial-intracranial arterial bypass to reduce the risk of ischemic stroke: results of an international randomized trial. *N Engl J Med* 1985; 313:1191–200.

29 American College of Cardiology (see No. 17).

30 Lu-Yao GL, Mclerran D, Wasson J, Wennberg JE. An assessment of radical prostatectomy: Time trends, geographic variation, and outcomes. *JAMA* 1993; 269:2633–6.
 Barry MJ, Mulley AG, Fowler FJ, Wennberg JE. Watchful waiting vs. immediate transurethral resection for symptomatic prostatism: the importance of patient preferences. *JAMA* 1988; 259:3010–17.
31 European Carotid Surgery Trialists' Collaborative Group. MRC European carotid surgery trial (see No. 15).
32 McNeil BJ, Pauker SG, Sox HC, Jr, et al. On the elicitation of preferences for alternative therapies. *N Engl J Med* 1982; 306:1259–62.
 Eddy DM. The challenge. *JAMA* 1990; 263:287.
33 Hatlie MJ. Climbing the learning curve: new technologies, emerging obligations. *JAMA* 1993; 270:1364–5.
34 Brook RH. Health services research: is it good for you and me? *Acad Med* 1989; 64:124–30.
 Tarlov AR, Ware JE, Greenfield S, Nelson EC, Perrin E, Zubkoff M. The medical outcomes study: an application of methods for monitoring the results of medical care. *JAMA* 1989; 262:925–30.
 Tarlov AR. Outcomes assessment and quality of life in patients with immunodeficiency virus infection. *Ann Int Med* 1992; 116:166–7.
35 Geigle R, Jones SB. Outcomes measurement: a report from the front. *Inquiry* 1990; 27:7–13.
 Brook RH, Kamberg CJ. General health status outcome measurement: a commentary on measuring functional status. *J Chronic Dis* 1987; 40 (suppl l):131S–136S.
 Lehr H, Strosberg M. Quality improvement in health care: is the patient still left out? *QRB* 1991; 17:326–9.
36 McNeil BJ, Weichselbaum R, Pauker SG. Speech and survival: trade-offs between quality and quantity of life in laryngeal cancer. *N Engl J Med* 1981; 305:982–7.
 Ware JE Jr, Brook RH, Davies AR, Lohr KN. Choosing measures of health status for individuals in general populations. *Am J Public Health* 1981; 71(6):620–5.
 Lohr KN. Outcome measurement: concepts and questions. *Inquiry* 1988; 25:37–50.
 Hollenberg NK, Testa M, Williams GH. Quality of life as a therapeutic endpoint: an analysis of therapeutic trials in hypertension. *Drug Safety* 1991; 6:83–9.
37 Eddy DM. Anatomy of a decision. *JAMA* 1990; 263:441–3.
38 Wortsman J. Letter to the Editor. *N Engl J Med* 1979; 300:928.
39 Barry MJ, Mulley AG, Fowler FJ, Wennberg JE. Watchful waiting (see No. 30).
40 McNeil B.J, Weichselbaum R, Pauker SG. (see No. 36).
41 Pauly MV. What is unnecessary surgery? *Milbank Q* 1979; 57:95–117.
 McNeil BJ, Weichselbaum R, Pauker SG. Fallacy of five-year survival in lung cancer. *N Engl J Med* 1978; 299:1397–1401.
 Danis M, Gerrity MS, Southerland LI, Patrick DL. A comparison of patient, family and physician assessments of the value of medical intensive care. *Crit Care Med* 1988; 16:594–600.
42 We are grateful to Gary A. Chase for providing this example.
43 Tomlinson T, Brody H. Futility and the ethics of resuscitation. *JAMA* 1990;

264:1276–80.
44 Meyer H. Cost-conscious hospitals set futile care rules. *AMNews* June 28, 1993, 3:20.
45 President's Commission for the Study of Ethical Problems in Medicine and Biomedical and Behavioral Research. *Securing Access to Health Care*, vol 1, *Report*. Washington, DC: US Government Printing Office, 1983.
46 Eddy DM. What care is 'essential'? What services are 'basic'? *JAMA* 1991; 265:782–8.
47 US Congress, Senate. Special Committee on Aging. Who lives, who dies, who decides: the ethics of health care rationing. Hearing, 19 Jun 1991. Washington: U.S. Government Printing Office; 1992.
Strosberg MA, Weiner JM, Baker R, Fein IA, eds. Rationing America's medical care: the Oregon plan and beyond. Washington: Brookings Institution; 1992.
48 Pellegrino ED. Rationing health care: the ethics of medical gatekeeping. *J Contemp Health Law and Policy* 1986 Spring; 2:23–45.
49 Hopkins A, Fitzpatrick R, Foster A, et al. p. 120 (see No. 4).
50 Callahan D. Medical futility, medical necessity: The problem without a name. *Hastings Center Rep* 1991:30–35.
51 Callahan D (see No. 50).

11

Recommendations for limiting iatrogenic harm

As we have noted, studies relating to the incidence of iatrogenic or comiogenic illness have suggested that perhaps one-quarter to one-half of such events are potentially preventable. The most convincing documentation for preventable or potentially preventable adverse drug events comes from the work of Leape and colleagues, initially in the large retrospective medical practice study of New York hospitals,[1] and more recently, in prospective studies of adverse drug events in Boston teaching hospitals.[2] These studies, together with others from the field of nosocomial infection control,[3] suggest that prevention strategies should involve attention to five broad but highly interrelated areas. These include the development of active surveillance methods, improvement in information technology, incorporation of systems analysis techniques, education, outcomes research, and implementation of continuous quality improvement. Of these, quality improvement has been discussed in previous chapters and will be addressed only in relation to the other strategies.

Surveillance strategies

Active surveillance methods have been used with considerable success to gather reliable information regarding incidence and causes of several major classes of iatrogenic illness, as well as to document the effectiveness of preventive strategies. In numerous studies, the use of active surveillance has identified a dramatically higher incidence of adverse drug reactions (ADRs) as compared to more traditional passive reporting approaches or retrospective chart reviews.[4] Active surveillance, particularly when combined with computerization of medical records/ordering and continuous quality improvement techniques, have led to a reduction in the incidence of specifically identified types of drug–drug interactions.[5] In the field of nosocomial infection control, epidemiologic methods focusing on complications in the patient population rather than on the performance of individual practitioners, have provided essential information on the different prevention strategies needed for bloodstream, surgical wound and urinary tract infections, and nosocomial pneumonias.[6]

The lessons learned from these approaches should, where possible, be generalized to other categories of medical harm as well as to other patient populations. Although there are at least ten times as many outpatient visits as hospital admissions in the United States annually,[7] there have been few systematic attempts to study adverse events in outpatient populations. Obstacles to the study of ambulatory populations include a paucity of recorded information; difficulty in defining the segment of care that may be the object of study; and uneven follow-up.[8] The centralized delivery of care in health maintenance organizations may remove some of these obstacles and thus provide an opportunity for addressing this gap in the literature on adverse patient outcomes.

Information technology

Improved accessibility to patient information by the health care team can serve both to identify and prevent potential adverse reactions especially to drug treatment.[9] For example, information provided at the time of drug ordering can help to educate providers about potential drug–drug, drug–food, and drug–disease interactions. The immediate availability of such information can also help to alert health care providers to potential treatment risks in individual cases. Provider accessibility to electronic medical records may also prevent complications resulting from the actions of multiple treating physicians who may be unaware of concurrent treatments provided by others. Instant access to information can also help to facilitate communication among health care providers and can be effectively used in conjunction with active surveillance techniques and systems analysis approaches to identify sources of treatment failures or treatment complications.[10] Improved information technology in the form of pharmacy databases can also alert pharmacists and patients to possibly preventable complications associated with multiple drug use.

Systems analysis

Systems analysis combined with continuous quality improvement (CQI) has been used in many industries to reduce error and improve outcomes.[11]

These strategies avoid the 'bad apple'[12] approach which targets individuals, and instead emphasize system design as a major determinant in patient outcomes. At the heart of system-focused CQI is a model of collective accountability. Everyone in the system is responsible for identifying potential systems breakdowns and focusing attention on necessary improvements.[13] Recently, investigators have used this approach to identify the relationship between harmful error and system failure in health care delivery.[14] Importantly, Leape et al. found that inadequacies in the availability of information regarding patients and proper use of drug therapies represented the single greatest system deficiencies related to ADRs.[15] Systems analysis and improved information technology could be used together to minimize adverse reactions. It has been shown, for example, that fewer prescribing errors are made if prescribing options are automatically limited to clinically appropriate alternatives.[16] This principle can be used in developing computerized drug ordering systems that limit a physician's drug-ordering options, both with regard to specific drug utilization and dosing alternatives.

System-focused CQI has also been implemented in hospital infection control.[17] Through the use of flow-charting and cause and effect diagramming, and improved educational methods, an infection control staff was able to reduce in-hospital exposures to tuberculosis.

Education

Overcoming the ethos of infallibility

As Leape has pointed out, the education and socialization of doctors has tended to emphasize perfectibility and infallibility.[18] This ethos is reflected in the models of legal accountability and quality assurance that focus exclusively on individual performance. As we have argued, the emphasis on individual agency, fails to capture the broader, system-dimensions of harmful error. Further, as sociologist Charles Bosk has observed, the inculcation of a sense of individual rather than corporate responsibility in medical training serves to insure that 'the physician's conscience . . . is the patient's only protection.'[19] If the physician's conscientiousness is supplanted by cowardice, greed, callousness, pride, or self-deception, the already vulnerable patient must bear the brunt.

McIntyre and Popper have argued that the ethos of infallibility in medicine is encouraged by the philosophy of science is the basis for medical practice and education.[20] According to these authors, medical science and practice are largely based on the assumption that scientific knowledge grows by the accumulation of objective truth and that deference should be given to authorities who display the most accumulated knowledge. On this traditional model of professionalism, authority is the ideal and is precisely understood to be free from error. This approach to learning, they argue, encourages intellectual dishonesty in 'authorities' who do not admit error and in students who hide ignorance rather than regard it as a basis for learning. In opposition to this view, McIntyre, Popper and other philosophers of science argue that, in fact, knowledge develops through error and correction rather than through accumulation.[21] In other words, fallibility is an inevitable and necessary feature of intellectual growth. The ethos that accompanies *this* view of scientific inquiry is one in which practitioners would recognize, acknowledge, and learn from their mistakes. In medical care, McIntyre and Popper propose that this new ethos would manifest itself in full and systematic recording of all medical and surgical errors. The mechanisms for identifying error – medical audits, peer review, and active surveillance – would not be implemented as disciplinary tools but as valuable forms of feedback. Such review would be required for improving all performance regardless of its quality.

This call for a new scientific and medical ethos – what McIntyre and Popper call an ethos of professional self-criticism – is echoed in the growing body of literature on continuous quality improvement. It also reflects the principle that formed the core of both Nightingale's and Codman's calls for reform – improvement can only follow from a clear understanding of deficiency.

In medical education, an ethos of self-criticism can be facilitated by forums for the discussion of error and fallibility.[22] These forums should have as their purpose quality improvement and also the moral development of the health care provider. Training for self-criticism and for uncertainty[23] can also be facilitated through philosophy of medicine and clinical ethics courses that emphasize the inevitability of error and the moral response to it.[24] This would alleviate the unrealistic pressures that health care providers labor under[25] and would invite a more authentic appreciation for providers as well as for patients of the complexities of the clinical situation.

Clinical education that is oriented to self-criticism and to uncertainty will also emphasize the centrality of informing patients about the nature and likelihood of the harms associated with clinical care.[26] Candid communication regarding the risks and uncertainties surrounding care invites the patient to become, as much as is possible, a full participant in that care.

As Guthiel and colleagues[27] observe, the acknowledgment of clinical uncertainty in the informed consent process, is not only valuable in itself, but may also be effective in reducing malpractice claims by disappointed patients.

In a discussion of medical fallibility it is important to point out the role that medical malpractice plays in discouraging medical professionals from reporting or disclosing bad outcomes. As we have discussed, medical malpractice is based on a model that emphasizes individual agency and accountability. Compensation under the theory of negligence depends upon the identification of an individual agent who, in failing to abide by established standards, caused patient harm. The fear of malpractice may not only encourage concealment of poor results but, in the process, limit the vital knowledge that can be gained from adverse outcome data.[28]

Even under current malpractice law, however, the argument for concealment of adverse events is untenable. As Couch et al.[29] have pointed out, actionable claims in medical malpractice are limited to claims of negligence. In other words, only those errors resulting from a violation of professional standards count as malpractice. This excludes unanticipated harms that result from reasonable and prudent medical care. Moreover, although it has traditionally been assumed that data collection on hospital-related complications presents a liability risk to hospitals, most legal experts and hospital administrators now take the opposite view. First, in most states in the United States, internal hospital committee records are considered privileged information and are not, therefore, discoverable in civil court proceedings. Secondly, based on the experience of hospital infection control, the presence of an effective surveillance system is now regarded as one of the best defenses against unwarranted claims.[30] Nevertheless, success in instilling an ethos of professional self-criticism and quality improvement, will undoubtedly depend on malpractice reform. As we suggested in Chapter 6, a no-fault (or strict liability) compensation scheme for medical injuries is an approach that might facilitate these goals. It would reduce or eliminate questionable strategies to maintain secrecy and immunity and would do so in a way that does *not* compromise the interests of individual patients in knowing about the quality of their care or in being compensated for adverse events.[31]

Evidence and outcomes

There is already some indication of a shift away from the 'authority-based' model of learning criticized by McIntyre and Popper. It comes in the form of what is known as 'evidence-based' learning or 'evidence-based' medicine.'[32] Briefly, evidence-based education stresses the need for evidence as the basis of clinical judgment and practice. While this approach does not reject the value or usefulness of didactic learning or clinical experience, it does stress that these important ingredients in clinical judgment must be supplemented by consultation with current literature about diagnostic and treatment options. This new paradigm places a much lower value on authority and a much higher value on the strength of evidence as it bears on a clinical problem. The key features of the evidence-based approach are MEDLINE training for clinicians, the encouragement of critical appraisal by role-models, and instruction on how to best evaluate published studies and their methodological criteria. Although this educational approach is relatively new, it does have the potential for making practitioners more aware of the clinical risks and benefits elucidated by studies of treatment options and the quality of evidence on which these assessments are based.

In the United States, there were more than 2.4 billion prescriptions dispensed in 1996,[33] and, as we know from empirical studies, the majority of medically-induced complications are attributable to the adverse effects of drugs. One area in which medical education might contribute to the reduction of comiogenic harm is in improved training in clinical pharmacology. Medical education relating to issues such as pharmacokinetics, pharmacodynamics, pharmacoepidemiology, and pharmacoeconomics is woefully inadequate. Physicians are often less than fully cognizant of the side effects of many of the drugs they prescribe and are commonly unaware of even well documented drug–drug interactions. One potential training approach would be to better integrate clinical pharmacology in the clinical training years, in addition to its more usual introduction in the preclinical period of training during the first two years of medical school. Regular 'rounds' by clinical pharmacologists may also provide educational opportunities for both medical students and staff physicians. A concept for developing centers of education and research in therapeutics has recently been proposed.[34] This could prove helpful by providing accurate and unbiased information regarding pharmacotherapeutics to practicing physicians on an ongoing basis.

Although this book has emphasized the roles and responsibilities of physicians, the development of new educational strategies for other health care professionals is also essential to comiogenic harm prevention. Systems analyses have identified drug administration errors by nurses as a significant factor contributing to ADRs in hospitalized patients.[35] These errors can be reduced by system improvement as well as by nurse education.

Because errors at the drug ordering stage have the potential to be intercepted by nurses or pharmacists, attention to this important preventive role can also be emphasized in provider education.

Expanding the evidentiary basis of practice

Health services research indicates that less than a third of medical treatments are substantiated by strong experimental evidence. Moreover, the evidence that is available tends to emphasize efficacy (the level of benefit achievable under ideal clinical conditions) rather than effectiveness (benefit achievable under 'normal' treatment conditions).[36] Compounding the problem, physicians often do not have the skills to interpret and evaluate the medical literature, or to apply it in their practices.[37] This state of affairs has prompted a call not only for more evidence-based education but also for research initiatives to improve the quality of information that guides medical practice.[38] A number of strategies have been suggested in meeting this goal. One federal initiative begun in 1988 is the Agency for Health Care Policy and Research's (AHCPR) Patient Outcomes Research Team (PORT) studies. PORT studies provide a hybrid evidence-based approach that also relies on meta-analysis and expert consensus to determine clinical appropriateness. Since 1988, AHCPR has used the PORT studies as a basis for 19 practice guidelines for treatment of low back pain, otitis media, heart failure, human immunodeficiency virus, and benign prostate hyperplasia, among others.

Brook has suggested that the mandate for an improved evidentiary basis for medicine should extend beyond national policy to all academic and professional medical organizations as well as to practicing physicians. These organizations, together with managed care plans, he argues,[39]

must explicitly alter the physician's role in society to include their responsibility to participate in the production of new knowledge about what does and does not improve health. All physicians should devote a portion of their time to this activity. Medical students should be educated about the importance of this function as well as about how to collect reliable data and how to follow patients to reach accurate conclusions as to outcome.

In essence, Brook is advocating collective action on the part of the health care profession and individual and institutional providers to determine the clinical value of drugs, tests, and procedures – that is, their value in achieving measurable clinical benefit and minimizing patient harm. A reliable evidentiary basis for treatment recommendations has the potential to limit comiogenic harms in a number of ways. Sound evidence may enhance the informed consent process, by making patients more aware of the risks and benefits associated with treatment options. It may help to prevent harms associated with both the overuse and the underuse of treatments, as well as to improve the safety and quality of the treatments that *are* provided. Without the availability of reliable evidence, there is legitimate concern that the pressure to contain costs may become the strongest force guiding health care decision making.

In this book we have argued that moral norms are the fundamental mechanisms of accountability in health care. With this in mind, we maintain that improvements in the evidentiary basis of medicine and in the quality of patient care demand not only collective effort but also collective accountability on the part of health care providers to the moral norms of patient benefit and the prevention of patient harm, to patient self-determination and to public policies that promote justice in the distribution of health care to those in need.

Endnotes

1 Leape LL, Lawthers AG, Brennan TA, Johnson WG. Preventing medical injury. *J Qual Impr (QRB)* 1993; 19(5):144–9.
2 Bates DW, Cullen DJ, Laird N, et al. Incidence of adverse drug events and potential adverse drug events. JAMA 1995; 294:29–34.
3 Crede W, Hierholzer WJ. Surveillance for quality assessment: I. Surveillance in infection control success reviewed. *Infect Control Hosp Epidemiol* 1989; 10:470–474.
   McGeer A, Crede W, Hierholzer WJ, Jr. Surveillance for quality assessment: II. Surveillance for noninfectious processes: Back to basics. *Infect Control Hosp Epidemiol* 1990; 11:36–41.
   Haley RW, Culver DH, White JW, et al. The efficacy of infection surveillance and control programs in preventing nosocomial infections in US hospitals. *Am J Epidemiol* 1985; 121:182–205.
4 Classen DC, Pestotnick SL, Evans RS, Burke JP. Computerized surveillance of adverse drug events in hospital patients. JAMA 1991; 266:2847–51.
5 Classen DC, Burke JP, Pestotnic SL, et al. Surveillance for quality assessment: IV. Surveillance using a hospital information system. *Infect Control Hosp Epidemiol* 1991; 12:239–44.
6 Haley RW. The development of infection surveillance and control programs. In Bennett JV, Brachman PS. *Hospital Infections*, 3rd edn. Boston: Little, Brown, 1992, p. 63–78.
7 United States Buerau of the Census. *Statistical Abstract of the US: 1995*, 11th edn. Washington, DC, 1995, Table No. 185: Hospital use rates by type of hospital.
8 Donabedian A. Evaluating the quality of medical care. In White KL, ed. *Health Services Research: An Anthology*. Washington, DC: PAHO, 1992, p. 345–65.
9 Kahn KL. Above all 'Do no harm': How shall we avoid errors in medicine?

JAMA 1995; 274:75–7.
10 Leape LL. Error in medicine. JAMA 1994; 272:1851–7.
11 Shewhart WA. *Statistical Method from the Viewpoint of Quality Control.*
    Washington, DC: Dept. of Agriculture, 1939.
    Deming WE. *Out of the Crisis.* Cambridge, MA: MIT Center for Applied
    Engineering Studies, 1986.
    Juran JM, Gryna FM, eds. *Juran's Quality Control Handbook*, 4th edn. New
    York: McGraw Hill, 1988.
12 Berwick DM. Continuous improvement as an ideal in health care. *N Engl J
    Med* 1989; 321(1):53–6.
13 See Moray N. Error reduction as a systems problem; Cook RI, Woods DD.
    Operating at the sharp end: The complexity of human error and Gaba D.
    Human error in dynamic medical domains. All in: Bogner MS (ed.). *Human
    Error in Medicine.* Hillsdale NJ: Erlbaum, 1994, pp. 67–92; 197–224; 225–310.
14 Leape LL. (see No. 10).
15 Leape LL, Bates DW, Cullen DJ, et al. for the ADE Prevention Study Group.
    Systems analysis of adverse drug events. *JAMA* 1995; 274:35–43.
16 Bates DW, Kuperman G, Teich JM. Computerized physician order entry and
    quality of care. *Qual Manage Health Care* 1994; 2:18–27.
17 Cook JD, Lewis L, Thomassen KA. The use of continuous quality
    improvement to achieve proper isolation of patients with suspected
    tuberculosis. *Am J Infect Control* 1995; 23(5):323–8.
18 Leape LL. (see No. 10).
19 Bosk CL. *Forgive and Remember: Managing Medical Failure.* Chicago:
    University of Chicago Press 1979, p. 192.
20 McIntyre N, Popper K. The Critical attitude in medicine: The need for a new
    ethics. *Br Med J* 1983; 287:1919–23.
21 Kuhn TS. *The Structure of Scientific Revolutions*, 2nd edn. Chicago:
    University of Chicago Press, 1970.
22 Levinson W, Dunn PM. Coping with fallibility. *JAMA.* 1989; 261:2252.
23 Fox R. Training for uncertainty. In Merton R, Reader G, Kendell P, eds. *The
    Student Physician.* Cambridge: Harvard University Press, 1957.
24 Meyer BA. A student teaching module: physician errors. *Fam Med* 1989;
    21(4):299–300.
    Fricchione GL. Facing limitation and failure: four literary portraits. *Pharos*
    1985; 48(4):13–18.
25 Dubovsky SL, Schrier RW. The mystique of medical training: Is teaching
    perfection in medical house-staff training a reasonable goal or a precursor of
    low self-esteem? *JAMA* 1983; 250:3067–58.
    Christensen JF, Levinson W, Dunn PM. The heart of darkness: the impact of
    perceived mistakes on physicians. *J Gen Intern Med* 1992; 7:424–31.
    Hilfiker D. Facing our mistakes. *N Engl J Med* 1984; 310:118–22.
26 For a caveat about sensitivity to cultural perceptions of truth-telling in
    medicine see our discussion in Chapter 5.
27 Guthiel TG, Bursztajn H, Brodsky A. Malpractice prevention through the
    sharing of uncertainty: Informed consent and the therapeutic alliance. *N Engl
    J Med* 1984; 311:49–51.
28 Couch NP, Tilney NL, Moore FD. The cost of misadventures in colonic
    surgery: a model for the analysis of adverse outcomes in standard procedures.
    Am J Surg 1978; 135:641–6.
29 Couch NP, Tilney NL, Rayner AA, Moore FD. The high cost of

low-frequency events: The anatomy and economics of surgical mishaps. *N Engl J Med* 1981; 304(11):634–7.

30 Haley RW, Gaynes RP, Arber RC, et al. Surveillance of nosocomial infections. In Bennett JV, Brachman PS. *Hospital Infections*, 3rd edn. Boston:Little, Brown, 1992, p. 85.

31 Weiler PC, Hiatt HH, Newhouse JP, et al. *A Measure of Malpractice: Medical Injury, Malpractice Litigation and Patient Compensation*. Cambridge, MA: Harvard University Press, 1993.

32 Woodward CA. Monitoring an innovation in medical education: The McMaster experience. In Ezzat ES, ed. *Innovation in Medical Education: An Evaluation of Its Present Status*. New York: Springer Publishing, 1990, pp. 27–39.

33 Buckley B. Top 200 drugs of 1996. *Pharmacy Times* 1997; 63(4):27–51.

34 Woosley RL. Centers for education and research in therapeutics. *Clin Pharm Therap* 1992; 55:249–55.

35 Leape LL, Bates DW, Cullen DJ, et al. (see No. 15).

36 Brook RH, Lohr KN. Efficacy, effectiveness, variations, and quality. Boundary-crossing research. *Med Care* 1985 May; 23(5):710–22.

37 Berwick D, Fineberg H, Weinstein M. When doctors meet numbers. *Am J Med* 1981; 71:991–8.

38 Roper WL, Winkenwerder W, Hackbarth GM, et al. Effectiveness in health care: An initiative to evaluate and improve medical practice. *N Engl J Med* 1988; 319:1197–202.

39 Brook RH. Quality of care: Do we care? *Ann Intern Med* 1991; 115:486–90 (p. 487).

Appendix

Table A.1. *Iatrogenic complications in the hospital setting**

Author (year)	Type of study	Number of patients affected (%)	Remarks
Barr[1] (1956)	unsystematic	500/1500 (5)	general hospital; restrictive definition
Schimmel[2]	prospective	198/1014 (19.5)	general medical service; restrictive definition
Reichel[3] (1965)	prospective	146/500 (29.2)	elderly population; general medical service; broad definition
McLamb and Huntley[4] (1967)	prospective	47/240 (19.5)	general medical service; broad definition
Ogilvie and Ruedy[5] (1967)	prospective	177/731 (24)	general medical service; broad definition
Steel, et al.[6] (1981)	prospective	290/815 (36)	general medical service including intensive care unit; somewhat restrictive definition
Couch et al.[7] (1981)	prospective	36/3612 (0.8)	general surgical service; highly restrictive definition
Jahnigen et al.[8] (1982)	prospective	93/222 (41.8)	elderly population; Veterans Hospital; broad definition
De la Sierra et al.[9] (1989)	not reported	295/1176 (25.1)	general medical service; broad definition
Harvard Medical Practice Study[10] (1991)	retrospective	1133/30195 (3.7)	multiple hospitals/services; highly restrictive definition

*If one averages the results from the broadest prospective studies,[2-6,8,9] using comparable populations during the period 1963–89, the mean incidence of iatrogenic illness in hospitalized patients is approximately 28%. It should be noted, however, that in most of these studies, the authors considered the reported data to represent conservative estimates of incidence, reflecting suboptimal surveillance and/or reporting mechanisms. Among these studies, the average incidence of major complications, that is, life-threatening or permanently disabling injury, was 5.7%. Importantly, the lowest reported incidence rates were found in studies that were either retrospective[10] or used highly restrictive definitions.[7,10] In the two studies evaluating elderly populations,[3,8] the average reported incidence of iatrogenic illness was somewhat higher (37%). One study reported a higher incidence in women; this is consistent with the literature on adverse drug reactions as a function of gender (see Chapter 8).

Table A.2. *Hospital admissions due to iatrogenic complications*

Author (year)	Type of study	Number of iatrogenic admissions (%)	Remarks
Trunet et al.[11] (1980)	prospective	41/325 (12.6)	ICU admissions; broad definition but excludes improper treatment
Lakshmanan, et al.[12] (1986)	prospective	45/834 (5.4)	medical service broad definition
Bigby, et al.[13] (1987)	prospective	47/686 (6.8)	ER admissions broad definition

ICU: intensive care unit; ER: emergency room.

Table A.3. *Adverse drug effects (ADE) in outpatients*

Author (year)	Type of study	Incidence of ADE (%)	Remarks
Stewart & Cluff[14] (1971)	retrospective	38/75 (50.6)	general medical clinic; survey; side effects at some time in the past; historical experience
Kellaway & McCrae[15] (1973)	prospective	63/200 (31.5)	acute medical ward discharges; WHO definition
Martys[16] (1979)	prospective	335/817 (41)	general practice; patients administered single drugs for first time, WHO definition
Klein, et al.[17] (1984)	patient perception	89/299 (30)	general medical clinic; 'broad' definition, but excluding treatment failures
Hutchinson, et al.[18]	prospective telephone surveillance	49/1026 (5)	internal medicine practice; excludes 19% 'possible' reactions
Chrischilles, et al.[19] (1992)	patient survey	381/3170 (10)	rural non-institutionalized elderly population; patient self-report; broad, non-standard definition
Schneider, et al.[20] (1992)	prospective	46/463 (10)	general medical practice 'restrictive' definition; excludes 11% 'possible' reactions

WHO: World Health Organization.

Table A.4. *Adverse drug effects (ADE) in the hospital setting*

Author (year)	Type of study	Incidence of ADE (%)	Severity of Complications (N, %)	Remarks
Schimmel[2] (1964)	prospective	103/1014 (10)	moderate 44 (4.3) major 14 (1.3)	medical service, univ. hospital broad definition
Cluff, et al.[21] (1965)	prospective	97/714 (13.6)	moderate 71 (9.9) severe 10 (1.4)	medical service, univ. hospital; restrictive definition includes documented/probable
Seidl, et al.[22] (1966)	prospective/ retrospective	38/267 (11.3)	not reported	medical service, univ. hospital restrictive definition
Ogilvie & Ruedy[23] (1967)	prospective	132/731 (18)	moderate 74 (10.1) major 67 (9.1)	medical service, teaching hospital; broad definition, includes diagnostic and therapeutic effects
Hoddinot et al.[24] (1967)	prospective	16/104 (15.4)	most reactions not serious	medical service, univ. hospital; restrictive definition; only probable reactions included
Simmons, et al.[25] (1968)	prospective	27/219 (12.3)	not reported	medical service, univ. hospital
Reidenberg[26] (1968)	retrospective	421/81,100 (0.49) 351/81,100 (0.41)	not reported	all services, univ. hospital
Borda[27] (1968)	prospective	291/830 (35)	moderate 159 (19) major 74 (8.9)	medical service, univ. hospital; 69% definite/probable active surveillance
Hurwitz & Wade[28] (1969)	not reported	118/1160 (10.2)	moderate 103 (8.8) severe 4 (0.34)	med-surg., psych wards, univ. hosp.; broad definition, but most were documented/probable
Wang & Terry[29] (1971)	prospective	128/8291 (1.5)	not reported	med-surg. ward, Veteran's Administration hospital; restrictive definition; no women
Smidt & McQueen[30] (1972)	retrospective	247/9104 (2.7)	moderate 117 (1.2) major 46 (0.5) fatal 8 (0.08)	all services, general hospital; higher incidence in medical services
Levy, et al.[31] (1973)	prospective	347/1239 (28)	moderate 133 (10.7) major 21 (1.6)	medical depts., univ. hospital; broad definition; 76% probable/definite
Levy, et al.[31] (1973)	prospective	3,329/11,891 (27)	moderate 1355 (11.3) major 376 (3.1)	medical depts., multiple sites; broad definition; 76% probable/definite
Burnum[32] (1976)	retrospective	24/276 (8.6)	not reported	all services, community hosp.
Schumock, et al.[33] (1991)	prospective	14/160 (8.75)	not reported	medical service, teaching hospital; ADR requires major change in patient management
Classen, et al.[34] (1991)	prospective, concurrent monitoring	648/36,653 (1.76)	moderate 600 (1.6) major 21 (1.6)	medical service, univ. hospital; may not include less severe
Leape, et al.[35] (1991)	retrospective	178/30,195 (0.6)	not reported	all services, 51 hospitals; restrictive definition (requiring prolongation of hospitalization or disability at discharge)
Bates, et al.[36] (1995)	prospective	297/4,031 (6.1)	moderate 30 (0.10) severe 13 (0.04)	11 med-surg. units in 2 hospitals; broad definition; active surveillance

Table A.5. *Drug-related hospital admissions*

Author (year)	Type of study	Number of drug-related admissions (%)	Remarks
Cluff, et al.[21] (1965)	prospective	28/714 (3.9)	restrictive definition; higher in women/elderly
Ogilvie & Ruedy[23] (1967)	prospective	48/731 (6.6)	broad definition
Hurwitz[37] (1969)	prospective	37/1268 (2.9)	details limited
Levy, et a.[31] (1973)	prospective	73/1239 (5.9) 797/11,891 (6.7)	from Israel and North America broad definition
Caranasos, et al.[38] (1974)	prospective	177/6063 (2.9)	restrictive definition; higher in women/elderly
Miller, et al.[39] (1974)	prospective	260/7017 (3.7)	restrictive definition
McKenney & Harrison[40] (1976)	prospective	17/216 (7.95)	broad definition
Burnum[32] (1976)	prospective	17/276 (6.1)	not defined
Ghose[41] (1980)	not reported	15/171 (8.8)	broad definition; excludes self-poisoning
Williamson & Chopin[42] (1980)	prospective	209/1998 (10.4)	restricted to elderly; England, Wales, Scotland
Bergman & Wiholm[43] (1981)	prospective	16/285 (5.6)	includes only definite/probable
Black & Somers[44] (1984)	retrospective	30/481 (6.2)	excludes self-poisoning
Lakshmanan, et al.[12] (1986)	prospective	35/834 (4.2)	broad definition
Ives, et al.[45] (1987)	retrospective	17/293 (5.8)	higher in elderly
Grymonpre, et al.[46] (1988)	prospective	83/718 (11.5)	broad definition; higher in women
Colt & Shapiro[47] (1989)	retrospective	23/244 (9.4)	higher in elderly
Bero, et al.[48] (1991)	retrospective	45/684 (7)	broad definition
Hallas, et al.[49] (1992)	prospective	212/1999 (10.6)	broad definition; includes therapeutic failures

Table A.6. *Deaths due to the administration of drugs*

Author (year)	Type of study	Number of drug-related deaths (%)	Remarks
Seidl, et al.[22] (1966)	prospective	8/714 (1.1)	medical wards, univ. hospital
Ogilvie & Ruedy[5] (1967)	prospective	17/739 (2.3)	medical service, general hospital
Shapiro, et al.[50] (1971)	prospective	27/6,199 (0.44)	medical wards, six hospitals
Smidt & McQueen[30] (1972)	prospective	8/9,104 (0.08)	all hospital services
Porter & Jick (1977)[51]	prospective	24/26,462 (0.09)	acute disease medical wards
Bates, et al.[36] (1995)	prospective	3/4031 (0.07)	med. surg. units, two tertiary care hospitals

References

1 Barr DP. Hazards of modern diagnosis and therapy – the price we pay. *JAMA* 1956; 159:1452–6.
2 Schimmel EM. The hazards of hospitalization. *Ann Intern Med* 1964; 60:100–10.
3 Reichel W. Complications in the care of five hundred elderly hospitalized patients. *J A, Geriatr Soc* 1965; 13:973–81.
4 McLamb JT, Huntley RR. The hazards of hospitalization. *South Med J* 1967; 60:469–72.
5 Ogilvie RI, Ruedy J. Adverse reactions during hospitalization I. *Can Med Ass J* 1967; 97:1445–50.
6 Steel K, Gertman PM, Crescenzi C, Anderson J. Iatrogenic illness on a general medical service at a university hospital. *N Engl J Med* 1981; 304(11):638–42.
7 Couch NP, Tilney NL, Rayner AA, Moore FD. The high cost of low-frequency events: The anatomy and economics of surgical mishaps. *N Engl J Med* 1981; 304(11):634–7.
8 Jahnigen D, Hannon C, Laxson L, et al. Iatrogenic disease in hospitalized elderly veterans. *J Am Geriatr Soc* 1982; 30(6):387–90.
9 De la Sierra A, Cardellach F, Cobo E., et al. Iatrogenic illness in a department of general internal medicine: A prospective study. *The Mount Sinai J Med* 1989; 56(4):267–71.
10 Brennan TA, Leape LL, Laird NM, et al. Incidence of adverse events and negligence in hospitalized patients. Results of the Harvard Medical Practice Study I. *N Engl J Med* 1991; 324(6):370–6.
11 Trunet P, LeGall JR, Lhoste F, et al. The role of iatrogenic disease in admissions to intensive care. *JAMA* 1980; 244:2617–20.
12 Lakshmanan MC, Hershey CO, Breslau D. Hospital admissions caused by iatrogenic disease. *Arch Intern Med* 1986; 146:1931–4.

13 Bigby J, Dunn J, Goldman L, et al. Assessing the preventability of emergency hospital admissions. *Am J Med* 1987; 83:1031–6.

14 Stewart RB, Cluff LE. Studies on the epidemiology of adverse drug reactions: VI: Utilization and interactions of prescription and non-prescription drugs in outpatients. *Johns Hopkins Med J* 1971; 129:319–31.

15 Kellaway GSM, McCrae E. Intensive monitoring for adverse drug effects in patients discharged from acute medical wards. *NZ Med J* 1973; 78:525–8.

16 Martys CR. Adverse reactions to drugs in general practice. *Br Med J* 1979; 2:1194–7.

17 Klein LE, German PS, Levine DM, et al. Medication problems among patients: a study with emphasis on the elderly. *Arch Int Med* 1984; 144:1185–8.

18 Hutchinson TA, Flegel KM, Kramer MS, et al. Frequency, severity and risk factors for adverse drug reactions in adult out-patients: A prospective study. *J Chron Dis* 1986; 39(7):533–42.

19 Chrischilles EA, Segar ET, et al. Self-reported adverse drug reactions and related resource use. *Ann Intern Med* 1992; 117:634–40.

20 Schneider JK, Mion LC, Frengley JD, et al. Adverse drug reactions in an elderly outpatient population. *Am J Hosp Pharm* 1992; 49:90–6.

21 Cluff LE, Thornton CF, Seidl LG, Smith J. Epidemiological study of adverse drug reactions. *Trans Assoc Am Phys* 1965; 78:255–68.

22 Seidl LG, Thornton GF, Smith JW, Cluff LE. Studies on the epidemiology of adverse drug reactions. III: Reactions in patients on a general medical service. *Bull Johns Hopkins Hosp* 1966; 119:299–315.

23 Ogilvie RI, Ruedy J. Adverse drug reactions during hospitalization II. *Can Med Assn J* 1967; 97:1450–7.

24 Hoddinott BC, Gowdey CW, Coulter WK, et al. Drug reactions and errors in administration on a medical ward. *Can Med Ass J* 1967; 97:1001–6.

25 Simmons M, et al. Adverse drug reactions during hospitalization (letter). *Can Med Assoc J* 1968; 98:175.

26 Reidenberg MM. Registry of adverse drug reactions. *JAMA* 1968; 203(1):31–4.

27 Borda IT, Slone D, Jick H. Assessment of adverse reactions within a drug surveillance Program. *JAMA* 1968; 205:645–7.

28 Hurwitz N, Wade OL. Intensive hospital monitoring of adverse reactions to drugs. *Br Med J* 1969; 1:531–6.

29 Wang RIH. Terry LC. Adverse drug reactions in a Veterans Administration Hospital. *J Clin Pharmacol* 1971; 11:14–18.

30 Smidt NA, McQueen EG. Adverse reactions to drugs: A comprehensive hospital inpatient survey. *NZ Med J* 1972; 76:397–401.

31 Levy M, Nir I, Birnbaum D, et al. Adverse reactions to drugs in hospitalized medical patients: A comparative study. *Isr J Med Sci* 1973; 9:617–26.

32 Burnum JF. Letter: Preventability of adverse drug reactions. *Ann Intern Med* 1976; 85(1):80–1.

33 Schumock GT, Thornton JP, et al. Comparison of pharmary-based concurrent surveillance and medical record retrospective reporting of adverse drug reactions. *AJHP* 1991; 48:1974–6.

34 Classen DC, Pestotnik SL, Evans RS, Burke JP. Computerized surveillance of adverse drug events in hospital patients. *JAMA* 1991; 266(20):2847–51.

35 Leape LL, Brennan TA, Laird N, et al. The nature of adverse events in hospitalized patients. Results of the Harvard Medical Practice Study II. *N Engl J Med* 1991; 324(6):377–84.

36 Bates DW, Cullen DJ, Laird N, et al. Incidence of adverse drug events and potential adverse drug events. *JAMA* 1995; 274:29–34.
37 Hurwitz N. Admissions to hospital due to drugs. *Br Med J* 1969; 1:539–40.
38 Caranasos GJ, Stewart RB, Cluff LE. Drug-induced illness leading to hospitalization. *JAMA* 1974; 228:713–17.
39 Miller RR. Hospital admissions due to adverse drug reactions. *Arch Intern Med* 1974; 134:219–223.
40 McKenney JM, Harrison WL. Drug-related hospital admissions. *Am J Hosp Pharm* 1976; 33(8):792–5.
41 Ghose K. Hospital bed occupancy due to drug related problems. *J Roy Soc Med* 1980; 73:853–6.
42 Williamson J, Chopin JM. Adverse reactions to prescribed drugs in the elderly: A multi-centre investigation. *Age Aging* 1980; 9:73–80.
43 Bergman U, Wiholm B-E. Drug-related problems causing admission to a medical clinic. *Eur J Clin Pharmac* 1981; 20:193–200.
44 Black AJ, Somers K. Drug-related illness resulting in hospital admissions. *J R Coll Physicians London* 1984; 18.40–1.
45 Ives TJ, Bentz EJ, Gwyther RE. Drug-related admissions to a family medicine inpatient service. *Arch Intern Med* 1987; 147:1117–20.
46 Grymonpre RE, Mitenko PA, Sitar DS, et al. Drug-associated hospital admissions in older medical patients. *J Am Geriatrics Soc* 1988; 36:1092–8.
47 Colt, HG, Shapiro AP. Drug-induced illness as a cause for admission to a community hospital. *J Am Geriatr Soc* 1989; 37:323–6.
48 Bero LA, Lipton HL, Bird JA. Characterization of geriatric drug-related hospital readmissions. *Med Care* 1991; 29(10):989–1003.
49 Hallas J, Gram LF, Grodum E, Damsbo N, et al. Drug related admissions to medical wards: a population based survey. *Br J Clin Pharmacol* 1992; 33(1):61–8.
50 Shapiro S, Slone D, Lewis GP, et al. Fatal drug reactions among medical inpatients. *JAMA* 1971; 216:467–72.
51 Porter J, Jick H. Drug-related deaths among medical in-patients. *JAMA* 1977; 237:879.

Bibliography

Abraham KS. Medical liability reform: a conceptual framework. *N Engl J Med* 1988; 260:68–72.

Ackerknecht EH. *Medicine at the Paris Hospital 1794–1848*. Baltimore: The Johns Hopkins Press, 1967.

Ackerknecht EH. *Therapeutics from the Primatives to the 20th Century*. New York: Hafner Press, 1973.

Ackerknecht EH. Zur Geschichte der iatrogenen Erkrankungen des Nervensystems. *Therapeutische Umschau* 1970; 27(6):345–6.

Ackerknecht EH. Zur Geschichte der iatrogenen Krankheiten. *Gesnerus* 1970; 27(1):57–63.

Albert RK, Condie F. Hand-washing patterns in medical intensive-care units. *N Engl J Med* 1981; 304:1465–6.

Allan EL, Barker KN. Fundamentals of medication error research. *Am J Hosp Pharm* 1990; 47(3):555–71.

American College of Cardiology/American Heart Association Task Force on Assessment of Diagnostic and Therapeutic Cardiovascular Procedures (Subcommittee on coronary artery bypass graft surgery). Guidelines and indications for coronary artery bypass graft surgery. *J Am Coll Cardiol* 1991; 17:543–89.

American College of Obstetricians and Gynecologists Committee on Ethics. Policy Statement, No. 170. *Physician Responsibility Under Managed Care: Patient Advocacy in a Changing Health Care Environment*. Washington, DC: ACOG, 1996.

American College of Obstetricians and Gynecologists Committee on Ethics. Policy Statement, No. 85. *Human immunodeficiency virus infection: Physician's responsibilities*. Washington, DC: ACOG, 1990.

American Hospital Association. *A Patient's Bill of Rights*. Chicago: American Hospital Association, 1973. Reprinted in Reich WT, ed., *The Encyclopedia of Bioethics*. New York: Simon and Schuster/Macmillan, 1995, p. 2619.

American Hospital Association. *Infection Control in Hospitals*. Chicago: American Hospital Association, 1968.

American Medical Association Council on Ethical and Judicial Affairs. Ethical issues in managed care. *JAMA* 1995; 273(4):330–335.

American Medical Association. *Code of Medical Ethics*, 2nd edn. New York: William Wood & Company, 1868.

American Medical Association. Principles of medical ethics, 1957. Reprinted in

Reich WT, ed., *The Encyclopedia of Bioethics*, vol V. New York: Simon and Schuster/Macmillan, 1995, pp. 2648–9.

Amundsen DW. Medical deontology and pestilential disease in the late Middle Ages. *J Hist Med All Sci* 1977; 32:403–21.

Anderson GM, Grumbach K, Luft HS, Roos LL, Mustard C, Brook R. Use of coronary artery bypass surgery in the United States and Canada. Influence of age and income. *JAMA* 1993; 269:1661–6.

Anderson RE, Fox RC, Hill RB. Medical uncertainty and the autopsy: Occult benefits for students. *Hum Pathol* 1990; 21(2):128–35.

Annas G. Reframing the debate on health care reform by replacing our metaphors. *N Engl J Med* 1995; 332:774–7.

Appelbaum PS, Lidz CW, Meisel A. *Informed Consent: Legal Theory and Clinical Practice*. New York: Oxford, 1986.

Asch DA, Parker RM. The Libby Zion case: One step forward or two steps backward? *N Engl J Med* 1988; 318:771–5.

Asken MJ, Raham DC. Resident performance and sleep deprivation: A review. *J Med Ed* 1983; 58:382–8.

Associated Press. Report details errors at Cancer Institute. *Washington Post*, May 31, 1995, p. A20.

Avorn J, Chren M, Hartley R. Scientific versus commercial sources of influence on the previous behavior of physicians. *Am J Med* 1982; 73:4–8.

Baier A. Trust and antitrust. *Ethics* 1986; 96:231–60.

Baker R, Porter D, Porter R. (eds.). *The Codification of Medical Morality: Historical and Philosophical Studies of the Formalization of Western Medical Morality in the Eighteenth and Nineteenth Centuries*, Vol. 1: *Medical Ethics and Etiquette in the Eighteenth Century*. Boston: Kluwer Academic Publishers, 1993.

Baker R. Deciphering Percival's code. In Baker R, Porter D, Porter R, eds. *The Codification of Medical Morality:Historical and Philosophical Studies of the Formalization of Western Medical Morality in the Eighteenth and Nineteenth Centuries*, Vol. 1: *Medical Ethics and Etiquette in the Eighteenth Century*. Boston: Kluwer Academic Publishers, 1993, pp. 179–211.

Barnett HJM, Haines SJ. Carotid endarterectomy for asymptomatic carotid stenosis. *N Engl J Med* 1993; 328:276–79.

Barr DP. Hazards of modern diagnosis and therapy – the price we pay. *JAMA* 1956; 159:1452–6.

Barry MJ, Mulley AG, Fowler FJ, Wennberg JE. Watchful waiting vs immediate transurethral resection for symptomatic prostatism: The importance of patient preferences. *JAMA* 1988; 259:3010–17.

Bates DW, Cullen DJ, Laird N, et al. Incidence of adverse drug events and potential adverse drug events: Implications for prevention. *JAMA* 1995; 274:29–34.

Bates DW, Kuperman G, Teich JM. Computerized physician order entry and quality of care. *Qual Manag Health Care* 1994; 2:18–27.

Bawkin H. The tonsil-adenoidectomy enigma. *J Pediatrics* 1958; 52:339–61.

Beaty HN, Petersdorf RG. Iatrogenic factors in infectious disease. *Ann Intern Med* 1966; 65:641–55.

Beauchamp TL, Childress JF. *Principles of Biomedical Ethics*, 4th edn. New York: Oxford University Press, 1994.

Beauchamp TL, Childress JF. *Principles of Biomedical Ethics*. New York: Oxford University Press, 1979.

Beauchamp TL, McCullough LB. *Medical Ethics: The Moral Responsibilities of Physicians.* Engelwood Cliffs, NJ: Prentice-Hall, 1984.

Bedell SE, Deitz DC, Leeman D, et al. Incidence and characteristics of preventable iatrogenic cardiac arrests. *JAMA* 1991; 265:2815–20.

Beecher HK. Ethics in clinical research. *N Engl J Med* 1966; 274:1354–60.

Beecher HK, Todd DP. A study of the deaths associated with anesthesia and surgery. *Ann Surg* 1954; 140:1–34.

Bergman U, Wiholm B-E. Drug related problems causing admission to a medical clinic. *Eur J Clin Pharmac* 1981; 20:193–200.

Bernstein SJ, Hilborne LH, Leape LL, et al. The appropriateness of use of coronary angiography in New York State. *JAMA* 1993; 269(6):766–9.

Bernstein SJ, McGlynn EA, Siu AL, et al. The appropriateness of hysterectomy. *JAMA* 1993; 269:2398–402.

Bero LA, Lipton HL, Bird JA. Characterization of geriatric drug-related hospital readmissions. *Med Care* 1991; 29(10):989–1003.

Berwick D, Fineberg H, Weinstein M. When doctors meet numbers. *Am J Med* 1981; 71:991–8.

Berwick DM. Measuring health care quality. *Pediatr Rev* 1988; 10(1):11–16.

Berwick DM. Continuous improvement as an ideal in health care. *N Engl J Med* 1989; 320(1):53–6.

Berwick DM. Health services research and quality of care. *Med Care* 1989; 27(8):763–71.

Berwick DM. Controlling variation in health care: A consultation from Walter Shewhart. *Med Care* 1991; 29(12):1212–25.

Berwick DM, Enthoven A, Bunker JP. Quality management in the NHS: The doctor's role I. *Br Med J* 1992; 304:235–9.

Bigby J, Dunn J, Goldman L, et al. Assessing the preventability of emergency hospital admissions. *Am J Med* 1987; 83:1031–6.

Black AJ, Somers K. Drug related illness resulting in hospital admissions. *J R Coll Physicians London* 1984; 18:40–1.

Blackman PH. How common is human error? Washington Post Health, April 21, 1992, p. 2.

Blake JB (ed.). *Safeguarding the Public: Historical Aspects of Medicinal Drug Control.* Baltimore: The Johns Hopkins Press, 1970.

Blake JB. Smallpox innoculation in colonial Boston. In Brieger G, ed., *Theory and Practice in American Medicine: Historical Studies from the Journal of the History of Medicine and the Allied Sciences.* New York: Science History Publications, 1976, pp. 107–23.

Bleuler E. *Textbook of Psychiatry* (trans., by A. A. Brill). New York: Macmillan, 1924.

Blumberg M. Provider price changes for improved health care use. In G Chacko, ed., *Health Handbook: An International Reference on Care and Cure* Amsterdam: North Holland, 1979, pp. 27–49.

Bogner MS (ed.). *Human Error in Medicine.* Hillsdale, NJ: Erlbaum, 1994.

Bolande RP. Ritualistic surgery – circumcision and tonsillectomy. *N Engl J Med* 1969; 280:591–6.

Borda IT, Slone D, Jick H. Assessment of adverse reactions within a drug surveillance Program. *JAMA* 1968; 205:645–7.

Bornstein NM, Norris JW. Evolution and management of asymptomatic carotid stenosis. *Cerebrovasc Brain Metab Rev* 1993; 5:301–13.

Bosk CL. *Forgive and Remember: Managing Medical Failure.* Chicago: University of Chicago Press, 1979, p. 192.

Bowman JG. Hospital standardization series: General hospitals of 100 or more beds, Report for 1919. *Bull Am Coll Surg* 1920; 4:3–36.

Brennan TA, Leape LL, Laird NM, Hebert L, Localio AR, Lawthers AG, Newhouse JP, Weiler PC, Hiatt HH. Incidence of adverse events and negligence in hospitalized patients. Results of the Harvard Medical Practice Study I. *N Engl J Med* 1991; 324(6):370–6.

Brennan TA. Ethics of confidentiality: The special case of quality assurance research. *Clin Research* 1990; 38(3):551–7.

Brieger G (ed.). *Medical America in the 19th Century: Readings from the Literature.* Baltimore: Johns Hopkins University Press, 1972.

Brieger G (ed.). *Theory and Practice in American Medicine: Historical Studies from the Journal of the History of Medicine and the Allied Sciences.* New York: Science History Publications, 1976.

Brieger GH. American surgery and the germ theory of disease. *Bull Hist Med* 1966; 40:135–45.

Brook RH, Kamberg CJ. General health status outcome measurement. A commentary on measuring functional status. *J Chronic Dis* 1987; 40 (supp. l): 131S–136S.

Brook RH. Health services research: Is it good for you and me? *Acad Med* 1989; 64:124–30.

Brook RH. Quality of care: Do we care? *Ann Intern Med* 1991; 115:486–90.

Brook RH, Lohr KN. Efficacy, effectiveness, variations, and quality. Boundary-crossing research. *Med Care* 1985; 23(5):710–22.

Buchanan AE. Philosophical foundations of beneficence. In Shelp EE, ed. *Beneficence in Health Care.* Dordrecht: D. Reidel, 1982.

Buckley B. Top 200 drugs of 1996. *Pharmacy Times* 1997; 63(4):27–51.

Bunker JP. Surgical manpower: A comparison of operation and surgeons in the United States and in England and Wales. *N Engl J Med* 1970; 282:135–44.

Bunker JP, Hinkley D, McDermott WV. Surgical innovation and its evaluation. *Science* 1978; 200:937–41.

Burns CR. *Medical Ethics in the U.S. Before the Civil War.* Ann Arbor: University Microfilms, 1973.

Burnum JF. Letter: Preventability of adverse drug reactions. *Ann Intern Med* 1976; 85(1):80–1.

Bush V. *Science, The Endless Frontier: A Report to the President on a Program for Postwar Scientific Research.* Washington, DC: National Science Foundation, 1960. (First pub. 1945.)

Butterfield LH (ed.). *Letters of Benjamin Rush,* vol. 2. Princeton: American Philosophical Assn., 1951.

Bynum WF, Porter R (eds.). *Companion Encyclopedia of the History of Medicine.* New York: Routledge, 1993.

Bynum WF. *Science and the Practice of Medicine in the Nineteenth Century* Cambridge: Cambridge University Press, 1994.

Callahan D. Medical futility, medical necessity: The problem without a name. *Hastings Center Rep* 1991; 21:30–5.

Canterbury v *Spence* No. 22099 US Ct of Appeals, DC Circuit, (May 19, 1972). 464 Fed Rep 2d 772.

Caplan A, Engelhardt HT, McCartney J. *The Concepts of Health and Disease.* Reading, MA: Addison-Wesley, 1981.

Caplan RA, Posner KL, Cheney FW. Effect of outcome on physician judgments of appropriateness of care. *JAMA* 1991; 265:1957–60.

Caranasos GJ, Stewart RB, Cluff LE. Drug-induced illness leading to hospitalization. *JAMA* 1974; 228:713–17.

Carlson R. A conceptualization of a no-fault compensation system for medical malpractice injuries. *Law and Society Review* 1973; 7:329–69.

Carmichael DH. Learning medical fallibility. *South Med J* 1985; 78:1–3.

Carrese JA, Rhodes LA. Western bioethics on the Navajo reservation. *JAMA* 1995; 274:826–9.

Carter KC, Tate GS. The earliest-known account of Semmelweis's initiation of disinfection at Vienna's Allgemeines Krankenhaus. *Bull Hist Med* 1991; 65:252–7.

Carter KC. On the decline of bloodletting in nineteenth century medicine. *J Psych Anthro* 1982; 5:219–34.

Cassedy JH. *American Medicine and Statistical Thinking.* Cambridge, MA: Harvard University Press, 1984.

Cassell EJ. *Talking with Patients,* Vol. 1: *The Theory of Doctor-Patient Communication.* Cambridge, MA: MIT Press, 1985.

Cassell J. Technical and moral error in medicine and in fieldwork. *Human Organization* 1981; 40(2):160–8.

Cavuto NJ, Woosley RL, Sale M. Pharmacies and the prevention of fatal drug interactions. *JAMA* 1996; 275:1086–8.

Centers for Disease Control. Proceedings of the International Conference on Nosocomial Infections. August 3–6. Atlanta: CDC, 1970.

Chalmers I. Minimizing harm and maximizing benefit during innovation in health care: Controlled or uncontrolled experimentation? *Birth* 1986; 13:155 –64.

Chalmers I. The Cochrane collaboration: Preparing, maintaining, and disseminating systematic reviews of the effects of health care. *Ann NY Acad Sci* 1993; 703:156–65.

Chalmers TC. Meta-analysis in clinical medicine. *Trans Am Clin Climatol Assn* 1987; 99:144–50.

Chandrasekar PH, Kruse JA, Matthews MF. Nosocomial infection among patients in different types of intensive care units at a city hospital. *Crit Care Med* 1986; 14:508–10.

Chassin M, Brook R, Park R, et al. Variations in the use of medical and surgical services by the Medicare population. *N Engl J Med* 1986; 314:285.

Chassin MR, Kosecoff J, Park RE, et al. Does inappropriate use explain geographic variations in the use of health care services? *JAMA* 1987; 258(18):2533–7.

Chassin MR, Kosecoff J, Solomon DH, Brook RH. How coronary angiography is used. Clinical determinants of appropriateness. *JAMA* 1987; 258:2543–7.

Chassin MR. Standards of care in medicine. *Inquiry* 1988; 25(4):437–53.

Chavigny KH, Helm A. Ethical dilemmas and the practice of infection control. *Law Med Health Care* 1982; 10:168–71,174.

Childress J. *Who Should Decide?: Paternalism in Health Care.* New York: Oxford, 1982.

Childress J. Hospital acquired infections: Some ethical issues. In RP Wenzel, ed. *Prevention and Control of Nosocomial Infections.* Baltimore: Williams and Wilkins, 1987, pp. 49–55.

Classen DC, Burke JP, Pestotnic SL, et al. Surveillance for quality assessment: IV. Surveillance using a hospital information system. *Infect Control Hosp*

Epidemiol 1991; 12:239–44.

Classen DC, Pestotnik SL, Evans RS, Burke JP. Computerized surveillance of adverse drug events in hospital patients. *JAMA* 1991; 266(20):2847–51.

Clinton JJ. From the agency for health care policy and research. *JAMA* 1991; 266:2057.

Cluff LE, Thornton G, Seidl L, et al. Epidemiological study of adverse drug reactions. *Trans Assoc Am Physicians* 1965; 78:255–68.

Cluff LE, Thornton CF, Seidl LG, Smith J. Epidemiological study of adverse drug reactions *Trans Assoc Am Phys* 1965; 78:255–68.

Codman EA. *A Study in Hospital Efficiency as Demonstrated by the Case Report of the First Five Years of a Private Hospital.* Boston: n.p., n.d probably 1916. (Reprinted Oakbrook Terrace, IL: Joint Commission on Accreditation of Health Care Organizations, 1996.)

Codman EA. A study in hospital efficiency as represented by product. *Trans Am Gynecol Soc* 1914; 39:60–100.

Codman EA. The product of the hospital. *Surg Gynecol Obstet* 1914; 18(4):491–6.

Codman EA. *The Shoulder* Malabar, FL: RE Kreiger. 1984 (First published 1934.)

Colt HG, Shapiro AP. Drug-induced illness as a cause for admission to a community hospital. *J Am Geriatr Soc* 1989; 37:323–6.

Committee on Infections within Hospitals, American Hospital Association. Statement on microbiological sampling in the hospital. *Hospitals* 1974; 48:125–6.

Cook JD, Lewis L, Thomassen KA. The use of continuous quality improvement to achieve proper isolation of patients with suspected tuberculosis. *Am J Infect Control* 1995; 23(5):323–8.

Cook RI, Woods DD. Operating at the sharp end: The complexity of human error. In Bogner MS, ed. *Human Error in Medicine.* Hillsdale NJ: Erlbaum, 1994, pp. 225–310

Cooper JB, Newbower RS, Kitz RJ. An analysis of major errors and equipment failures in anesthesia management. Considerations for prevention and detection. *Anesthesiology* 1984; 60:34–42.

Cotton P. Determining more good than harm is not easy. *JAMA* 1993; 270:153–8.

Couch NP, Tilney NL, Moore FD. The cost of misadventures in colonic surgery: a model for the analysis of adverse outcomes in standard procedures. *Am J Surg* 1978; 135:641–6.

Couch NP, Tilney NL, Rayner AA, Moore FD. The high cost of low-frequency events: The anatomy and economics of surgical mishaps. *N Engl J Med* 1981; 304(11):634–7.

Crawshaw R, Rogers DE, Pellegrino ED, et al. Patient–physician covenant. *JAMA* 1995; 273:1553.

Crede W, Hierholzer WJ. Surveillance for quality assessment: I. Surveillance in infection control success reviewed. *Infect Control Hosp Epidemiol* 1989; 10:470–4.

Crossen HS. Abdominal surgery without detached pads or sponges. *Am J Obstet* 1909; 59:58–75, 250–284.

Curran WJ. Governmental regulation of the use of human subjects in medical research: The approach of two federal agencies. *Daedalus* 1969; 98:542–94.

Danis M, Gerrity MS, Southerland LI, Patrick DL. A comparison of patient, family and physician assessments of the value of medical intensive care. *Crit*

Care Med 1988; 16:594–600.

Dans PE. Clinical peer review: Burnishing a tarnished icon. *Ann Intern Med* 1993; 118(7):566–8.

Danzon PM. *New Evidence on the Frequency and Severity of Medical Malpractice Claims.* Santa Monica: RAND, 1986

DATTA Report. Laminectomy and microlaminectomy for treatment of lumbar disk herniation. *JAMA* 1990; 264:1469–72.

DATTA report. Reassessment of automated percutaneous lumbar diskectomy for herniated disks. *JAMA* 1991; 265:2122–3, 2125.

Davies DM. *Textbook of Adverse Drug Reactions.* 4th edn. Oxford: Oxford University Press, 1991.

Davis FD. *Phronesis and the Physician: A Defense of the Practical Paradigm of Clinical Rationality.* (Doctoral dissertation). Georgetown University, Washington, DC, April, 1996.

De la Sierra A, Cardellach F, Cobo E, et al. Iatrogenic illness in a department of general internal medicine: A prospective study. *The Mount Sinai J Med* 1989; 56(4):267–71.

Dearden CH, Rutherford WH. The resuscitation of the severely injured in the accident and emergency department – a medical audit. *Injury* 1985; 16:249–52.

Deming WE. *Out of the Crisis.* Cambridge, MA: MIT Center for Applied Engineering Studies, 1986.

DeMott RK, Sandmire HF. The Green Bay cesarean section study. I. The physician factor as a determinant of cesarean birth rates. *Am J Obstet Gynecol* 1990; 162(6):1593–9.

DeVille KA. *Medical Malpractice in Nineteenth-Century America: Origins and Legacy.* New York: NYU Press, 1990.

Dixon RE. Costs of nosocomial infections and benefits of infection control programs. In Wenzel RP, ed., *Prevention and Control of Nosocomial Infections.* Baltimore: Williams and Wilkins, 1987, pp. 19–25.

Dixon RE. Effect of infections on hospital care. *Ann Intern Med* 1978; 89:749–53.

Doctor who cut off wrong leg is defended by colleagues. *New York Times,* September 17, 1995, p. A28.

Doebbeling BN, Stanley GL, Sheetz CT, et al. Comparative efficacy of alternative hand-washing agents in reducing nosocomial infections in intensive care units. *N Engl J Med* 1992; 327(2):88–93.

Donabedian A. The epidemiology of quality. *Inquiry* 1985; 22:282–92.

Donabedian A. The quality of care. How can it be assessed? *JAMA.* 1988; 260(12):1743–8.

Donabedian A. Contributions of epidemiology to quality assessment and monitoring. *Infect Control Hosp Epidemiol* 1990; 11:117–21.

Donabedian A. The seven pillars of quality. *Arch Pathol Lab Med.* 1990; 114(11):1115–18.

Donabedian A. Evaluating the quality of medical care. In White KL, ed., *Health Services Research: An Anthology.* Washington, DC: PAHO, 1992, pp. 345–65.

Dowling HF. *Fighting Infection: Conquests of the Twentieth Century.* Cambridge, MA: Harvard University Press, 1977.

Doyle JC. Unnecessary hysterectomies: Study of 6,248 operations in thirty-five hospitals during 1948. *JAMA* 1952; 151(5):360–5.

Doyle JC. Unnecessary ovariectomies. *JAMA* 1952; 148:1105–11.

Dubois RW, Brook RH. Preventable deaths: Who, how often and why? *Ann Intern Med* 1988; 109:582–9.

Dubovsky SL, Schrier RW. The mystique of medical training: Is teaching perfection in medical house-staff training a reasonable goal or a precursor of low self-esteem? *JAMA* 1983; 250:3067–58.

Earle AS. The germ theory in America: Antisepsis and asepsis (1867–1900). *Surgery* 1969; 65:508–22.

Eddy DM. Clinical policies and the quality of clinical practice. *N Engl J Med* 1982; 307:343–7.

Eddy DM. Variations in physician practice: The role of uncertainty. *Health Affairs* 1984; 3(4): 74–89.

Eddy DM. Anatomy of a decision. *JAMA* 1990; 263:441–3.

Eddy DM. The challenge. *JAMA* 1990; 263:287.

Eddy DM. What care is 'essential'? What services are 'basic'? *JAMA* 1991; 265:782–8.

Eddy DM. Three battles to watch in the 1990s. *JAMA* 1993; 270:520–6.

Edelstein L. The Hippocratic physician. In Tempkin O, Tempkin CL, eds. *Ancient Medicine: Selected Papers of Ludwig Edelstein* . Baltimore: The Johns Hopkins Press, 1967.

Eickhoff TC. Microbiological sampling *Hospitals* 1970; 44:86–7

Eickhoff TC. The third dicennial international conference on nosocomial infections: Historical perspective: The landmark conference in 1970. *Am J Med* 1991; 91:3B–5S.

Eickhoff TC, Brachman PW, Bennett JV, et al. Surveillance of nosocomial infections in community hospitals. I. Surveillance methods, effectiveness and initial results. *J Infect Dis* 1969; 120(3):305–17.

Eisenberg J. *Doctor's Decisions and the Cost of Medical Care*. Ann Arbor, MI: Health Administration Press, 1986.

Eliason EL, McLaughlin C. Post-operative wound complications. *Ann Surg* 1934; 100:1159–76.

Emanuel EJ, Emanuel LL. What is accountability in health care? *Ann Intern Med* 1996; 124:229–39.

Emerson R, Creedon JJ. Unjustified surgery dilemma: second opinion versus preset criteria. *NY State J Med* 1977; 77:779–85.

Engelhardt HT, Jr. *The Foundations of Bioethics*, New York: Oxford, 1986.

Engelhardt HT, Jr. *The Foundations of Bioethics*, 2nd edn. New York: Oxford, 1996.

Engelhardt HT, Jr., Rie MA. Morality for the medical-industrial complex: A code of ethics for the mass marketing of health care. *N Engl J Med* 1988; 319:1086–9.

European Carotid Surgery Trialists' Collaborative Group. MRC European Carotid Surgery Trial: interim results for symptomatic patients with severe (70–99%) or with mild (0–29%) carotid stenosis. *Lancet* 1991; 337:1235–43.

Faden RR, Beauchamp TL. *A History and Theory of Informed Consent*. New York: Oxford University Press, 1986.

Feinberg J. *The Moral Limits of the Criminal Law*, vol. 1: Harm to Others. New York: Oxford, 1984.

Feinstein A. *Clinical Judgment*. Baltimore: Williams and Wilkins, 1967.

Feinstein A. *Clinimetrics* New Haven: Yale University Press, 1987.

Ferguson RP. Iatrogenesis: The hidden and general dangers. *Hosp Prac* 1989; 24:89–94.

Fink A, Brook RH, Kosecoff J, Chassin M, Solomon DH. The sufficiency of the clinical literature for learning about the appropriate use of six medical and surgical procedures. *West J Med* 1987; 147:609–15.

Fleming C, Wasson JH, Albertsen PC, Barry MJ, Wennberg JE. A decision analysis of alternative treatment strategies for clinically localized prostate cancer. *JAMA* 1993; 269:2650–8.

Fox R. 'Training for uncertainty' In , Merton R, Reader G, Kendell P, eds. *The Student Physician*. Cambridge: Harvard University Press, 1957.

Franklin GM, Haug J, Heyer N, McKeefrey SP, Picciano J. Outcome of lumber fusion in Washington state worker's compensation. *Spine* 1994; 19:1897–903.

Franks P, Clancy CM, Nutting PA. Gatekeeping revisited: protecting patients from overtreatment. *N Engl J Med* 1992; 327(6):424–9.

Freeman R. Intrapartum fetal monitoring: A disappointing story. *N Engl J Med* 1990; 322(9):624–6.

Freeman WK, Schaff HV, Orszulak TA, Tajik AJ. Ultrasonic aortic valve decalcification: serial Doppler echocardiographic follow-up. *J Am Coll Cardiol* 1990; 16:623–30.

French PA (ed.). *The Spectrum of Responsibility*. New York: St. Martin's Press, 1991.

Fricchione GL. Facing limitation and failure: four literary portraits. *Pharos* 1985; 48(4):13–18.

Fuchs VR, Garber AM. The new technology assessment. *N Engl J Med* 1990; 323:673–7.

Gaba D. Human error in dynamic medical domains. In Bogner MS, ed. *Human Error in Medicine*. Hillsdale NJ: Erlbaum, 1994, pp. 197–224.

Gambone JC, Reiter RC, Lench JB. Quality assurance indicators and short-term outcome of hysterectomy. *Obstet Gynecol* 1990; 76:841–5.

Garipey TP. The introduction and acceptance of Listerian antisepsis in the United States. *J Hist Med Allied Sci* 1994; 49:167–206.

Garner JS and the Hospital Infection Control Practices Advisory Committee. Guideline for isolation precautions in hospitals. *Am J Infect Control* 1996; 24:24–52.

Gartry DS, Kerr MG, Marshall J. Excimer laser photorefractive keratectomy. *Ophthalmology* 1992; 99:1209–19.

Geigle R, Jones SB. Outcomes measurement: A report from the front. *Inquiry* 1990; 27:7–13.

Gerteis M, Edgman–Levitan S, Daley J, Delbanco T (eds.). *Through the Patient's Eyes: Understanding and Promoting Patient-Centered Care*. San Fransisco: Jossey-Bass, 1993.

Ghose K. Hospital bed occupancy due to drug related problems. *J Roy Soc Med* 1980:73: 853–6.

Gill TM, Feinstein AR. A critical appraisal of the quality of quality-of-life measurements. *JAMA* 1994; 272:619–26.

Glass RM. The patient–physician relationship: *JAMA* focuses on the center of medicine. *JAMA* 1996; 275:147–8.

Goff BH. An analysis of wound union. *Surg Gyn Obstet* 1925; 41:728–39.

Goldberg HI. Ethical issues in administrative continuous improvement. *Med Care* 1990; 28:822–33.

Goldman D, Larson E. Hand-washing and nosocomial infections. *N Engl J Med* 1992; 327:120–2.

Goodin R. *Protecting the Vulnerable.* Chicago: University of Chicago Press, 1985.

Gordon A. (ed.) A treatise on the epidemic of puerperal fever in Aberdeen (1795), reprinted in *Essays on the puerperal fever and other diseases peculiar to women selected from the writings of British authors previous to the close of the eighteenth century.* Fleetwood Churchill. London: Sydenham Society, 1849, pp. 445–500.

Gorovitz S, MacIntyre A. Toward a theory of medical fallibility. *J Med Phil* 1976; 1:51–71.

Gray BH. *The Profit Motive and Patient Care: The Changing Accountability of Doctors and Hospitals.* Cambridge, MA: Harvard University Press, 1991.

Gray D, Hampton JR, Bernstein S, et al. Audit of coronary angiography and bypass surgery. *Lancet* 1990; 335:1317–20.

Green JW, Wenzel RP. Postoperative wound infection: A controlled study of the increase duration of hospital stay and direct costs of hospitalization. *Ann Surg* 1977; 185:264–8.

Greenfield S, Kaplan S, Ware JE, Jr. Expanding patient involvement in care: Effects on patient outcomes. *Ann Intern Med* 1985; 102:520–8.

Greenfield S, Kaplan SH, Ware JE, Jr, et al. Patients' participation in medical care: effects on blood sugar control and quality of life in diabetes. *J Gen Intern Med* 1988; 3:448–57.

Greenfield S, Nelson EC. Recent developments and future issues in the use of health status assessment measures in clinical settings. *Med Care* 1992; 30:MS23–MS41.

Greenspan AM, Kay HR, Berger BC, et al. Incidence of unwarranted implantation of permanent cardiac pacemakers in a large medical population. *N Engl J Med* 1988; 318:158–63.

Gregory J. *Lectures on the Duties and Qualifications of a Physician* Philadelphia: M. Carey & Son, 1817.

Grimes DA. Technology Follies: The uncritical acceptance of medical innovation. *JAMA* 1993; 269:3030–3.

Grymonpre RE, Mitenko PA, Sitar DS, et al. Drug-associated hospital admissions in older medical patients. *J Am Geriatrics Soc* 1988; 36:1092–8.

Guadagnoli E, McNeil BJ. Outcome research: Hope for the future or the latest rage? *Inquiry* 1994; 31:14–24.

Guyatt GH, Cook DJ. Health status, quality of life, and the individual. *JAMA* 1994; 272:630–1.

Haley RW. Measuring the costs of nosocomial infections: Methods for estimating economic burden on the hospital. *Am J Med* 1991; 91(3B):32S–38S.

Haley RW. The development of infection surveillance and control programs. In Bennett JV, Brachman PS. *Hospital Infections*, 3rd edn. Boston:Little, Brown, 1992, pp. 63–78.

Haley RW, Culver DH, White JW, et al. The efficacy of infection surveillance and control programs in preventing nosocomial infections in US hospitals. *Am J Epidemiol* 1985; 121:182–205.

Haley RW, Gaynes RP, Aber RC, Bennett JV. Surveillance of nosocomial infections. In Bennett JV, Brachman PS, eds. *Hospital Infections* 3rd edn. Boston:Little, Brown, 1992, pp. 79–108.

Haley RW, Shactman RH. The emergence of infection surveillance and control programs in US hospitals: An assessment. *Am J Epidemiol* 1980; 111:574–91.

Haley RW, White JW, Culver DH, et al. The financial incentive for hospitals to prevent nosocomial infections under the prospective payment system. An empirical determination from a nationally representative sample. *JAMA* 1987; 257(12):1611–14.

Hall v. *Hilburn* 466 So 2d 856, 873 (Miss 1985).

Hallas J, Gram LF, Grodum E, Damsbo N, et al. Drug related admissions to medical wards: a population based survey. *Br J Clin Pharmacol* 1992; 33(1):61–8.

Hamborg CJ. Medical utilization review: The new frontier for medical malpractice claims? *Drake Law Rev* 1992; 41:113–38.

Hatlie MJ. Climbing the learning curve: new technologies, emerging obligations. *JAMA* 1993; 270:1364–5.

Healy B. Women's health, public welfare. *JAMA* 1991; 226(4):566–8.

Heilbrunn JZ, Rolph J. *Cesarean Sections as Defensive Medicine.* Santa Monica, CA: RAND, 1993.

Herwaldt LA. Ethical aspects of infection control. *Infect Control Hosp Epidemiol* 1996; 17:108–13.

Hiatt HH, Barnes BA, Brennan TA, et al. A study of medical injury and medical malpractice: An overview. *N Engl J Med* 1989; 321:480–4.

Hilborne LH, Leape LL, Bernstein SJ, et al. The appropriateness of use of percutaneous transluminal coronary angioplasty in New York State. *JAMA* 1993; 269(6):761–5.

Hilfiker D. Facing our mistakes. *N Engl J Med* 1984; 310:118–122.

Himmelfarb G. *The De-Moralization of Society.* New York: Knopf, 1995

Hippocrates. Epidemics I. In *Hippocrates,* trans., WHS Jones. Loeb Classical Library. Cambridge, MA: Harvard University Press, 1923–1988.

Hippocrates. The Oath. In *Hippocrates* (trans., WHS Jones). Loeb Classical Library. Cambridge, MA: Harvard University Press, 1923–88.

Hoddinott BC, Gowdey CW, Coulter WK, et al. Drug reactions and errors in administration on a medical ward. *Can Med Ass J* 1967; 97:1001–6.

Hollenberg NK, Testa M, Williams GH, et al. Quality of life as a therapeutic endpoint: an analysis of therapeutic trials in hypertension. *Drug Safety* 1991; 6:83–9.

Holmes OW. The contagiousness of puerperal fever. *N Engl Q J Med* 1843:1–23. (Reprinted in *Medical Classics,* vol. 1. Baltimore: Williams and Wilkins, 1937).

Holmes OW. Currents and counter-currents in medical science. Annual Address before the Massachusetts Medical Society, May 30, 1860. In *Medical Essays 1842–1882.* Boston: Houghton Mifflin, 1911.

Holmes OW. Homeopathy and its kindred delusions. In *Medical Essays 1842–1882.* Boston: Houghton Mifflin, 1911.

Hooker W. *Physician and Patient; Or a Practical View of the Mutual Duties, Relations, and Interests of the Medical Profession and the Community.* New York: Baker and Scribner, 1849.

Hopkins A, Fitzpatrick R, Foster A, et al. What do we mean by appropriate health care? *Quality in Health Care* 1993; 2:117–23.

Horwitz NH, Rizzoli HV. *Postoperative Complications of Extracranial Surgery.* Baltimore: Williams and Wilkins, 1987.

Hume D. *A Treatise of Human Nature.* L A Selby-Bigge, P Nidditch, eds. Oxford: Clarendon Press, 1978.

Hurwitz N. Admissions to hospital due to drugs. *Br Med J* 1969; 1:539–40.

Hutchinson TA, Flegel KM, Kramer MS, et al. Frequency, severity and risk factors for adverse drug reactions in adult out-patients: A prospective study. *J Chron Dis* 1986; 39(7):533–42.

Illich I. *Medical Nemesis: The Expropriation of Health.* New York: Pantheon Books; 1976.

In the Matter of Karen Quinlan: The Complete Briefs, Oral Arguments, and Opinions in the Superior Court of New Jersey (vol. I) and in the *New Jersey Supreme Court*, vol. II. Arlington, VA: University Publications of America, 1976.

Inglehart JK. Medicare begins prospective payment of hospitals. *N Engl J Med* 1982; 368:1482–3.

Inlander CB, Levin LS, Weiner E. *Medicine on Trial.* New York: Prentice Hall, 1988.

International drug monitoring – the role of the hospital. World Health Organization Drug Intelligence. *Clin Pharm* 1970; 4:101.

Ives TJ, Bentz EJ, Gwyther RE. Drug related admissions to a family medicine inpatient service. *Arch Intern Med* 1987; 147:1117–20.

Jahnigen D, Hannon C, Laxson L, et al. Iatrogenic disease in hospitalized elderly veterans. *J Am Geriatr Soc* 1982; 30(6):387–90.

Jellinek MS, Todres ID, Catlin EA, Cassem EH, Salzman A. Pediatric intensive care training: confronting the dark side. *Crit Care Med* 1993; 21(5):775–9.

Joint Commission on the Accreditation of Hospitals. *Accreditation Manual for Hospitals.* Oakbrook Terrace, IL: JCAH, 1970.

Joint Commission on Accreditation of Healthcare Organizations. The agenda for change. *Agenda Change Update* 1987; 1:1–3.

Joint Commission on Accreditation of Health Care Organizations. *Accreditation Manual for Hospitals.* Oakbrook Terrace, IL. JCAHO, 1993.

Jonsen AR. Do no harm: Axiom of medical ethics. In Spicker S, Engelhardt HT, Jr., eds. *Philosophical Medical Ethics: Its Nature and Significance.* Dordrecht: Kluwer, 1977, pp. 27–41.

Juran JM, Gryna FM (eds.). *Juran's Quality Control Handbook*, 4th edn. New York: McGraw Hill, 1988.

Kahn KL. Above all 'Do no harm': How shall we avoid errors in medicine? *JAMA* 1995; 274:75–6.

Kane RL. Iatrogenesis: Just what the doctor ordered. *J Community Health* 1980; 5:149–58.

Karch FE, Lasagna L. Adverse drug reactions: A critical review *JAMA* 1975; 234:1236–41.

Katz J. Informed consent – a fairy tale? In Walters L, Beauchamp TL, eds. *Contemporary Issues in Bioethics*, 2nd edn. Belmont, CA: Wadsworth, 1982.

Katz J. Why doctors don't disclose uncertainty. *Hastings Cent Rep* 1984; 14:35–44.

Keeler EB, Brodie M. Economic incentives in the choice between vaginal delivery and cesarean section. *Milbank Q* 1993; 71:365–404.

Keeton P, Keeton R, Sargentich L, Steiner H. *Tort and Accident Law.* St. Paul:West Publishing Co., 1983.

Keeton P. Compensation for medical accidents. 121 U. PA. Law Rev. 590: (1973).

Kellaway GSM, McCrae E. Intensive monitoring for adverse drug effects in patients discharged from acute medical wards. *N Z Med J* 1973; 78:525–8.

Kessler DA (for the Working Group). Introducing MedWatch: A new approach to reporting medication and device adverse effects and product problems. *JAMA* 1993; 269:2765–8.

Klein LE, German PS, Levine DM, et al. Medication problems among patients: A study with emphasis on the elderly. *Arch Int Med* 1984; 144:1185–8.

Kleinman A. *The Illness Narratives: Suffering, Healing and the Human Condition.* New York: Basic Books, 1988.

Klicka KS. Control of Surgery. *Mod Hosp* 1948; 71:84–6.

Knowles J, (ed.). *Doing Better and Feeling Worse: Health Care in the United States.* New York: W.W. Norton, 1977.

Konold DE. *A History of Americal Medical Ethics: 1847–1912.* Madison: State Historical Society of Wisconsin. 1962.

Kramer MS, Leventhal JM, Hutchinson TA, et al. An algorithm for the operational assessment of adverse drug reactions. *JAMA* 1979; 242:623–32.

Krause EA. *Power and Illness: The Political Sociology of Health and Medical Care.* New York: Elsevier, 1977.

Kudlien F. Medical ethics and popular ethics in Greece and Rome. *Clio Med* 1970; 5:91–121.

Kuhn TS, *The Structure of Scientific Revolutions*, 2nd edn. Chicago: University of Chicago Press, 1970.

Kurz A, Sessler DI, Lenhardt R, et al. Perioperative normothermia to reduce the incidence of surgical-wound infection and shorten hospitalization. *N Engl J Med* 1996; 334:1209–15.

L'Abbé KA, Detsky AS, O'Rourke K. Meta-analysis in clinical research. *Ann Intern Med* 1987; 107:224–33.

Laffel G, Berwick DM. Quality in health care. *JAMA* 1992; 268(3):407–9.

Laffel G, Blumenthal D. The case for using industrial quality management science in health care organizations. *JAMA* 1989; 83:1031–7.

Laine C, Davidoff F. Patient-centered medicine: A professional evolution. *JAMA* 1996; 275:152–6.

Lakshmanan MC, Hershey CO, Breslau D. Hospital admissions caused by iatrogenic disease. *Arch Intern Med* 1986; 146:1931–4.

Larson E, Kretzer EK. Compliance with handwashing and barrier precautions. *J Hosp Infect* 1995; 30(supp.):88–106.

Larson E. A causal link between handwashing and risk of infection? Examination of the evidence. *Infect Control* 1988; 9:28–36.

Larson E. Innovations in health care: Antisepsis as a case study. *Am J Pub Health* 1989; 79:92–9.

Lawrence G. Surgery (traditional). In Bynum WF, Porter R, eds. *Companion Encyclopedia of the History of Medicine.* New York: Routledge, 1993, ch. 41.

Leape LL. Unnecessary surgery. *Annu Rev Publ Health* 1992; 13:363–83 (see p. 370).

Leape LL. Error in medicine. *JAMA* 1994; 272:1851–7.

Leape LL. Translating medical science into medical practice: Do we need a National Medical Standards Board? *JAMA* 1995; 273(19):1534–7.

Leape LL, Brennan TA, Laird N, et al. The nature of adverse events in hospitalized patients. *N Engl J Med* 1991; 324:377–84.

Leape LL, Bates DW, Cullen DJ, et al for the ADE Prevention Study Group. Systems analysis of adverse drug events. *JAMA* 1995; 274:35–43.

Leape LL, Brennan TA, Laird N, et al. The nature of adverse events in hospitalized patients. Results of the Harvard Medical Practice Study II. *N Engl J Med* 1991; 324(6):377–84.

Leape LL, Lawthers AG, Brennan TA, Johnson WG. Preventing medical injury. *Qual Review Bull* 1993; 19(5):144–9.

Leape L, Park RE, Solomon DH, et al. Relation between surgeons' practice volumes and geographic variation in the rate of carotid endarterectomy. *N Engl J Med* 1989; 314:653–7.

Leape LL, Park RE, Solomon DH, et al. Does inappropriate use explain small area variations in the use of health care services? *JAMA* 1990; 263:669–72.

Lehr H, Strosberg M. Quality improvement in health care: is the patient still left out? *QRB* 1991; 17:326–9.

Lembcke PA. Measuring the quality of medical care through vital statistics based on hospital service areas I. Comparative study of appendectomy rates. *Am J Pub Health* 1952; 42:276–86.

Lembcke PA. Evolution of the medical audit. *JAMA* 1967; 199:534–50.

Levey M. *Medical Ethics of Medieval Islam, With Special Reference to Al-Ruhawi's Practical Ethics of the Physician.* Philadelphia: American Philosophical Society, 1967.

Levin LS. Aim and scope of the journal. *Iatrogenics* 1991; 1:i.

Levinson W, Dunn PM. Coping with fallibility. *JAMA.* 1989; 261:2252.

Levy M, Lipshitz M, Eliakim M. Hospital admissions due to adverse drug reactions. *Am J Med Sci* 1979; 277:49 56.

Levy M, Nir I, Birnbaum D, et al. Adverse reactions to drugs in hospitalized medical patients: A comparative study. *Isr J Med Sci* 1973; 9:617–26.

Lewis CE. Variations in the incidence of surgery. *N Engl J Med* 1969; 281:880–4.

Lipp M. *The Bitter Pill: Doctors, Patients and Failed Expectations.* New York: Harper and Row; 1980.

Lister J. On the antiseptic principle in the practice of surgery. *Lancet* 1867; 1:741–5.

Lister J. Effects of the antiseptic system of treatment upon the salubrity of a surgical hospital. *Lancet* 1870; 1:4 6, 40–2.

LoGerfo JP. Organizational and financial influences on patterns of surgical care. *Surg Clin N Am* 1982; 62:677–84.

LoGerfo JP, Efird RA, Diehr PK, Richardson WC. Rates of surgical care in prepaid group practices and the independent setting. *Med Care* 1979; 17:1–10.

Lohr KN. Outcome measurement: concepts and questions. *Inquiry* 1988; 25:37–50.

Lomas J, Enkin M, Anderson GM, et al. Opinion leaders vs. audit and feedback to implement practice guidelines: Delivery after previous cesarean section. *JAMA* 1991; 265:2202–7.

Lu-Yao GL, Mclerran D, Wasson J, Wennberg JE. An assessment of radical prostatectomy: Time trends, geographic variation, and outcomes. *JAMA* 1993; 269:2633–6.

MacKeigan LD, Pathak DS. Overview of health-related quality-of-life measures. *Am J Hosp Pharm* 1992; 49:2236–45.

Manuel BM. Professional liability: A no-fault solution. *N Engl J Med* 1990; 322(9): 627–31.

Martys CR. Adverse reactions to drugs in general practice. *Br Med J* 1979; 2:1194–7.

Marwick C. Federal agency focuses on outcomes research. *JAMA* 1993; 270:164–5.

Mathieu D. *Preventing Prenatal Harm: Should the State Intervene?* Dordrecht:

Kluwer, 1991.

Mayberg MR, Wilson SE, Yatsu F, et al. Carotid endarterectomy and prevention of cerebral ischemia in symptomatic carotid stenosis. *JAMA* 1991; 266:3289–94.

McCarthy EG, Finkel ML. Second opinion elective surgery programs: Outcome status over time. *Med Care* 1978; 16:984–94.

McCarthy EG, Widmer GW. Effects of screening by consultants on recommended elective surgical procedures. *N Engl J Med* 1974; 291:1331–5.

McCullough LB, Chervenak FA. *Ethics in Obstetrics and Gynecology.* New York: Oxford University Press, 1994.

McGeer A, Crede W, Hierholzer WJ, Jr. Surveillance for quality assessment. II. Surveillance for noninfectious processes: Back to basics. *Infect Control Hosp Epidemiol* 1990; 11:36–41.

McGettigan P, Chan R, McManus J, et al. Sources of drug information in prescribing in general practice. *Br J Clin Pharmacol* 1994; 7:512–13.

McIntyre N, Popper K. The critical attitude in medicine: The need for a new ethics. *Br Med J* 1983; 287:1919–23.

McKenney JM, Harrison WL. Drug-related hospital admissions. *Am J Hosp Pharm* 1976; 33(8):792–5.

McLamb JT, Huntley RR. The hazards of hospitalization. *South Med J* 1967; 60:469–72.

McLaughlin CP, Kaluzny AD. Total quality management in health: Making it work. *Health Care Mgmt Rev* 1990; 15:7–14.

McNeil BJ, Pauker SG, Sox HC, Jr, et al. On the elicitation of preferences for alternative therapies. *N Engl J Med* 1982; 306:1259–62.

McNeil BJ, Weichselbaum R, Pauker SG. Fallacy of five-year survival in lung cancer. *N Engl J Med* 1978; 299:1397–401.

McNeil BJ, Weichselbaum R, Pauker SG. Speech and survival: Trade-offs between quality and quantity of life in laryngeal cancer. *N Engl J Med* 1981; 305:982–7.

Mechanic D. Trust and informed consent to rationing. *Milbank Q* 1994; 72:217–23.

Meigs C. *On the Nature, Signs, and Treatment of Childbed Fever.* Philadelphia, 1859.

Meinhard v. *Salmon.* 164 N.E. 545, 546 (N.Y. 1928).

Meleney FL. Infection in clean operative wounds. A nine-year study. *Surg Gyn Obstet* 1935; 60:264–75.

Melmon KL. Preventable drug reactions – causes and cures. *N Engl J Med* 1971; 284:1361–8.

Meyer BA. A student teaching module: Physician errors. *Fam Med* 1989; 21(4):299–300.

Meyer H. Cost-conscious hospitals set futile care rules. *Am Med News* June 28, 1993, 3:20.

Meyler L. *Side-Effects of Drugs.* Amsterdam: Elsevier, 1952, p. vi.

Miller F. Hysterectomy: Therapeutic necessity or surgical racket? *Am J Obstet Gyn* 1946; 51:804–10.

Miller RR. Hospital admissions due to adverse drug reactions. *Arch Intern Med* 1974; 134:219–23.

Millman M. *The Unkindest Cut: Life in the Backrooms of Medicine.* New York: William Morrow & Co Inc; 1977.

Mills DH, Boyden JS, Rubsamen DS. *Medical Insurance Feasibility Study.* San

Francisco, California Medical Association, 1977.

Mintz M. *By Prescription Only: A Report on the Roles of the U.S. F.D.A., the A.M.A., the P.M.A. and Others in Connection with Irrational and Massive Use of Prescription Drugs That May be Worthless, Injurious, or Even Lethal,* 2nd edn. Boston: Beacon Press, 1967.

Mitchell JB, Cromwell J. Variations in surgical rates and the supply of surgeons. In Rothberg DL, ed. *Regional Variations in Hospital Use.* Lexington, MA: Lexington books, 1982.

Mizrahi T. Managing medical mistakes: ideology, insularity and accountability among internists'-in-training. *Soc Sci Med* 1984; 19:135–46.

Modell W. Editorial. *Clin Pharm Ther* 1960; 1(1):1–2.

Mohr, JC. *Medical Jurisprudence in Nineteenth-Century America.* New York: Oxford University Press, 1993.

Moore FD. Social biology and applied sociology: Cannon and Codman Fifty years later. *Harvard Med Alum Bull* 1975; 493:12–21.

Morain C. Looking for more controls on managed care in California. *Am Med News* 1995, May 8; 5:6.

Moray N. Error reduction as a systems problem. In Bogner MS ed. *Human Error in Medicine.* Hillsdale NJ: Erlbaum, 1994, pp. 67–92

Morreim EH. Am I my brother's warden? Responding to the unethical or incompetent colleague. *Hast Ctr Rep* 1993; 23(3):19–27.

Morreim EH. *Balancing Act: The New Medical Ethics of Medicine's New Economics.* Washington, DC: Georgetown University Press, 1995.

Moser RH. *Diseases of Medical Progress.* Springfield, Ill: Chas. Thomas, 1959, 2nd edn, 1969.

Moser RH. Diseases of medical progress. *N Engl J Med* 1956; 255:606–14.

Naranjo CA, Busto U, Sellers EM, et al. A method for estimating the probability of adverse drug reactions. *Clin Pharmacol Ther* 1981; 30:239–45.

National Women's Health Resource Center. *Forging a Women's Health Research Agenda.* Washington, DC: National Women's Health Resource Center, 1991.

Neuhauser D. Ernest Amory Codman, MD, and end results of medical care. *Int J Technol Assess Health Care* 1990; 6:307–25.

Nicolson M. The art of diagnosis: Medicine and the five senses. In Bynum WF, Porter R, eds. *Companion Encyclopedia of the History of Medicine* New York: Routledge, 1993, ch. 35.

Nightingale F. *Introductory Notes on Lying-In Institutions.* London: Longman, Green, 1871.

Nightingale F. *Notes on Hospitals.*, 3rd edn. London: Longman, Green, 1863.

North American Symptomatic Carotid Endarterectomy Trial Collaborators. Beneficial effect of carotid endarterectomy in symptomatic patients with high-grade carotid stenosis. *N Engl J Med* 1991; 325:445–53.

Nuland, SB. *Doctors: The Biography of Medicine.* New York: Vintage, 1988.

Nutton V. Humoralism. In Bynum WF, Porter R, eds. *Companion Encyclopedia of the History of Medicine.* New York: Routledge, 1993, ch. 14.

Oberman L. Prescription for professionals: better approach could prevent patient injuries. *Am Med News* 1993; 3:27.

Office of Technology Assessment. *Assessing the Efficacy and Safety of Medical Technologies.* Washington DC: US Government Printing Office, 1978.

Office of Technology Assessment. *The Impact of Randomized Clinical Trials on Health Policy and Medical Practice.* Washington, DC: US Government

Printing Office, 1983.

Ogilvie RI, Ruedy J. Adverse reactions during hospitalization I. *Can Med Ass J* 1967; 97:1445–50.

Ogilvie RI, Ruedy J. Adverse drug reactions during hospitalization II. *Can Med Ass J* 1967; 97:1450–7.

Orton DI, Gruzelier JH. Adverse changes in mood and cognitve performance of house officers after night duty. *Br Med J* 1989; 298:21–3.

Oxford English Dictionary, Supplement, vol. II, Oxford: Clarendon Press, 1976.

Park RE, Fink A, Brook RH, Chassin MR, et al. Physician ratings of appropriate indications for six medical and surgical procedures. *Am J Public Health* 1986; 76:766–72.

Patterson JE, Vecchio J, Pantelick EL, et al. Association of contaminated gloves with transmission of *Acinetobacter calcoaceticus* var. *anitratus* in an intensive care unit. Am J Med 1991; 91(5):479–83.

Paul-Shaheen P, Clark JD, Williams D. Small area analysis: a review and analysis of the North American literature. *J Health Polit Policy Law* 1987; 12:741–809.

Pauly MV. What is unnecessary surgery? *Milbank Q* 1979; 57:95–117.

Peabody, FW. The care of the patient. *JAMA* 1927; 88:877–82.

Pear R. Doctors say HMOs limit what they can tell patients. *New York Times* December 21, 1995, pp. A1, B13.

Pear R. The tricky business of keeping doctors quiet. *New York Times* September 22, 1996, p. E7.

Pearson KC, Kennedy DC. Adverse drug reactions and the Food and Drug Administration. *J Pharm Pract* 1989; 2:209–10.

Peebles RJ. Second opinions and cost-effectiveness: The questions continue. *Am Coll Surg Bull* 1991; 76:18–25.

Pellegrino ED, Thomasma DC. *For the Patient's Good: The Restoration of Beneficence in Health Care.* New York: Oxford, 1988.

Pellegrino ED. Beneficence, scientific autonomy and self-interest: Ethical dilemmas in clinical research. *Cambridge Quarterly Health Care Eth* 1992; 1:361–9.

Pellegrino ED. Toward a reconstruction of medical morality: The primacy of the act of profession and the fact of illness. *J Med Phil* 1979; 4:32–55.

Pellegrino ED. Rationing health care: the ethics of medical gatekeeping. *Contemp Health Law and Policy.* 1986; 2:23–45.

Pellegrino ED. Is truth telling to the patient a cultural artifact? *JAMA* 1992; 268:1734–5.

Pellegrino ED. Managed care and managed competition: Some ethical reflections. *Calyx* 1994; 4:1–5.

Pellegrino ED. Words can hurt you: Some reflections on the metaphors of managed care. *J Am Bd Fam Prac* 1994; 7:508.

Percival T. *Medical Ethics or A Code of Institutes and Precepts adapted to the Professional Conduct of Physicians and Surgeons.* Manchester: S. Russell, 1803.

Pernick M. *A Calculus of Suffering: Pain, Professionalism and Anesthesia in Nineteenth Century America.* New York: Columbia University Press, 1985.

Pernick MS. The patient's role in medical decision making: A social history of informed consent in medical therapy. In President's Commission for the Study of Ethical Problems in Medicine and Biomedical and Behavioral Research. *Making Health Care Decisions*, vol. 3. Washington, DC: USGPO,

1982.

Pernick MS. The calculus of suffering in nineteenth-century surgery. *Hastings Ctr Rep* 1983; 13:28.

Porter J, Jick H. Drug related deaths among medical in-patients. *JAMA* 1977; 237:879.

Preger L. *Iatrogenic Diseases*. Boca Raton: CRC Press, 1986.

President's Commission for the Study of Ethical Problems in Medicine and Biomedical and Behavioral Research. *Securing Access to Health Care*, vol. 1, *Report*. Washington, DC: US Government Printing Office, 1983.

Preston TA. *The Clay Pedestal*. Seattle: Madrona Publishers, 1986.

Prosser TR, Kamysz PL. Multidisciplinary adverse drug reaction surveillance program. *Am J Hosp Pharm* 1990; 47:1334–9.

Public health: Surveillance, prevention and control of nosocomial infections. *Morb Mort Week Rep* 1992; 41:783–7.

Ratzan RM, Ferngren GB. A Greek progymnasma on the physician-poisoner. *J Hist Med Allied Sci* 1993; 48:157–70.

Rawlins MD. Clinical pharmacology: Adverse Reactions to drugs. *Br Med J* 1981, 282:974–6.

Reich WT (ed.). *The Encyclopedia of Bioethics*, New York: Simon and Schuster/Macmillan, 1995.

Reichel W. Complications in the care of five hundred elderly hospitalized patients. *J Am Geriatr Soc* 1965; 13:973–81.

Reidenberg MM. Registry of adverse drug reactions. *JAMA* 1968; 203(1):31–4.

Reiser SJ. The era of the patient: Using the experience of illness in shaping the missions of health care. *JAMA* 1993; 269:1012–17.

Reiser SJ. The science of diagnosis: Diagnostic technology. In Bynum WF, Porter R, eds. *Companion Encyclopedia of the History of Medicine*. New York: Routledge, 1993, ch. 36 (pp. 826–51).

Relman A. Assessment and accountability: The third revolution in medical care. *N Engl J Med* 1988; 319:1220–2.

Relman AS. Salaried physicians and economic incentives. *N Engl J Med* 1988; 319:784.

Reverby S. Stealing the golden eggs: Ernest Amory Codman and the science and management of medicine. *Bull Hist Med* 1981; 55:156–71.

Reynolds RA, Rizzo JA, Gonzales ML. The cost of medical professional liability. *JAMA* 1987; 257:2776–81.

Rice TH. The impact of changing Medicare reimbursement rates on physician-induced demand. *Med Care* 1983; 21:803–15.

Rich S. Managed care, once an elixir, goes under legislative knife: cost-cutting feared harmful to patients. *Washington Post* September 25, 1996, p. A1.

Richmond PA. American attitudes toward the germ theory of disease (1860–1880). *J Hist Med and Allied Sci* 1954; 9:428–54.

Risse G. Medical care. In Bynum WF, Porter R, eds. *Companion Encyclopedia of the History of Medicine*. New York: Routledge, 1993, ch 4 (pp. 45–77).

Robertson G. Fraudulent concealment and the duty to disclose medical mistakes. *Alberta Law Rev* 1987; 25(2): 215–23.

Robins N. *The Girl Who Died Twice: Every Patient's Nightmare: The Libby Zion Case and the Hidden Hazards of Hospitals*. New York: Delacorte Press, 1995.

Rodwin MA. Strains in the fiduciary metaphor: Divided physician loyalties and obligations in a changing health care system. *Am J Law and Med* 1995; 21:241–2.

Roos NP. Hysterectomy. Variations in rates across small areas and across physicians' practices. *Am J Public Health* 1984; 7:327–35.

Roos NP, Roos LL Jr. Surgical rate variations: Do they reflect the health or socioeconomic characteristics of the population? *Med Care* 1982; 20:945–58.

Roos NP, Roos LL Jr, Henteleff PD. Elective surgical rates – do high rates mean lower standards?: Tonsillectomy and adenoidectomy in Manitoba. *N Engl J Med* 1977; 297:360–5.

Roper WL, Winkenwerder W, Hackbarth GM, et al. Effectiveness in health care: an initiative to evaluate and improve medical practice. *N Engl J Med* 1988; 319:1197–202.

Rosenberg CE. Florence Nightingale on contagion: The hospital as moral universe. In Rosenberg CE, ed. *Healing and History*. New York: Dawson, 1979.

Rosenberg CE. The therapeutic revolution. In Vogel MJ, Rosenberg CE, eds. *The Therapeutic Revolution: Essays in the Social History of Medicine*. Philadelphia: University of Pennsylvania Press, 1979.

Rosenberg CE. *The Care of Strangers: The Rise of America's Hospital System*. New York: Basic Books, 1987.

Rothman DM. *Strangers at the Bedside: A History of How Law and Bioethics Transformed Medical Decision-Making*. New York: Basic Books, 1991.

Rothstein WG. *American Physicians in the Nineteenth Century: From Sects to Science*. Baltimore: Johns Hopkins Press, 1992.

Rush B. Lecture XII: On the opinions and modes of practice of Hippocrates. In *Sixteen Introductory Lectures*. Philadelphia: Bradford and Innskeep, 1811.

Rutkow IM, Zuidema GD. Unnecessary surgery: An update. *Surgery* 1978; 84:671–78.

Sackett DL. Rules of evidence and clinical recommendations on the use of antithrombotic agents. *Chest* 1989; 95(Suppl. 2):2s–4s.

Sagoff M. *The Economy of the Earth*. New York: Cambridge University Press, 1988.

Salgo v. *Leland Stanford Jr. University Board of Trustees*, 317 P.2d 170, (Cal Ct App 1957).

Salz JJ, Maguen E, Nesburn AB, et al. A two-year experience with excimer laser photorefractive keratectomy for myopia. *Ophthalmology* 1993; 100:873–82.

Sandalulescu C. 'Primum non nocere': Philological commentaries on a medical aphorism. *Acta-Antigua Hungarica* 1965; 13:827–32

Savitt TL. *Medicine and Slavery: The Disease and Health Care of Blacks in Antebellum Virginia*. Urbana: University of Illinois Press, 1978.

Schadewaldt H. Hospitalinfektionen im Wandel. *Zentralbl Bakteriol Mikrobiol Hyg* 1986; 183:91–102.

Schimmel EM. The physician as pathogen. *J Chronic Dis* 1963; 16:1–4.

Schimmel EM. The hazards of hospitalization. *Ann Intern Med* 1964; 60:100–10.

Schloendorff v. *Society of New York Hospitals*. 211 N.Y. 125, 105 N.E. 92 (1914).

Schneider JK, Mion, LC, Frengley JD, et al. Adverse drug reactions in an elderly outpatient population. *Am J Hosp Pharm* 1992; 49:90–6.

Schoenbaum SC. Toward fewer procedures and better outcomes. *JAMA* 1993; 269:794–6.

Schroeder SA, Marton KI, Strom BL. Frequency and morbidity of invasive procedures: A report of a pilot study from two teaching hospitals. *Arch Intern Med* 1978; 138:1809–11.

Schumock GT, Thornton JP, Witte KW, et al. Comparison of pharmacy-based concurrent surveillance and medical record retrospective reporting of adverse drug reactions. *Am J Hosp Pharm* 1991; 48:1974–6.

Searle J. How to derive 'ought' from 'is'. *Phil Review* 1964; 73:43–58.

Seckler SG, Spritzer RC. Disseminated disease of medical progress. *Arch Intern Med* 1966; 117:447–50.

Seidl LG, Thornton GF, Smith JW, Cluff LE. Studies on the epidemiology of adverse drug reactions. III: Reactions in patients on a general medical service. *Bull Johns Hopkins Hosp* 1966; 119:299–315.

Selwyn S. Hospital infection: The first 2500 years. *J Hosp Inf* 1991; 18(supp):5–64.

Semmelweis I. *The Etiology, Concept, and Prophylaxis of Childbed Fever.* (Ed. and trans. K. C. Carter.) Madison: University of Wisconsin Press, 1983.

Shapiro S, Slone D, Lewis GP, et al. Fatal drug reactions among medical inpatients. *JAMA* 1971; 216:467–72.

Sharpe VA. *How the Liberal Ideal Fails as a Foundation for Medical Ethics or Medical Ethics 'In a Different Voice'.* (Dissertation). Georgetown University, Washington, DC, 1991.

Sharpe VA. Justice and care: The implications of the Kohlberg-Gilligan debate for medical ethics. *Theoretical Medicine* 1992; 13:295–318.

Sharpe VA, Faden AI. Appropriateness in patient care: A new conceptual framework. *Milbank Q* 1996; 74:115–38.

Shaw GB. *The Doctor's Dilemma: A Tragedy.* New York: Brentano's, 1923, p. v

Shewhart WA. *Statistical Method from the Viewpoint of Quality Control.* Washington, DC: Dept. of Agriculture, 1939.

Shryock RH. *The Development of Modern Medicine.* New York: Knopf, 1947.

Shryock RH. *Medicine and Society in America: 1660–1860.* New York: New York University Press, 1960.

Shryock RH. The history of quantification in medical science. *Isis* 1961; 52:215–37.

Silverman M, Lee P. *Pills, Profits and Politics* Berkeley: University of California Press, 1974.

Silverman WA. The lesson of retrolental fibroplasia. *Sci Am* 1977; 236(6):100–7.

Simmons M, Parker, JM, Gowdy CW, et al. Adverse drug reactions during hospitalization. *Can Med Ass J* 1968; 98:175.

Simpson JY. Our existing system of hospitalism and its effects. *Edinburgh Med J* 1869; 14:816–30, 1084–115; 15:523–32.

Simpson JY. Some propositions on hospitalism. *Lancet* 1869; 2:295–7, 332–5, 431 433, 475–8, 535–8, 698–700.

Simpson JY. *Anaesthesia, Hospitalism, Hermaphrodism and a Proposal to Stamp Out Small-pox and other Contagious Diseases.* Edinburgh: Adam & Charles Black, 1871.

Siu AL, Sonnenberg FA, Manning WG, et al. Inappropriate use of hospitals in a randomized trial of health insurance plans. *N Engl J Med* 1986; 315:1259–66.

Small v. *Howard* 128 Mass 131 (1880).

Smidt NA, McQueen EG. Adverse reactions to drugs: A comprehensive hospital inpatient survey. *N Z Med J* 1972; 76:397–401.

Smith CR, Petty BG. Specific complications of medical management. In Harvey A, RJ Johns, eds. *The Principles and Practices of Medicine*, 21st edn. Norwalk, CT: Appleton-Century-Crofts, 1984

Smith R. The ethics of ignorance. *J Med Ethics* 1992; 18:117–18,134.

Spain DM. *The Complications of Modern Medical Practice: A Treatise on*

Iatrogenic Diseases. New York: Grune and Stratton, 1963.

Stamm WE: Infections related to medical devices. *Ann Intern Med* 1978; 89:764–8.

Starr P. *The Social Transformation of American Medicine.* New York: Basic Books, 1982.

Starr P. Look who's talking health care reform now. *New York Times Magazine* September 3, 1995.

Steel K, Gertman PM, Crescenzi C, Anderson J. Iatrogenic illness on a general medical service at a university hospital. *N Engl J Med* 1981; 304(11):638–42.

Steel K. Iatrogenic disease on a medical service. *J Am Geriatr Soc* 1984; 32(6):445–9.

Stewart RB, Cluff LE. Studies on the epidemiology of adverse drug reactions: VI: Utilization and interactions of prescription and non-prescription drugs in outpatients. *Johns Hopkins Med J* 1971; 129:319–31.

Stroman DF. *The Quick Knife: Unnecessary Surgery.* New York: Kennikat, 1979.

Strosberg MA, Weiner JM, Baker R, Fein IA (eds.). Rationing America's medical care: the Oregon plan and beyond. Washington: Brookings Institution, 1992.

Sullivan RB. Sanguine practices: A historical and historiographic reconsideration of heroic therapy in the age of Rush. *Bull Hist Med* 1994; 68:225.

Tancredi LR, Barondess JA. The problem of defensive medicine. *Science* 1978; 200:879–82.

Tarlov AR, Ware JE, Greenfield S, Nelson EC, Perrin E, Zubkoff M. The medical outcomes study: An application of methods for monitoring the results of medical care. *JAMA* 1989; 262; 925–30.

Tarlov AR. Outcomes assessment and quality of life in patients with immunodeficiency virus infection. *Ann Int Med* 1992; 116:166–7.

Temin P. *Taking Your Medicine: Drug Regulation in the United States.* Cambridge, MA: Harvard University Press, 1980.

The EC/IC Bypass Study Group. Failure of extracranial-intracranial arterial bypass to reduce the risk of ischemic stroke: results of an international randomized trial. *N Engl J Med* 1985; 313:1191–200.

Todd JW. The errors of medicine. *Lancet* 1970; 1:665–70.

Tomlinson T, Brody H. Futility and the ethics of resuscitation. *JAMA* 1990; 264:1276–80.

Trunet P, LeGall JR, Lhoste F, et al. The role of iatrogenic disease in admissions to intensive care. *JAMA* 1980; 244:2617–20.

Truog RD, Brett AS, Frader J. The problem with medical futility. *N Engl J Med* 1992; 326:1560–4.

Turner JA, Ersek M, Herron L, Haselkorn J, Kent D, et al. Patient outcomes after lumbar spinal fusion. *JAMA* 1992; 268:907–11.

United States Congress, House Subcommittee on Oversight and Investigation. *Cost and Quality of Health Care: Unnecessary Surgery.* Washington DC: USGPO, 1976.

United States Congress. Senate. Special Committee on Aging. *Who lives, who dies, who decides: the ethics of health care rationing.* Hearing, 19 Jun 1991. Washington: U.S. Government Printing Office; 1992.

United States Department of Health, Education and Welfare. *Task Force on Prescription Drugs: Report and Recommendations.* Committee Print of the US Congress, Senate Subcommittee on Monopoly of the Senate Select Committee on Small Business, 90th Congress, 2nd session, 1968.

United States Department of Health and Human Services, Ethics Advisory Board. The request of the Centers for Disease Control for a limited exemption from the freedom of information act. Washington, DC: US Government Printing Office, 1980.

United States Preventive Services Task Force. *Guide to Cinical Preventive Services: An Assessment of the Effectiveness of 169 Interventions.* Baltimore: Williams and Wilkins, 1989.

Vayda E, Anderson GD. Comparison of provincial surgical rates in 1968. *Can J Surg* 1975; 18:18–26.

Vayda E, Barnsley JM, Mindell WR, Cardillo B. Five-year study of surgical rates in Ontario's counties. *Can Med Ass J* 1984; 131:111–15.

Veatch RM. *A Theory of Medical Ethics.* New York: Basic Books, 1981.

Vernon DTA, Blake RL. Does problem based learning work? A meta-analysis of evaluative research. *Acad Med* 1993; 68:550–63.

Vogel MJ, Rosenberg CE (eds.). *The Therapeutic Revolution: Essays in the Social History of Medicine.* Philadelphia: University of Pennsylvania Press, 1979.

Walco GA, Cassidy RC, Schecter NL. Pain, hurt, and harm: The ethics of pain control in infants and children. *N Engl J Med* 1994; 331:541–4.

Waltz JR. The rise and gradual fall of the locality rule in medical malpractice litigation. *De Paul Law Review* 1969; 18:406–20.

Wang RIH, Terry LC. Adverse drug reactions in a Veteran's Administration Hospital. *J Clin Pharmacol* 1971; 11:14–18.

Ward GG. Audits measure our results. *Mod Hosp* 1947; 69:86.

Ware JE Jr, Brook RH, Davies AR, Lohr KN. Choosing measures of health status for individuals in general populations. *Am J Public Health* 1981; 71(6):620–5.

Warner JH. Ideals of science and their discontents in late 19th century American medicine. *Isis* 1991; 82:454–78.

Warner JH. *The Therapeutic Perspective: Medical Practice, Knowledge and Identity in America 1820–1885.* Cambridge, MA: Harvard University Press, 1986.

Weiler PC, Hiatt HH, Newhouse JP, et al. *A Measure of Malpractice: Medical Injury, Malpractice Litigation and Patient Compensation.* Cambridge, MA: Harvard University Press, 1993.

Weiler PC, *Medical Malpractice on Trial.* Cambridge MA: Harvard University Press, 1991.

Weinert HV, Brill R. Effectiveness of a hospital tissue committee in raising surgical standards. *JAMA* 1952; 150:992–6.

Weisman CS, Morlock LL, Teitelbaum MA, Klassen AC, Celantano DD. Practice changes in response to the malpractice litigation climate: results of a Maryland physician study. *Med Care* 1989; 27:16–24.

Wennberg J, Gittelsohn A. Small-area variations in health care delivery. *Science* 1973; 182:1102–8.

Wennberg J, Gittelsohn A. Variations in medical care among small areas. *Sci Am* 1982; 246:120–34.

Wennberg JE, Barnes BA, Zubkoff M. Professional uncertainty and the problem of supplier induced demand. *Soc Sci Med* 1982; 16:811–24.

Wennberg JE, Blowers L, Parker R, et al. Changes in tonsillectomy rates associated with feedback and review. *Pediatrics* 1977; 59:821–6.

Wennberg JE, Bunker JP, Barnes B. The need for assessing the outcome of common medical practices. *Ann Rev Publ Health* 1980; 1:277–95.

Wennberg JE, Freeman JL, Culp WJ. Are hospital services rationed in New York or over-utilized in Boston? *Lancet* 1987; 1:1185–9.

Wenzel RP, Osterman CA, Hunting KJ. Hospital acquired infections II. Infection rates by site, service and common procedures in a university hospital. *Am J Epidemiol* 1976; 104:645–51.

Wenzel RP, Pfaller, MA. Infection control: The premier quality assessment program in United States hospitals. *Am J Med* 1991; 91(Supp. 3B): 27S–31S.

Wenzel RP, Thompson RL, Landry SM, et al. Hospital-acquired infections in intensive care unit patients: An overview with emphasis on epidemics. *Infect Control* 1983; 4:371–5.

White FMM. Nosocomial infection control: Scope and implications for health care. *Am J Infect Control* 1981; 9:66.

Whorton JC. 'Antibiotic abandon': The resurgence of therapeutic rationalism. In Parascondola J, ed. *The History of Antibiotics: A Symposium*. Madison, WI: American Institute of the History of Pharmacy, 1980.

Wickline v. *State of California* 228 Cal. Reptr. 661 (Cal. App.2Dist.1986).

Williams REO. Summary of the conference. In Brachman PS, Eickhoff TC, eds. *Proceedings of the International Conference on Nosocomial Infections.* Chicago: AHA, 1971, pp. 318–21.

Williamson J, Chopin JM. Adverse reactions to prescribed drugs in the elderly: A multi-centre investigation. *Age Aging* 1980; 9:73–80.

Wilson IB, Cleary PD. Linking clinical variables with health-related quality of life. *JAMA* 1995; 273:59–65.

Winslow CM, Kosecoff JB, Chassin M, et al. The appropriateness of performing coronary artery bypass surgery. *JAMA* 1988; 260(4):505–9.

Wise RI, Ossman EA, Littlefield DR. Personal reflections on nosocomial staphylococcal infections and the development of hospital surveillance. *Rev Infect Dis* 1989; 11:1005–19.

Wolf SM. Health care reform and the future of physician ethics. *Hastings Ctr Rep* 1994; 24:36.

Woodward CA. Monitoring an innovation in medical education: The McMaster experience. In Ezzat ES, ed. *Innovation in Medical Education: An Evaluation of Its Present Status.* New York: Springer Publishing, 1990, pp. 27–39.

Woolf SH. Practice guidelines, a new reality in medicine. *Arch Intern Med* 1992; 152:946–52.

Woosley RL. Centers for education and research in therapeutics. *Clin Pharm Therap* 1992; 55:249–55.

Wortsman J. Letter to the Editor. *N Engl J Med* 1979; 300:928.

Wu AW, Folkman S, McPhee SJ, Lo B. Do house officers learn from their mistakes? *JAMA* 1991; 265(16):2089–94.

Zimmerman M. Sharing responsibility. In French PA, ed., *The Spectrum of Responsibility*. New York: St. Martin's Press, 1991, pp. 275–86.

Index